Human Medical Experimentation

Human Medical Experimentation

From Smallpox Vaccines to Secret Government Programs

FRANCES R. FRANKENBURG, EDITOR

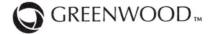
GREENWOOD™

An Imprint of ABC-CLIO, LLC

Santa Barbara, California • Denver, Colorado

Library of Congress Cataloging-in-Publication Data

Names: Frankenburg, Frances Rachel, editor.
Title: Human medical experimentation : from smallpox vaccines to secret
   government programs / Frances R. Frankenburg, editor.
Description: Santa Barbara, California : Greenwood, [2017] | Includes
   bibliographical references and index.
Identifiers: LCCN 2016032025 | ISBN 9781610698979 (hardcopy : alk. paper) |
   ISBN 9781610698986 (e-book)
Subjects: | MESH: Human Experimentation—history | Research
   Personnel—history | Government Programs—history | Biography
Classification: LCC R853.H8 | NLM WZ 112 | DDC 174.2/8—dc23
LC record available at https://lccn.loc.gov/2016032025

ISBN: 978-1-61069-897-9
EISBN: 978-1-61069-898-6

21 20 19 18 17   1 2 3 4 5

This book is also available as an eBook.

Greenwood
An Imprint of ABC-CLIO, LLC

ABC-CLIO, LLC
130 Cremona Drive, P.O. Box 1911
Santa Barbara, California 93116-1911
www.abc-clio.com

This book is printed on acid-free paper ∞

Manufactured in the United States of America

Contents

Preface

This encyclopedia covers some of the key events and people involved in the history of experimentation on humans. The goal is to provide a readable reference for those wanting to learn more about the experiments themselves as well as the researchers who explore health and illness by carrying out tests on human subjects. The descriptions of the Nazi experimentation on concentration camp victims have been seared into the minds of many, yet human experimentation is more than that; it is part of the history of improvements in medicine.

The book is divided into six sections, or eras: pre-1800s, 1800s, 1900s pre–World War II, World War II, Cold War, and post–Cold War. Four of the six eras are denoted by their relationship to wars. This designation reflects the disconcerting fact that military conflict and new weaponry often spur on medical research. Each section begins with an introduction and a timeline. The entries are arranged alphabetically. Entries in the last era cover some general subjects to do with the modern practice of human experimentation, such as institutional review boards (IRBs), the evolving understanding of informed consent, and the increase in regulation. For each era, documents that describe some incidents in vivid and direct language are included. A bibliography ends each time period.

The encyclopedia is not comprehensive and does not have to be read from cover to cover. Rather, it is designed to be an accessible reference that can be consulted according to the reader's interests. Experimentation on humans can be unethical, but when performed properly, the investigation of physiology and illness carried out directly on humans illustrates the ingenuity and determination of researchers who are driven to make discoveries and to help others.

ACKNOWLEDGMENTS

I am grateful to the following: Gregory Acampora, Arthur Anderson, Ross Baldessarini, Ruth Becker, Sanford Becker, Juan Bilbao, Alan Cole, Gary Cole, Lucy Cole, Charles Drebing, Charles Frankenburg, Reuven Frankenburg, Shoshana Frankenburg, Michelle Gelfand, Larry Herz, James Hudson, Tiffany Lago, Jennifer O'Leary, Joel Paris, Heather Rodino, Carol Sawka, Mary Seeman, Maxine Taylor, Catherine Zahn, and Mary Zanarini.

Introduction

People experiment on others so that they can understand human bodies or learn how better to treat illnesses. Medical experiments can prove or refute theories about the body, illness, or cures, thereby advancing science and improving our lives. Sometimes, however, experimentation can lead the researcher to place the value of the research above the comfort or safety of the experimental subject. While an experiment may promise to increase medical knowledge, it may not offer any immediate benefit to the subject—and may also put that person at risk of discomfort or harm. Human experimentation is thus marked by tension between three competing values: scientific inquiry, the drive to help people, and respect for the subject. Experimentation has led to much progress in medicine, but it has also resulted in abuses—at times troubling, at times lethal and even criminal—when respect for the subject has been disregarded.

Human experimentation has a brief history. In the ancient past, people who wanted to control their health and avoid illness resorted to rituals, superstitions, and incantations. It was not until people had acquired some understanding of human biology that they became able and willing to experiment on themselves or others.

THE EXPERIMENTERS

Those who have performed medical experiments throughout history have usually been young, intelligent, curious, educated, wealthy, and mostly male. They have not always been scientists or physicians. For example, in 1660, a small group of men from a variety of occupations began meeting at Gresham College in London and formed the Royal Society to promote experimental knowledge. (The first women were not elected until 1945.) Christopher Wren (1632–1723), the architect who designed St. Paul's Cathedral, was one of the founders of the society and performed the first successful injection of laudanum into a blood vessel in a hind leg of a dog in 1665.

The goal of the society was to spread knowledge so that people could benefit from the advances of others. One example was the work by the first American "colonial" to be elected to the society: Cotton Mather (1663–1728), the Puritan preacher of Massachusetts. Mather read a letter that Emanuel Timonius, a physician from Constantinople, had sent to the society, in which he described inoculation against smallpox. Then Mather's Guaramantese slave told him about the same practice in Africa. Mather used this information to promote inoculations against smallpox—an early experiment in preventive medicine.

Sometimes, however, important discoveries are not so easily disseminated and require the intervention of others who recognize their importance. One such instance was the cure for scurvy, which was discovered through what is now one of the best-known experiments in medicine. The experimenter was British navy physician James Lind (1716–1794), and the subjects were sailors who had a restricted diet. Lind described his discovery that citrus fruits could cure scurvy in an opaque way in a lengthy book. His cure would not have been known about were it not for another physician, Gilbert Blane (1749–1834), who read Lind's book and understood the importance of Lind's work better than Lind did himself.

Although it seems obvious that an experimenter should transmit what he has learned so that others can build on his work, occasionally a modicum of ignorance can be helpful. Frederick Banting (1891–1941), the Canadian codiscoverer of insulin, knew little about others performing similar experiments in diabetes when he began his Nobel Prize–winning work, and this may have been helpful in that he underestimated how difficult his work would be. Walton Lillehei (1918–1999), the great cardiac surgeon of Minnesota, advised his students not to read the works of others so that they would not repeat their mistakes.

AMBITION AND RIVALRY

Experimentation can be fueled by ambition and rivalry. The French scientist Louis Pasteur (1822–1895) and the German physician and bacteriologist Robert Koch (1843–1910), founders of microbiology, were bitter rivals—each detested the country of the other. Pasteur performed a risky experiment with a relatively untested rabies vaccine on an eight-year-old boy. He did so out a desire to help the boy, but his interest in proving the superiority of France may have also played a part. Max von Pettenkofer (1818–1901), a respected German physician, experimented on himself when he drank a vial of live cholera bacilli to try to prove Koch—his countryman but rival—wrong in his theory that cholera bacilli caused cholera. (He survived.)

Another great rivalry existed between Jonas Salk (1914–1995), Albert Sabin (1906–1993), and Hilary Koprowski (1916–2013), each of whom wanted to be the first virologist to design an effective polio vaccine. Carrying out experiments and trials on institutionalized children, their own children, prisoners, and huge numbers of schoolchildren and people in Europe and the Belgian Congo, each introduced an effective polio vaccine to the world.

The discovery of anesthesia, one of the greatest boons to suffering humanity, is the story of four Americans performing experiments on themselves and others in a spirit of competition that brought out the worst in some of them. They wanted to abolish dental and surgical pain, but they also wanted public and financial recognition.

The urge to be the first to come up with a procedure or treatment can lead to desperate experiments that can exacerbate pain and suffering. The clearest such examples may come from psychiatry. Until the 1950s, there was no treatment for schizophrenia. In efforts to help people with this devastating illness, an amazing number of therapies were tried, from the benign, such as "moral therapy"; to the harmful, such as removal of teeth or other organs at the hands of psychiatrist Henry Cotton (1876–1933); or to repetitive or regressive electroconvulsive therapies designed to make patients forget their psychotic symptoms. These patients became incontinent and so confused that they could not feed themselves. But these therapies were less harmful than lobotomies, in which physicians, intent on curing the patient, cut into the frontal lobes of the brain.

MILITARY CONFLICTS AND MEDICINE

Many have noted the paradox that the understanding of wound healing, nutritional deficiencies, and infectious diseases has often been helped by military conflicts. Indeed, Hippocrates (ca. 460 BCE–ca. 370 BCE) advised those who wanted to learn surgery to follow armies. In 1537, while on the battlefields of Turin in the Italian Piedmont, Ambroise Paré (1510–1590), a young and inexperienced French barber-surgeon, devised new ways of treating wounds. At that time, the standard treatment included pouring boiling oil over wounds. When the supply of boiling oil was exhausted, Paré experimented—anxiously—with gentler methods and advanced the art of wound healing.

Other medical experiments arising from wars have in turn influenced the course of world events. James Lind, mentioned above, discovered the cure for scurvy while working with the British navy as they fought the French. His 1747 discovery and Gilbert Blane's later appreciation of it improved the health of the English sailor and may have thus protected Britain from Napoleon's invasion.

The experiments of U.S. Army physician Walter Reed (1851–1902) with yellow fever resulted from the 1898 Spanish-American War and the American acquisition of Cuba. The United States was determined to prevent yellow fever, rampant in Cuba, from sickening American troops and spreading northward. Reed's experiments showed that the mosquito transmitted the viral illness. A few years before Reed's work, French diplomat Ferdinand De Lesseps (1805–1894), having carved out the 105-mile Suez Canal between the Red Sea and the Mediterranean Sea in 1869, began to build a canal through Panama. Twenty-five thousand men died in the French attempt to build this canal, many because of malaria or yellow fever.

In 1905, the United States succeeded in building the canal, largely because William Gorgas (1854–1920), an American physician who was the chief sanitary officer for the American canal project, appreciated the importance of Reed's yellow fever experiments in Cuba. Gorgas undertook a huge project to eradicate mosquitoes. "Mosquito brigades" drained pools and swamps, cut brush and grass, oiled wet areas, spread larvicides, and screened openings. This effort required trains, earthmovers, geologists, surveyors—and the determination of U.S. president Theodore Roosevelt (1858–1919)—but without the work of Gorgas, the canal could not have been built.

Humans are ingenious in devising ways of hurting others, and emperors, generals, and physicians alike have been fascinated by biological warfare. Spreading infections to the enemy is a venerable practice, going back at least to 1155, when Emperor Barbarossa (1122–1190) poisoned Italian water wells with corpses. In Japan, Shirō Ishii (1892–1951), a physician, organized and put into practice a massive and clandestine program in biological warfare. Ishii studied bacteriology in the West and then masterminded terrible experiments in biological warfare as director of the infamous Unit 731, where experiments on Chinese and prisoners of war were performed. He poisoned water wells in China with cholera and typhus microbes and dispersed infectious microorganisms. Altogether, he was responsible for the deaths of as many as 400,000 people in China.

During the Cold War, the American Central Intelligence Agency (CIA) was also concerned with biological warfare. To understand the dispersion of microbes, they sprayed San Francisco with bacteria. In a similar way, British researchers at Porton Down sprayed the English countryside with zinc cadmium sulfide.

Chemical warfare also has a long history. In the fifth century BCE, the Spartans burned wood that had been soaked in pitch and sulfur so that the smoke would poison the Athenians. Defying The Hague Conventions of 1899 and 1907 prohibiting the use of poison gases, the Germans, using their industrial and chemical prowess, began to use lethal gases against the Allied troops in the trenches in France in 1915. Scottish physiologist and physician John Scott Haldane (1860–1936) and his son, John Burdon Sanderson Haldane (1882–1964), a British scientist and geneticist, experimented on themselves to investigate the toxicity and identity of these gases and then to construct better gas masks. (Allied troops also used poison gases.)

The atomic bombs used during World War II unleashed a new set of weapons and with them an astounding series of experiments in the United States. At that time, the medical effects of exposure to radiation and elements such as plutonium and uranium were unknown, and this uncertainty led to many experiments. Between 1945 and 1947, researchers injected 18 American patients with plutonium without their knowledge. In one case, a patient was injected with plutonium and then asked to collect his urine and feces for the next 20 years so that his excreta could be measured for radioactivity. Soldiers in Nevada were exposed to atomic explosions. Many other people, from pregnant women in Nashville to patients dying from brain tumors at the Massachusetts General Hospital (MGH), were also exposed to radiation.

The CIA jumped with alacrity onto yet another form of warfare—mind-controlling drugs. During the Cold War, an operation called MKULTRA was involved with exposing the CIA's own agents to lysergic acid diethylamide (LSD). There is a shameful history of psychiatrists, partly paid by the CIA, who experimented on their own patients in the United States and Canada with psychoactive drugs or other treatments, often causing irreversible harm.

War, or the threat of war, with its high passions and demonization of the enemy, has also been the background for experimentation that was as much about cruelty as discovery. The clearest examples of this are, of course, the Nazis' cruel experiments on prisoners of concentration camps and other individuals that they deemed less than human and the activities of the Japanese Unit 731 in the years preceding and during World War II. As one of the principles of warfare or hostility between countries is secrecy, undoubtedly there are medical experiments that took place of which we know very little. This may be particularly true for countries without autonomy of the professions or a free press, such as Stalinist Russia or present-day North Korea. In some cases, the interest of the researchers in making medical discoveries to help their own compatriots is complemented by their sadism, and experimentation becomes torture.

THE SUBJECTS OF EXPERIMENTS AND THE DIFFERENCE BETWEEN THERAPEUTIC AND NONTHERAPEUTIC EXPERIMENTS

A key component of the human experiment is, of course, the person undergoing the experiment. Subjects are chosen or volunteer for a variety of reasons, often because they are ill and hope to receive a possible benefit from an experimental treatment. For example, the first people who received insulin or heart transplants, experimental procedures at the time, were looking for effective new treatments for themselves. The distinction between therapeutic experiments—those intended to help the person involved, but also to yield information—and other experiments, where the intention is not to help the subject but to gain knowledge, is sometimes difficult to find.

This division can be particularly blurred with respect to surgical or technological innovation. The patients who are the first to be treated with a new procedure are subjects to an experiment of sorts, and they do not always do well. For example, the construction of the first dialyzer, or artificial kidney, began with impressive ingenuity but no clinical success. Dialysis is the artificial removal of waste products from the blood, a process usually carried out by kidneys.

During the German occupation of the Netherlands in World War II, Dutch physician Willem Kolff (1911–2009) filled cellophane sausage casings with blood, added a kidney waste product called urea, and agitated the contraption in a bath of saltwater. In five minutes, all the urea had moved into the saltwater. He used a water-pump coupling from Ford Motor engines, orange juice cans, and a clothes washing machine. The first 15 patients with kidney disease who were connected to Kolff's dialyzer died. Yet, after that agonizing beginning, dialysis has turned out to be a successful procedure that prolongs the lives of those without functioning kidneys. Kolff also worked on the membrane oxygenator for the heart bypass machines and, with Robert Jarvik (b. 1946), an American physician, scientist, and entrepreneur, on the first artificial heart. (While dialysis is now common, the implantation of an artificial heart is still unusual.)

The first person who received a heart transplant lived only 18 days after surgery. American physician and researcher Thomas Starzl (b. 1926) attempted the first liver transplant in 1963, but the first successful one was not performed until 1967.

Liver transplants were not considered to be a clinically accepted treatment until 1983—meaning that all of the liver transplants carried out in those 20 years were experimental. The issue of informed consent in these therapeutic experiments is complex. Some of the patients thought that they were getting the most up-to-date treatment; others agreed to be the subjects of experiments, and others were too ill to have any understanding of what they were undergoing.

A researcher who decides to experiment on himself (there are few women in this category) finds a convenient, willing, informed, and perhaps accurate observer who does not need to be paid and who can give informed consent. Moreover, the experimenter can then tell other subjects that he too has undergone the experiment. Koprowski, mentioned above in reference to polio vaccines, administered Colorado tick fever, polio, and rabies vaccines to himself. Waldemar Haffkine (1860–1930), a physician and microbiologist, experimented with plague and cholera vaccines, using himself as the first subject in each case.

Similarly, the researcher may use an extension of himself—family members. Some vaccine developers, for example, gave their own children their newly developed vaccines as a way of both testing them and assuring an anxious public that they were sure of the safety of the vaccine. Presumably, the children assented, and their parents—the experimenting father—gave implicit consent. Jonas Salk, John Kolmer (1886–1962), and others first vaccinated their own children to test the safety of their vaccines.

The Haldane father-and-son team in Great Britain, mentioned earlier, are an example of researchers who experimented on themselves, their family, and their friends. The father, J. S. Haldane, experimented on himself to understand the mechanisms involved in breathing and gas exchange in the lungs. He recruited colleagues and also his two children to help him in these experiments, sometimes putting his young son at some risk. This son, J. B. S. Haldane, also grew up to experiment on himself and on colleagues, including a former Spanish premier and a wife-to-be. The Haldanes investigated the effects of extreme environmental stresses and in so doing made advances in a number of scientific fields and improved the safety of those working in mines, on submarines, at high altitudes, and those exposed to poisonous gases.

William Halsted (1852–1922), a medical and surgical pioneer, transfused his sister who was hemorrhaging after giving birth in what has been called one of the first emergency transfusions. A few months later, he removed his mother's gallstones—one of the first times that this had ever been done. These therapeutic experiments contributed to the greater body of medical knowledge. (He also experimented with cocaine and developed a lifelong addiction.)

Some of the self-experimentation was in the areas of physiology. German physician Werner Forssmann (1904–1979) catheterized his own heart in 1929 and received the Nobel Prize in Physiology or Medicine for this experiment in 1956.

In contrast to these examples of researchers experimenting upon themselves, there is a long and dispiriting list of vulnerable populations that have been experimented upon. Researchers cannot always resist the idea of using captive groups of people, such as prisoners, aboriginal people, children, and the ill, because they are easy to control, monitor, and follow. These groups have often been subjected to experiments without their consent.

Prisoners have sometimes been rewarded for their participation in experiments. British and American researchers in the Philippines took advantage of the huge Bilibid Prison in Manila to perform a number of experiments. The prisoners who signed consent for the amoebic dysentery experiments received nothing, but in other Bilibid experiments involving beriberi, tropical medicine researcher Richard Strong (1872–1948) and B. C. Crowell paid prisoners with cigars and cigarettes. In the United States, Mississippi prisoners who volunteered for pellagra experiments were promised pardons.

Prisoners were subjected to many medical procedures by Leo Stanley (1886–1976), chief surgeon at San Quentin prison, between 1913 and 1951. Without, it seems, any checks on what he was doing, he carried out experiments in an attempt to forestall the aging process by implanting testicles from executed prisoners or animals into some of the living inmates.

Experimentation on prisoners is now viewed with disfavor. But some note that prisoners enjoyed the sense of altruism and argue that they should be allowed to participate in experiments if they desire. Nathan Leopold (1904–1971), the infamous murderer, was proud that he volunteered for malaria experiments while a prisoner at Stateville penitentiary in Illinois.

Another vulnerable population subjected to human experimentation was the poor black sharecroppers in Macon County, Alabama, who were enrolled in the Tuskegee Study of Untreated Syphilis without being told that they had syphilis; they received no or inadequate treatment. In another case, Canadian nutritionists deliberately maintained some aboriginal schoolchildren on vitamin-deficient diets.

Mentally ill people who cannot give consent have often been the subjects of experimentation. A mentally ill man brought by the Rome police to two Italian psychiatrists, Ugo Cerletti (1877–1963) and Lucio Bini (1908–1964), in 1938 was the first person to undergo electroconvulsive therapy. He did not give consent, but he did make a complete recovery. Nutrition scientists from beriberi researchers in Kuala Lumpur to pellagra researchers in Mississippi to vitamin researchers at Elgin State Hospital in Ohio have manipulated the diets of the mentally ill to establish our basic nutritional requirements.

Researchers used institutionalized children in experiments involving vaccines, from polio to hepatitis. Young boys at the Fernald State School in Massachusetts were given radioisotopes in their oatmeal, and their parents were sent a letter telling them that if they didn't object the experimenters will assume consent. Koprowski was criticized for called mentally retarded children "volunteers." English physician and gadfly Maurice Pappworth (1910–1994) wrote a book in 1967 detailing disturbing experiments, many of them on ill children, that were performed by English physicians in a cavalier way. As was the case with the mentally ill and sailors, researchers have also used children in orphanages to establish some of our nutritional needs. For example, American physician and epidemiologist Joseph

Goldberger (1874–1929) advanced our understanding of the role of niacin deficiency in pellagra by manipulating diets of orphanages in Jackson, Mississippi. In vitamin D experiments that took place in Berlin, Kurt Huldschinsky (1883–1940) used mercury vapor lamps on orphans to cure their rickets. Harriette Chick (1875–1977) showed that either vitamin D or sunlight could treat rickets in children in Viennese orphanages. Alfred Hess (1875–1933) induced scurvy and rickets in orphans in New York in the early 20th century.

Pharmaceutical companies tested new drugs on prisoners until the 1970s. Now they often test new drugs in third-world countries, where the populations may be desperate for medical attention and may be relatively unsophisticated when it comes to taking new medicine or trusting people in white coats. Trials of antibiotics in Nigeria to treat meningitis and attempts in Zimbabwe to slow down the spread of HIV from pregnant women to their children have been controversial.

Some of these experiments on the vulnerable were done in secret—such as the ones in Nazi Germany and, even more so, those in World War II–era Japan. But most of the other experiments were not. Indeed, one of the purposes of many experiments is to produce publications. For example, the 13 publications stemming from the Tuskegee study unapologetically referred to the study as one of untreated syphilis in American Negroes.

Today, some people volunteer to participate in experiments or clinical trials and, depending on the unpleasantness, inconvenience, or dangerousness of the experiment, these "professional guinea pigs" can make thousands of dollars. Others who have the illness being studied appreciate the opportunity to get the newest treatment and volunteer to be subjects. Even if subjects do not benefit from the new treatment, at least they can benefit from additional care and attention from the clinical trial staff. (This benefit was used to justify the Tuskegee study, although, of course, the subjects did not actually get treatment.)

Others choose to be subjects in experiments or clinical trials for altruistic reasons. The young men who volunteered for starvation experiments in Minnesota during World War II; the British conscientious objectors who were exposed to scurvy and vitamin deficiencies at Sorby in Sheffield, England; and the Seventh-day Adventists who volunteered in the 1950s to be exposed to Q fever and tularemia as part of Operation Whitecoat in Fort Detrick, Maryland, all wanted to avoid military service, but they also wanted to help their country and advance the science of medicine.

* * * * *

The experiments described in this encyclopedia offer moments in medical history that lend themselves to storytelling. The actual process of medical discovery is somewhat different, consisting of incremental steps and replication of the work of others, and is often lengthened by detours and dead ends. Yet, experimentation on humans remains one of the most fascinating parts of medical progress, involving fraught decisions and ethically complex situations. As the episodes detailed in the following pages show, while human experimentation is often based on altruistic motives, it sometimes illuminates the darker sides of the human psyche.

Era 1: Pre–19th Century

INTRODUCTION

For much of human history, the workings of the body and illnesses were seen as mysterious or magical processes or events were properly the subject of prayer or ritual. But beginning with Hippocrates (ca. 460–ca. 370 BCE), the father of scientific medicine, physicians (and others) instead began looking at the body, along with its illnesses, as something to be observed and understood. Later, the influential Greco-Roman physician Galen (ca. 131–ca. 201 CE) experimented on animals—but not on humans. For the succeeding centuries, until the 1800s, human experimentation—interfering with human bodies to try to understand how they work and help healing—happened only occasionally and usually on a small scale.

Galen believed in direct observation and experimentation, but for many hundreds of years, few actually made such independent observations. Galen's ideas and the concept of health as a balance of the humors finally began to be challenged during the Renaissance—more than 1,400 years after his death. Theophrastus Bombastus von Hohenheim (1493–1541), now known as Paracelsus, was a German-Swiss alchemist who scorned the reverence paid to Galen's work. He burned Galen's books in the Basel town square and mocked his colleagues for following outmoded practices. Paracelsus thought that diseases were the result of either chemical imbalances or poisons. His interest in chemistry was part of the long tradition of alchemy and the search for the philosopher's stone that could transform base metals into gold and silver. Although he had beliefs that seem to us to be unscientific, such as the belief in the supremacy of the trio of salt, sulfur, and mercury, he did help to pave the way for rejection of unproven dogma.

Francis Bacon (1561–1626) was another major influence on the development of modern medicine and experimentation. Not a physician, Bacon was a lawyer who encouraged others to observe nature closely. He emphasized the importance of the replication of scientific experiments and of sharing the results of observation and experimentation with others. This approach led to the establishment of the Royal Society in London in 1660, an early scientific society associated with many discoveries in medicine and science. For example, Anton van Leeuwenhoek (1632–1723), a draper and microscopist, began writing letters to the society in 1673 describing what he had seen with his handcrafted microscopes and continued to do so for the next 50 years. At the end of the 18th century, letters published by the Royal Society helped to popularize smallpox variolation.

French barber-surgeon Ambroise Paré (1510–1590) cured wounds by experimenting with gentler techniques when the usual boiling oil was not available. In

Padua, Italy, Andres Vesalius (1514–1564), a Belgian physician, observed human anatomy himself and corrected some of Galen's errors. The British physician William Harvey (1578–1657) also studied in Padua. Interested in the heart and blood, Harvey examined cold-blooded animals and humans and showed that the blood circulates rather than being used up, as Galen had incorrectly thought. Harvey's work marked the beginning of modern scientific medicine.

By the 1700s, the first experiments with a semblance of scientific methodology took place in England. James Lind (1716–1794) carried out one of the first controlled clinical trials and in so doing discovered the cure for scurvy, improving the health of the British navy and thus allowing a prolonged and successful naval blockade of the French. Edward Jenner (1749–1823), an English doctor, listened to the accounts of English country dairymaids, and in 1796 vaccinated his gardener's young son, James Phipps, with cowpox from a dairymaid's pustule and then inoculated him two months later with smallpox—and James stayed well. Jenner was not the first to use cowpox to protect against smallpox, but he repeated his vaccination in many others and described his work at length and clearly. Jenner became a hero throughout the world, even to his country's archenemy, Napoleon. His small experiment had had far-reaching effects.

TIMELINE

ca. 460–ca. 370 BCE	Life of Hippocrates, the father of scientific medicine.
ca. 131–ca. 201 CE	Life of Galen of Pergamum, an influential Greco-Roman physician who dissects humans and experiments on animals.
1510–1590	Life of Ambroise Paré, the "gentle surgeon" who experiments with the treatment of wounds.
1561–1636	Life of Santorio Sanctorius, an Italian physician who experiments on himself to study "insensible perspiration."
1628	William Harvey (1578–1657) publishes *De Motu Cordis*, the first widely accepted and correct account of the circulation of the blood.
June 1667	In France, Jean-Baptiste Denys (1643–1704) transfuses blood from sheep to a 15-year-old boy.
November 1667	In England, Richard Lower (1631–1691) transfuses blood from sheep into Arthur Coga.
1718	Lady Mary Wortley Montagu (1689–1762) arranges for her five-year-old son to be inoculated against smallpox in Turkey.
1721	During a smallpox epidemic in Boston, Cotton Mather (1663–1728) and Zabdiel Boylston (1679–1766)

introduce inoculation against smallpox to America and meet with opposition.

1728–1793   Life of John Hunter, a British surgeon who advances the science of medicine by many experiments on animals and himself.

1747   James Lind (1716–1794) performs the first controlled clinical trial and finds the cure for scurvy on HMS *Salisbury*.

1796   Edward Jenner (1747–1823) vaccinates his gardener's son against smallpox using the relatively benign cowpox.

REFERENCE ENTRIES

GALEN OF PERGAMON

Galen was the most influential Greco-Roman physician, and his work became medical dogma for 15 centuries in the Western world. As surgeon to the gladiators, he became familiar with the human body. He also worked with animals, dissecting Barbary apes, dogs, pigs, goats, and stags and experimenting on live animals. From both his animal experiments and his encounters with wounded gladiators, Galen extrapolated to describe human anatomy and physiology. Yet, because he was not allowed to dissect human bodies, let alone perform experiments on them, much of his work was later shown to be mistaken.

Galen (ca. 131–ca. 201 CE) was born in the Anatolian city of Pergamon (sometimes Pergamum), which boasted the finest library in the world after Alexandria's. Galen's father was a successful architect who paid for his son's extensive education and left him with enough money to lead a comfortable life of study and writing.

In addition to its library, Pergamon had one of the world's finest Asclepiad medical schools, and Galen began studying there at an early age, finishing his first medical studies by the age of 20. He then went to Alexandria, where he trained for an additional 12 years, concentrating on anatomy. After travels to Smyrna and Corinth, Galen returned to Pergamon, where he practiced and was surgeon to the gladiatorial school for several years. He moved to Rome in 164 CE and remained there for more than 20 years, earning a reputation as the most successful practitioner of his time.

Galen published many books, only a few of which survive. He wrote 9 books on anatomy, 17 on physiology, 6 on pathology, 14 on therapeutics, and 30 on pharmacy. All were written in Greek.

Unlike Hippocrates, who was primarily an observer, Galen was an avid dissector and experimenter. He dissected thousands of animals, concentrating on apes for postmortem studies and pigs and dogs for live dissections but applying himself to whatever species came his way, even camels and elephants. He was one of the first to experiment on living organisms and disproved Aristotle's contention that the brain served only to cool the blood and that the heart was the seat of emotion and thought.

Galen's experiments and discoveries were wide-ranging and innovative for his time. He cut the spinal cord in a variety of places to produce different forms of paralysis. He stopped vocalization by cutting the recurrent laryngeal nerve in a live pig. He demonstrated that an excised heart would continue to beat and an excised muscle would contract. He proved that if one severed an optic nerve, blindness resulted.

Galen served as a military surgeon with Marcus Aurelius. He identified and differentiated degenerative and traumatic aneurysms. He controlled bleeding by finding the end of the severed vessel and twisting or tying it on itself or by suturing it with silk. (This was the first surgical use of the rare material that had been imported from the Orient to make the wardrobes of Roman women.)

Galen combined his experimental findings with the philosophy of Hippocrates and Pythagoras into a fanciful physiological system. Because he dissected animals and not humans, he made a number of anatomic errors, which persisted in the medical literature for 15 centuries after his death. Although he wrote that the student should always confirm what is taught, for the next 1,400 years, many people preferred to believe what Galen had written without making their own observations or performing their own experiments.

Jack E. McCallum

HARVEY, WILLIAM

William Harvey, a 17th-century English physician who performed many simple and safe experiments on humans, overthrew 1,400 years of mistaken theories about the heart and circulation based on the writings of the Greco-Roman physician Galen. He elucidated the true nature of the cardiovascular system, and his work ushered in the beginning of modern scientific medicine.

Harvey (1578–1657), born in Kent, England, was the oldest of seven children. He graduated from Cambridge at the age of 20 and from 1599 to 1602 studied with Fabrizio d'Acquapendente (1537–1619) at the renowned medical school in Padua, Italy. After his studies, he returned to England and lectured and cared for patients at St. Bartholomew's Hospital in London for the next 30 years. For some years, he was physician to King James I.

Harvey's greatest accomplishment was his discovery of the circulation of blood, which overturned many beliefs that had held for the previous 1,400 years. Galen (ca. 131–ca. 201 CE) had taught that blood was continuously formed in the liver and that veins carried the nutrient-dense blood to the tissues. He thought that the blood ebbed and flowed in the veins and was used up in the tissues, while the arteries, in contrast, carried a different substance, a vital spirit, to the tissues. Harvey's work corrected many of these errors.

One of the reasons it took so long to understand the circulatory system was that warm-blooded animals' hearts beat rapidly, which made circulation of the blood difficult to study. Harvey overcame this problem by examining cold-blooded animals, particularly snakes, whose hearts beat more slowly. He also examined the hearts of dying animals because the heart slows down as an animal approaches death. Harvey saw that the left ventricle of the heart pumped blood out through the aorta and into the arteries to all parts of the body and that the blood traveled through the veins back to the right ventricle. The right ventricle then pumped the blood into the lungs and back to the left ventricle. By showing that more blood left the heart than could possibly be generated by the liver or absorbed by the rest of the body, he argued that the blood was not used up—it was endlessly circulated. He could not ascertain *how* the blood moved from arteries through the body tissue to the veins (since capillaries could not be seen without the aid of microscopes), but even so, he was certain that the blood circulated.

An important part of Harvey's discovery was his comprehension of the purpose of valves in veins, which was aided by some simple human experiments. D'Acquapendente had described valves in the walls of veins but had not understood their function. Harvey tied ligatures (what we might call tourniquets) of varying pressure on people's arms. (Ligatures were used in those days to facilitate bleeding—then a common medical procedure.) Tightly tied ligatures stopped the flow of arterial blood to the arm. A ligature tied less tightly allowed arterial blood to flow into the arm, but prevented venous blood, under lesser pressure, from flowing out of the arm. The veins in the arm would become engorged with blood, and this allowed for easy bloodletting. The blood in the veins can be "milked" toward the heart and away from the valves; the valves prevent the blood from flowing back from the heart. In other words, blood in the veins is always flowing toward the heart. The illustrations derived from these experiments demonstrate the function of the valves and the direction of the blood flow in the veins.

Harvey's experiments must have been mildly and briefly painful, but otherwise their impact on the subject would have been trivial. Harvey did not perform any experiments (that we know of) on human hearts or human circulatory systems, other than the simple maneuvers described above. Nonetheless, these maneuvers and his examination of the circulatory systems of many cold-blooded animals allowed him to draw the correct conclusions about the human heart and circulation. (Harvey also showed that the arterial pulse, previously thought by Galen to be due to the artery itself, was actually due to the pumping of the heart's ventricles.)

Harvey published his findings in 1628 in a short monograph, written in Latin, published in Frankfurt, and dedicated to King Charles I of England. This book, *Exercitatio anatomica de motu cordis et sanguinis in animalibus* (*Concerning the Motion of the Heart and Blood*), often referred to as *De Motu Cordis*, is one of the most important books in the history of medicine.

Harvey's application of physical principles to a biological problem was the beginning of modern scientific medicine, and his work helped to end the 1,400-year-long dependence on Galenic medicine. Galen had urged people to experiment; Harvey did just that, and his work showed that Galen's conclusions could be challenged.

Harvey's last years were plagued by gout and kidney stones. He died following a stroke at age 79.

Frances R. Frankenburg

HIPPOCRATES OF COS

Hippocrates was the father of scientific medicine. He is credited with separating physicians and the practice of medicine from priests and religion. He did not conduct experiments, but his observational approach was the foundation for future experimentation.

Little is actually known of Hippocrates (ca. 460–ca. 370 BCE), although multiple admiring references from his Athenian contemporaries survive and leave no doubt that he played a key role in the development of Greek medicine. He was born on the island of Cos and was said to have been the son of Heraclides, a Coan physician who legend said was descended in a direct line of 18 generations from Aesculapius (sometimes Asclepius), the ancient Greco-Roman god of medicine. Hippocrates's mother was Phenarete (sometimes Praxithea), who was said to be descended through 19 generations from Hercules. Hippocrates was educated by his father, his uncle Gorgias the Sophist, and the philosopher Democritus.

After completing his education, Hippocrates traveled widely before coming to Athens, where he was a contemporary and acquaintance of Sophocles, Socrates, Plato, Euripides, Aristophanes (who satirized him), Herodotus, and Thucydides. He treated patients during the Great Plague of Athens. He later served as court physician to Persian emperor Artaxerxes (although he remained a loyal Greek) before returning to Thessaly, where he died between 85 and 104 years of age.

The oath bearing his name is the oldest and most durable statement of medical ethics, but probably originated in the Pythagorean School of southern Italy. The Hippocratic corpus, the authorship of which is not clear, organizes Greek medical knowledge, which had previously been largely aphoristic, and provides vivid case descriptions and detailed instructions for caring for specific illnesses and injuries. Later scholars' enthusiasm for fifth-century BCE Greek civilization enhanced Hippocrates's reputation.

Hippocrates's descriptions of surgery, particularly of wounds and orthopedic injuries, were the best available before those of Aulus Cornelius Celsus (ca. 25 BCE–ca. 50 CE) (a Roman writer who compiled and summarized much of the existing medical theory and practice). He recommended trepanation to relieve pressure from head injury (albeit for the wrong reasons), knew how to align clavicle fractures, and provided excellent descriptions of reducing dislocations and fixing long bone fractures. Many of the wounds he saw were inflicted in battle. In fact, Hippocrates said the only appropriate training for a surgeon was to find an army and follow it.

Hippocrates's observations, recommendations, and diagnoses were many. He recognized the physical manifestations of liver injury and dehydration. He described opposite-side paralysis from a brain injury, thought that fevers were often beneficial, associated the wasting of syphilitic tabes with sexual activity, and provided the first descriptions of human anthrax. Hippocrates recommended irrigating wounds with wine and clean water and insisted that physicians wash their hands with hot water and work only with the best available natural or artificial light, preferably with trained assistants in a room dedicated to surgical procedures. These descriptions and treatments continued to be referred to well into the 17th century and are valuable as primary examples of observation and clinical diagnosis rather than as works in experimental medicine. Hippocrates was an unusually honest observer (60 percent of his 42 cases died) who considered the ability to predict an outcome at least as important as effecting a cure.

Unlike the descriptive and surgical works, the theoretical portions of the Hippocratic corpus were based on error and persisted for centuries. Illness and response to trauma were assumed to be a function of imbalance among the four humors: black bile, yellow bile, blood, and phlegm, based on the four essential elements (earth, air, fire, and water). Treatments designed to restore balance, such as bleeding and purging, continued well into the 19th century.

Hippocrates's fame is due to his independence from religious beliefs and his dependence on observation. He recommended that the physician pay attention to the whole person—his or her diet, occupation, travel, and so on. He did not believe that prayer, visions, miracles, or rituals affected physical health. He rejected the theory that epilepsy was a "sacred disease." His emphasis on gathering information and making observations was essential for future experimenters.

Jack E. McCallum

HUNTER, JOHN

John Hunter was a British surgeon and polymath who took surgery from a technical exercise to a science. He gave a subject both syphilis and gonorrhea while investigating venereal diseases, and it is possible that the subject in this experiment was himself.

John Hunter (1728–1793) was born in the village of East Kilbride, near Glasgow, Scotland. His father was a moderately successful farmer, and John was the youngest of 10 children, including William—10 years John's senior—who became London's premier anatomist and was the father of obstetrics as a medical specialty.

Unlike his older brother, John Hunter did not attend university. In 1748, he moved to London and took a job helping his brother prepare anatomical specimens, a job he kept for the next 11 years. He worked with the grave snatchers, or body robbers, of the day to obtain corpses for dissection. He first studied surgery in the summer of 1749 under William Cheselden, a prominent surgeon famous for the speed of his procedures. Hunter also studied for short periods at Chelsea Hospital, St. Bartholomew's Hospital, and St. George's Hospital, where he became house surgeon in 1756. Throughout that time, he continued to teach anatomy with his brother.

Hunter served as a staff surgeon in the British army from 1760 to 1763 and participated in the invasion and occupation of Belle Isle in 1761. The British suffered a large number of casualties, and because Hunter was one of only three surgeons in the force, he acquired a unique expertise in treating gunshot wounds. Barber-surgeon Ambroise Paré's recommendation that such wounds be opened widely and the projectile removed seemed to Hunter to cause more harm than benefit, and he recommended that no gunshot wound be enlarged except as needed to manage an associated injury. To the horror of his colleagues—and the ultimate benefit of his patients—he left most wounds unexplored, later publishing his experience in the monumental *Treatise on the Blood, Inflammation, and Gunshot Wounds* published in 1794. He accompanied the British army to Portugal and then returned to London and private practice in 1763.

Hunter was knowledgeable in many other areas. He was an avid naturalist, and his extensive publications resulted in his being elected fellow of the Royal Society in 1767. He wrote about geology, embryology, and comparative anatomy. His medical career progressed also, and in 1768, he became a member of the Corporation of Surgeons and attending surgeon to St. George's Hospital. He wrote extensively on medical problems, including transplantation of teeth, tendon repair (a subject that got his interest after he ruptured his own Achilles tendon while dancing), the pathology of shock, artificial feeding through a flexible tube, forced respiration, and treatment of arterial aneurysm by high ligation of the feeding vessel.

He continued to teach surgery, and his pupils included Edward Jenner (1747–1823), who would go on to pioneer the smallpox vaccine. His reputation continued to grow, and in 1776, he was named surgeon extraordinary to King George III and, in 1790, inspector of hospitals and surgeon general of the British army.

Hunter collected anatomical curiosities, both animal and human. His collection survives as the basis of London's Hunterian Museum, and it secured Hunter's reputation as the founder of experimental and surgical pathology.

In addition to his surgical advancements, Hunter is also remembered for an experiment, possibly involving himself as the subject. While investigating venereal diseases, he inoculated a subject with material discharged from a patient with gonorrhea to test the theory that gonorrhea and syphilis were different forms of the same illness. Many assume that the subject was John Hunter himself, although there is no definitive proof. The assumption is due to the fact that he made detailed descriptions of the subject's penile sores and then rashes typical of a syphilitic illness. Hunter cured the subject—or himself—with mercury. He then married. This timing of the marriage was significant because he had been engaged for some time, and the delay of his marriage was another hint that he was the experiment's subject and had not wanted to marry until he was no longer actively ill. In any event, Hunter's deduction, that gonorrhea and syphilis were the same illness, was mistaken. He seems not to have realized that the original patient from whom the discharge was acquired could have been infected with both illnesses.

From the age of 45, Hunter suffered from bouts of severe chest and back pain, often accompanied by the loss of pulses in his arms. The episodes were often brought on by his bad temper. During a board meeting in which he was vigorously advocating the admission of two questionably qualified students to St. George's, he abruptly died. Although it has been widely stated that his chest pains were angina pectoris from coronary artery disease, his autopsy and symptoms were most compatible with a syphilitic aortic aneurysm.

After Hunter's death, his brother-in-law, Sir Everard Home, assumed the role of successor and plagiarized a number of his unpublished papers. Home ultimately burned all of Hunter's surviving manuscripts in an evident attempt to hide the theft. Virtually all that was left of Hunter's legacy were his published works and his museum.

Jack E. McCallum

JENNER, EDWARD

The pioneer of the smallpox vaccine, Edward Jenner, practiced medicine in the English countryside. He inoculated his gardener's son with cowpox and then smallpox, and his experiments led to the disappearance of this feared disease.

Cowpox is a mild illness that can affect cows or humans, and in the 18th century, it was not unusual for English dairy workers and farmers to contract it. There was a widely held belief in those rural areas that people who developed cowpox would not subsequently become ill from smallpox. Indeed, those who had been ill with cowpox cared for those with smallpox, knowing that they put themselves in no danger.

The idea of deliberately giving people cowpox to protect them from smallpox had occurred to several people before Edward Jenner tried it. The first person might have been Benjamin Jesty (1737–1816), a farmer who scratched cowpox material into his wife and two children in 1774. Jesty's two children were later inoculated with smallpox and did not become ill. In Europe, Peter Plett (1766–1823), a tutor in Holstein, administered cowpox lymph to three of his students. In a later smallpox epidemic, they also did not become ill. He reported his findings to the University of Kiel but was not taken seriously.

Edward Jenner (1747–1823) was an English physician and a student of John Hunter (1728–1793), an eminent English surgeon. Jenner was born in Berkeley, Gloucestershire, and was brought up by his older brother after being orphaned at the age of 5. He showed an early interest in science and was apprenticed to a country surgeon at the age of 13. Eight years later, he went to London and studied with Hunter. After two years, he returned to Berkeley to practice medicine.

Jenner was aware of the theory that cowpox protected people from smallpox, and in May 1796, during an outbreak of cowpox, he decided to test this theory. He transferred lymph from a cowpox pustule on the arm of dairymaid Sarah Nelmes, who had caught the illness from a cow named Blossom, into the arm of an eight-year-old boy, James Phipps, the son of his gardener. The boy became mildly ill for a day or so. Six weeks later, Jenner deliberately exposed Phipps to smallpox via variolation (the scratching or rubbing the material from one person's smallpox pustules into the skin of another person). He did not become ill. Jenner's results demonstrated the safety of cowpox, its efficacy against smallpox, and also that cowpox could be transmitted from cow to person, and then from person to person. In 1798, Jenner privately published a pamphlet, "An Inquiry into the Causes and Effects of the Variolae Vaccinae, a Disease Discovered in Some of the Western Counties of England, Particularly Gloucestershire, and Known by the Name of Cow Pox." In this pamphlet, Jenner described the successful vaccinations of Phipps and others.

Jenner has been celebrated not so much for his observation and experiment—neither of which was unique—but for his clearheaded appreciation of the importance of his experiment on James Phipps. Following Phipps's vaccination, Jenner spent decades publicizing, explaining, and facilitating vaccinations. He was helped in this work by his position as a physician, his connection with Hunter, and his conviction of its importance. He provided the vaccine to anyone who requested it.

Jenner used the word *vaccine*, coming from the Latin *vaccinus*, meaning of or from the cow. As we now know, the vaccination of people or animals means that they are exposed to the microbe that causes the illness; another substance related to the illness, such as a toxin; or a microbe that leads to a similar illness. This exposure leads to the development of protective antibodies.

Jenner's discovery was met with excitement and relief. The advantage of vaccination over variolation was that it did not lead to smallpox and was therefore safer. Variolation was outlawed in 1840, and vaccination against smallpox became compulsory in England as of 1853. Jenner was acclaimed even by England's enemy—Napoleon. His discovery was also met with disbelief and mockery. Cartoonists of the time drew cows growing out of the arms of people who had been vaccinated. An anti-vaccine movement—still strong today—was born. At the time, it was difficult to ensure the purity or strength of the early vaccines. In some cases, children became septic or, in one terrible episode, syphilitic because of contaminated vaccines. These complications strengthened the anti-vaccine movement.

Benjamin Waterhouse (1754–1846), a physician and Harvard professor, was the first American to perform a vaccination. He vaccinated his five-year-old son, Daniel, in 1800 and then persuaded President Thomas Jefferson (1743–1826) of the values of this practice.

The nature of the vaccinia virus, the microorganism in the smallpox vaccine, remains mysterious, as genetic testing shows that it is distinct from the organisms that cause cowpox and smallpox. Nonetheless, there is little doubt that vaccination against smallpox with the vaccinia virus is successful. Indeed, the use of the smallpox vaccine throughout the world led to an impressive accomplishment: the elimination of the disease.

In 1977, a man in Somalia became the last recorded natural case of smallpox. He had worked as a vaccinator and became ill with the disease. He had been reluctant to be vaccinated himself, fearing the pain of the procedure. (He recovered and went on to urge the vaccination of others against polio, telling his own story to people who were afraid to be vaccinated.) In 1978, a laboratory accident led to one fatal case of smallpox in England.

In 1980, the World Health Organization declared smallpox to be eradicated. This is one of the few contagious illnesses, perhaps the only one, which might have been conquered. However, the existence of smallpox stocks in some countries tempers our hope that smallpox has been eradicated.

Frances R. Frankenburg

LIND, JAMES

One of the most celebrated experiments in the history of Western medicine was one performed by James Lind in 1747 in which he showed that citrus fruits cured scurvy.

Scurvy is an illness caused by insufficient vitamin C, or ascorbic acid, which leads to fatigue, rashes, and swollen and bleeding gums. James Lind (1716–1794), the man associated with discovering the cure for scurvy, was born in Edinburgh, Scotland, and trained there at the College of Surgeons. He became a physician in the British Royal Navy in 1739. In the 1700s, because the English navy was an integral part of the defense of England against France and Spain, the health of the English seaman became a matter of national importance.

In 1747, Lind was serving as naval surgeon on the HMS *Salisbury*. He saw many cases of scurvy and became interested in the illness, aware that many theories existed about its cause and treatment. He had no strong beliefs about these theories himself, so he decided to test six current ones. (Large ships were a good "laboratory" for experiments because sailors were a "captive" group.) Lind took 12 sailors with scurvy, moved them into the sick bay of the *Salisbury*, and fed them the diet provided to all sailors: gruel for breakfast, mutton broth and pudding for lunch, and barley with sage for supper. Lind supplemented this diet in six different ways, each of which had been described as an effective cure for scurvy, and gave each supplement to two ill sailors. The six different treatments were (1) one quart of cider, (2) 25 drops of elixir of vitriol (sulfuric acid) three times a day, (3) two spoonfuls of vinegar three times a day, (4) half a pint of seawater, (5) two oranges and one lemon for six days, and (6) an "electuary" (a pasty mix of medicinal substances) the size of a nutmeg made up of garlic, mustard seed, balsam of Peru, dried radish root, and gum myrrh (a resin), along with barley water treated with tamarinds and cremor tártoro (cream of tartar, a leftover substance from winemaking). The men eating the citrus fruit became well within six days and actually helped to care for the other men who remained ill.

Lind's findings advanced medical science in two important ways. First, he performed one of the first controlled clinical trials. The word "controlled" means that Lind, without perhaps realizing how important this was, treated all of the sailors in the same way, except for the experimental variable. Thus, it was clear that whichever pair of sailors did best did so because of their particular treatment. Later researchers came to believe that it was also important that trials be randomized and double blind. In randomized trials, the subjects are assigned to a particular treatment by chance, making bias less likely.

As far as we know, Lind had no particular reason for assigning each treatment to each sailor and no particular reason to assume that any of the particular treatments was more likely to work than the others, so one could argue that Lind's study was randomized—although perhaps not in the sense that studies are randomized today, in which subjects are assigned treatments based on numbers picked randomly by computer programs. However, Lind's study—although a majestic feat—was not double blind: both he (the experimenter) and the sailors (the subjects) knew what the assigned treatment was for each pair of soldiers.

Second, he demonstrated that the cure for scurvy was citrus fruit. Lind's careful experiment proved that a plentiful supply of fresh citrus fruit would help to keep sailors, and others on restricted diets, free from scurvy.

In 1748, Lind retired from the navy and wrote the 400-page *Treatise on the Scurvy*, published in 1753, in which he reviewed the previous literature on scurvy and described his own powerful and convincing trial. It should have been a landmark work, but, famously, nothing happened. Why did the publication of this book cause so little stir? The problem was that he had produced a massive tome that was impossible to read, and what was worse, he hid the description of his experiment in five paragraphs in the middle of the book. Lind did not, out of modesty or uncertainty, highlight his own simple and convincing trial. And he only suggested hesitantly and with much qualification that the navy use "rob," a heated and condensed form of citrus juice, to treat scurvy.

Scientists are sometimes accused of improving their results or making too much of them. If there is any scientist innocent of this, it must be James Lind. A task of any researcher is to doubt his or her own findings, and to look for alternative explanations. James Lind would certainly go on to do this.

In 1758, Lind was put in charge of the large naval hospital at Haslar, Portsmouth, and was responsible for the care of thousands of scurvy patients. In 1772, Lind produced a third edition of the *Treatise* in which he reported on his experience at Haslar. He was confused and overwhelmed as he reviewed his own work. He became convinced that scurvy was due to putrefaction and then the blocking of perspiration. He recommended that lemon juice be mixed with wine and sugar. (This led to an effervescent drink that was helpful for the digestive system.) He did continue to use lemons, and sometimes with success, but lost his conviction that citrus fruits were the cure.

Some have suggested that the sick sailors at Haslar knew that citrus fruits would help them, so all of Lind's Haslar experiments were ruined by sailors managing to get hold of citrus fruit. This would mean that comparisons between different treatment groups would be misleading. Additionally, perhaps some sailors were ill with other diseases. Another possibility is that the lemon juice at Haslar was adulterated or spoiled. On the HMS *Salisbury*, Lind used actual fruit. The change from fruit to fruit juice was sometimes accompanied by a loss of the active vitamin.

Regardless of these doubts and confusions, Lind continues to be credited with the discovery of the cure for scurvy thanks to his original 1747 experiment. The person who discerned the importance of this experiment was Gilbert Blane (1749–1834)—not an experimenter but a physician, who persuaded the navy to improve the diet of its sailors. The British navy, then scurvy-free, was able to defeat the French navy and thus save Britain from a Napoleonic invasion.

Frances R. Frankenburg

PARÉ, AMBROISE

Ambroise Paré, known as "the gentle surgeon," experimented with ways of treating wounds that did not involve boiling oil—a common practice in his day. He also wrote in French, instead of Latin, so that his fellow barber-surgeons could learn from his experiences.

Ambroise Paré (1510–1590) was born in France in the village of Bourgon Hersent, near Laval, and went to Paris at the age of 19 as a barber-surgeon's apprentice. (Barber-surgeons were medical practitioners who had little formal training, performed many types of surgeries, and were not as highly regarded as physicians.) He served as a wound-dresser at the Parisian hospital, the Hôtel Dieu, before becoming an army surgeon in 1536, and later, surgeon to four kings.

Citing the Hippocratic doctrine that diseases caused by iron are best cured by fire—compounded by the belief that gunpowder was itself a poison—16th-century military surgeons treated gunshot wounds with a combination of red-hot cauteries and boiling elder oil. In 1537, after a battle during the French campaign in the Piedmont, Paré ran out of oil and was forced to substitute a mixture of egg yolks, oil of roses, and turpentine to irrigate wounds. Unable to use the entire standard treatment, he also elected to forgo the cautery. The following morning, he found that wounds treated with the new mixture lacked the typical inflammation and, in subsequent days, went on to heal better than those given the usual treatment. With this evidence, Paré had the audacity to question papal physician Giovanni de Vigo's assertion that gunshot wounds contained an innate poison that had to be burned out.

Paré had experimented out of necessity, not to test a theory, but nonetheless stumbled on an important finding. His fame lies in his willingness to use his consequent observation. At the time of Paré's battlefield experiment, he was a young barber-surgeon who had not yet passed his exams. He was brave enough to publish his evidence, which contradicted the beliefs of the time. (It is not difficult to imagine that other doctors might have hesitated to believe their own eyes, even if they had made the same observation as Paré because of their deference to the authorities of the time.)

Paré also reintroduced the use of ligatures, described centuries before by Aulus Cornelius Celsus (ca. 25 BCE–ca. 50 CE) (a Roman writer who compiled and summarized much of the existing medical theory and practice). Ligatures are ties around blood vessels that made it possible to control vessels too large to cauterize, which, in turn, made it possible to amputate well above the necrotic areas of a gangrenous limb and thereby significantly improve the patient's chances of survival.

He had other accomplishments. He created a series of surgical instruments adorned with such decorations as a carving of a beautiful woman languishing on the handle of his amputation knife. Paré was probably one of the first clinicians of that time to recognize that flies carry infectious disease, and he was one of the first to successfully reimplant avulsed teeth.

In 1552, he became surgeon-in-ordinary to the French king Henry II and continued in that capacity through the reigns of three more monarchs. He became particularly close to Charles IX, for whom he held the rank of principal surgeon.

Paré's works include a 1545 treatise on gunshot wounds and a 10-volume treatise on surgery (1564). Paré was ridiculed by his colleagues for writing in vernacular French rather than Latin, including having the temerity to translate Andreas Vesalius's work on anatomy from Latin into French. (Barber-surgeons were not typically able to read Latin.) But the fact that Paré did know Latin and chose instead to write in French meant that he helped to disseminate medical knowledge to the community of barber-surgeons. He was also adored by French soldiers for his skill in treating battlefield injuries and his compassion. He wrote "*Je le pansai, Dieu le guérit*" ("I bandaged him and God healed him").

Paré died in 1590 and was buried at Saint-André-des-Arcs in Paris.

Jack E. McCallum

SANTORIO SANCTORIUS

Santorio Sanctorius was an Italian physician interested in metabolism. He is best known for carrying out a 30-year-long experiment on himself in which he weighed everything that he ate and excreted, attributing the difference between the two amounts to what the Greco-Roman physician Galen called "insensible perspiration."

Santorio Sanctorius (1561–1636)—also known as Santorio Santorio, Sanctorio Sanctorio, Santorio Santorii, and other combinations—was born in Capodistria (now Koper, Slovenia), then a Venetian town on the Adriatic. He studied medicine at the famed University of Padua—one of the birthplaces of measurement and quantification—from which he obtained his medical degree in 1582. For the next several years, Sanctorius worked in Croatia and thereabouts before setting up a medical practice in Venice in 1599.

In 1611, Sanctorius turned his attentions to teaching and research, returning to the University of Padua as a professor of medical theory. He formed friendships with his colleagues at Padua, including the astronomer Galileo Galilei (1564–1642) and the anatomist Fabrizio d'Acquapendente (1537–1619). In 1624, he moved to the University of Venice, where he remained until his death in 1636.

Sanctorius studied metabolism and invented instruments. In 1614, he published *De Statica Medicina* (*On Medical Measurement*), possibly the first systematic study of basal metabolism. He modified the pendulum, the motion of which had been described by Galileo, and created a device to measure the pulse, the pulsilogium.

In another modification of Galileo's work, he attached a numerical scale to Galileo's thermoscope—which indicated differences in temperature—thereby creating a forerunner to today's thermometer.

Sanctorius, however, is perhaps best known for a 30-year-long study of his own metabolism. He designed a large scale on which he could eat and study while being weighed continually. The difference between the weight of what he ate and any stool or urine was the weight of his "insensible perspiration." The concept of insensible or undetectable perspiration had been proposed by Galen (ca. 131–ca. 201 CE) more than a thousand years before, but Sanctorius was the first person, as far we know, to measure this phenomenon. When we perspire, if the moisture evaporates before we feel it on our skin, we are not aware of it, and it is thus known as "insensible." (The term sometimes includes evaporation from the lungs.) Sanctorius recorded how the amounts of his insensible perspiration changed with age, activity, and environmental conditions. He concluded that insensible perspiration was vital to our health and more important than the more easily understood excreta, that it mostly happened after a meal, and that it was a sign of "robustness." Sanctorius had thus measured something we do not always feel. The water loss may be insensible, but that did not mean it could not be measured.

The experiment of Sanctorius is an example of self-experimentation without intervention—just decades of observation. His ability to tolerate the tedium and the unpleasantness of the work was remarkable, and his experiment has not been repeated.

Frances R. Frankenburg

SMALLPOX INOCULATION

Early attempts to prevent smallpox in the Western world include experiments by an English aristocrat on her own children and then by others on royal and orphaned children and prisoners. Physicians disapproved of some of the early champions of inoculation against smallpox.

Smallpox, known as the "the scourge of mankind," is caused by the *Variolae major* virus. The illness has no animal reservoirs, affecting only humans. It has an incubation period of 7 to 10 days, and the first symptoms are chills, fevers, headaches, and backaches. Two or three days later, small red spots appear on the face and extremities, and lesions develop in the mouth and throat. The spots become pustules, which last for several weeks before scabbing over and leaving deep scars. It has no treatment and a fatality rate of about 30 percent. Those who survive are often left with disfiguring scars or blindness.

The disease was epidemic in Europe and Asia for centuries and was particularly devastating when introduced to the native populations of the Americas at the time of the European conquests. These conquests were helped by the spread of infectious illnesses, among them smallpox, which had higher fatality rates than in other areas of the world.

While there is no treatment for smallpox, for many centuries there was at least a way of preventing it for most people. In areas where smallpox was endemic, some people practiced a type of early vaccination known as *inoculation*. The word comes from the Latin *inoculare*, meaning "to graft." Inoculation, also known as *variolation*, involved scratching or rubbing the material from one person's smallpox pustules into the skin of an uninfected person to cause a milder case of the illness and thus immunity to its severer forms.

Variolation was practiced in parts of Africa and Asia and became known to Europeans, thanks to Lady Mary Wortley Montagu (1689–1762), the wife of the English ambassador to the Ottoman Empire. While in Turkey, she became aware of the beauty of the women of the harems. One story, popularized by Voltaire (1694–1778), is that their beauty was due to inoculation. He wrote that Circassians were poor and wanted to sell their children to rich men, some of them owners of harems. To get a good price, they were careful to inoculate their children so that they would not later become scarred by smallpox.

Whether or not this is true, Lady Montagu recognized that smallpox was less serious in Turkey than it was in England. She had been ill with smallpox herself and as a result had disfiguring scars on her face. Not wanting her own children to suffer the same fate, in 1718, she arranged for the inoculation of her five-year-old son. A Turkish (or Greek; accounts differ) woman inoculated him awkwardly with a rusty needle; the family's Scottish surgeon, Charles Maitland, who was traveling with them, inoculated him again in the other arm. The Montagu family and Maitland returned to England, enthusiastic about this practice.

An unexpected consequence of the boy's variolation followed upon their arrival in England. Lady Montagu's son was enrolled in English boarding schools, which he disliked. Perhaps showing some of his mother's indomitable spirit, he often ran away from the schools, but he was easily recognized by his two distinctive variolation scars and brought back.

In 1721, Maitland inoculated Lady Montagu's four-year-old daughter, as well as six prisoners, all of whom survived. One prisoner, a woman, was deliberately exposed to smallpox and proved to be immune. Maitland then inoculated 10 orphaned children. The next year, he inoculated two daughters of the Princess of Wales. Following the inoculations of both the vulnerable (children, prisoners, and orphans) and the royal, variolation spread throughout England and then Europe.

At the same time, variolation was beginning in America. One of the people involved in the American story was Cotton Mather (1663–1728), a Puritan minister better known for his fiery sermons and involvement in the 1692–1693 Salem witchcraft affair. He was given a "gift" of an African man to serve as his slave, and this man told him about inoculations. After reading a report about inoculations by physician Emanuel Timonius in Turkey, Mather wrote,

> Many months before I met with any intimations of treating the smallpox with the method of inoculation, anywhere in Europe; I had from a servant of my own, an

account of its being practised in Africa. Enquiring of my Negro man Onesimus, who is a pretty intelligent fellow, whether he ever had the smallpox, he answered, both yes and no; and then told me that he had undergone an operation, which had given him something of the smallpox, and would forever preserve him from it; adding that it was often used among the Guaramantese and whoever had the courage to use it was forever free from the fear of the contagion. He described the operation to me, and showed me in his arm the scar which it had left upon him; and his description of it made it the same that afterwards I found related unto you by your Timonius.[1]

A smallpox epidemic began in Boston in 1721. Mather urged the 10 physicians of Boston to inoculate the population; all but one scoffed: Zabdiel Boylston. Boylston (1679–1766) inoculated his son and two of his own slaves. This experiment was greeted with outrage: Boylston had to hide for a couple of weeks, and a grenade was thrown into Mather's house—he welcomed the possibility of becoming a martyr. To some, Boylston's experiment seemed risky, not to mention an interference with divine providence. In addition, the idea that Mather could have learned something from a slave offended many. Mather replied,

> Here we have a clear Evidence, that in Africa, where the Poor Creatures dye of the Small Pox in the common way like Rotten Sheep, a Merciful GOD has taught them a wonderful Preservative. It is a Common Practice, and is attended with Success. I have as full Evidence of this, as I have that there are Lions in Africa. And I don't know why 'tis more unlawful to learn of Africans, how to help against the Poison of the Small Pox, than it is to learn of our Indians, how to help against the Poison of a Rattle Snake.[2]

Mather has been called the first physician of the United States and the inoculations in Boston the "earliest important experiment in preventive medicine in America."[3]

Observers noted that fatality of natural smallpox was about eight times greater than the mortality of smallpox following inoculation. Nonetheless, inoculation was not without risk, as it did sometimes lead to smallpox itself and had about a 2 percent fatality rate. It also could introduce smallpox into a community that otherwise might not have experienced this illness.

In 1724, Boylston published a book, *An Historical Account of the Small-pox Inoculated in New England upon All Sorts of Persons, Whites, Blacks, and of All Ages and Constitutions*. Variolation became accepted but disappeared once the safer practice of vaccination was developed.

Frances R. Frankenburg

References
1. Boylston, "The Origins of Inoculation," 310.
2. Brown, "The African Connection," 2,248.
3. Blake, "The Inoculation Controversy in Boston," 489.

TRANSFUSION

Experiments with blood transfusions began in the 1600s, after one notable failed experiment on the pope in 1492. The mere fact that transfusions were being performed in the 1600s was extraordinary because scientists and physicians did not yet understand the origin or function of blood. They knew that blood had an obvious connection with life itself as the loss of large quantities of blood so quickly led to death, but they didn't know why blood was so essential to life. They also didn't know, for example, about the existence of oxygen or hemoglobin, the pigment that carries oxygen. There was no way of quantifying blood volume, measuring red blood cells, or storing blood. The danger of incompatible blood types (even the existence of blood types) was not recognized, and the process of coagulation was not understood. Given this lack of knowledge, it is not surprising perhaps that these early and dangerous experiments, although they caused a flurry of excitement, did not actually lead to medical progress. In fact, transfusions did not become safe and viable until the early 20th century.

The earliest reference to blood transfusion involves Pope Innocent VIII in 1492. He was debilitated from a recent stroke, and three young clerics volunteered to have blood removed and given to him. It is likely that the pope actually drank the blood rather than receiving it intravenously. Neither he nor his donors survived the experiment.

Transfusion in the modern sense became possible thanks to work by English physician William Harvey (1578–1657). He demonstrated that blood circulated from the heart to the arteries and then back to the heart through the veins. In 1665, English surgeon John Wilkins (1614–1672) and, shortly thereafter, Richard Lower (1631–1691), a physician, successfully transfused blood collected from one dog into the vein of another.

It was the French physician Jean-Baptiste Denys (1643–1704) who carried out the first blood transfusions from animal to human in four men. The transfusions were somewhere between experimental and therapeutic. The first, of about 12 ounces of blood, was on June 15, 1667, from the carotid artery of a sheep to a 15-year-old boy. The boy had been ill for a couple of months and, as was the custom of the time, had been bled repeatedly. He seemed to benefit from the transfusion. The second recipient was a healthy 45-year-old man who also survived the transfusion. The third person was less fortunate: Swedish statesman Baron Gustaf Bonde was very ill. He received two transfusions and died shortly afterward.

In the winter of 1667, Denys performed his last animal-to-human transfusion. The subject was a highly agitated and mentally ill young man, Antoine Mauroy. This time, Denys used calf's blood. At first, Mauroy seemed to improve and he disappeared for a few weeks, but then he once again became mentally ill. Mauroy's wife insisted that he receive another transfusion; whether he did is not clear. In any event, he died a few days later. Mauroy's wife blamed Denys for her husband's death, and Denys was charged with murder. He was acquitted, and Mauroy's wife was accused of causing his death. But, as a result, the judge forbade more blood transfusions in France.

Later that same year, Lower transfused about eight or nine ounces of blood from a sheep into a 22-year-old man, Arthur Coga, a man described as eccentric but healthy and able to understand the procedure. He tolerated the procedure well and was paid.

These early transfusions were the subject of much publicity and competition between the English and the French. Publications sprang up within weeks of the events but did not lead to much progress.

In 1795, Philadelphia physician Philip Syng Physick (1768–1837) successfully transfused blood from one person to another, but he did not publish the results of his experiment, and the practice did not become general. The next documented transfusion was in 1818, when English obstetrician James Blundell (1790–1878) saved an exsanguinating patient by giving her blood collected from her husband. Twenty-two years later, he and an assistant, Samuel Armstrong Lane, repeated the experiment on a patient bleeding to death from hemophilia.

Transfusion remained impractical throughout the 19th century because of difficulties with clotting and the deterioration of collected blood as well as lack of knowledge of blood typing. Milk (obtained from cows, goats, and humans) was even tried as a substitute for blood but had a high rate of unacceptable complications, and that practice was replaced with the first saline transfusion in 1884.

The modern era of transfusion began in 1901 when Karl Landsteiner discovered the three major blood groups—A, B, and O—for which he was awarded the 1930 Nobel Prize in Physiology or Medicine. In 1908, Alexis Carrel (1873–1944) successfully transfused blood directly from the artery of a donor to the recipient's vein, thus avoiding the problem of clotting.

The clotting problem was partially solved in 1915 when Richard Lewisohn of New York's Mount Sinai Hospital discovered that the addition of sodium citrate to whole blood kept it from clotting. The following year, Francis Rous and J. R. Turner developed a citrate-glucose combination that allowed blood to be stored for several days.

Transfusions are now an accepted part of medical practice and usually consist of selected blood components rather than whole blood.

Jack E. McCallum

DOCUMENTS

AMBROISE PARÉ AND THE TREATMENT OF GUNSHOT WOUNDS (1537)

Ambroise Paré, the "gentle surgeon," knew that the standard teaching of how to treat gunshot wounds was boiling oil. He confirmed this with his colleagues. While serving with the French army in Piedmont as a young barber-surgeon in 1537, the supply of oil was exhausted, and so Paré devised an alternative treatment that turned out to be successful. He had the courage and appreciation of the importance of what he had done to publish his observations, which contradicted the received wisdom. He wrote about his experiment in vernacular French rather than the usual academic Latin.

Now I was at this time a fresh-water soldier; I had not yet seen wounds made by gunshot at the first dressing. It is true I had read in John de Vigo, first book, *Of Wounds in General,* eighth chapter, that wounds made by firearms partake of venenosity, by reason of the powder; and for their cure he bids you cauterize them with oil of elders scalding hot, mixed with a little treacle. And to make no mistake, before I would use the said oil, knowing this was to bring great pain to the patient, I asked first before I applied it, what the other surgeons did for the first dressing; which was to put the said oil, boiling well, into the wounds, with tents and setons; wherefore I took courage to do as they did. At last my oil ran short, and I was forced instead thereof to apply a digestive made of the yolks of eggs, oil of roses, and turpentine. In the night I could not sleep in quiet, fearing some default in not cauterizing, that I should find the wounded to whom I had not used the said oil dead from the poison of their wounds; which made me rise very early to visit them, where beyond my expectation I found that those to whom I had applied my digestive medicament had but little pain, and their wounds without inflammation or swelling, having rested fairly well that night; the others, to whom the boiling oil was used, I found feverish, with great pain and swelling about the edges of their wounds. Then I resolved never more to burn thus cruelly poor men with gunshot wounds.

Source: Stephen Paget, *Ambroise Paré and His Times, 1510–1590* (New York: G. P. Putnam's Sons, 1899), 33–34.

WILLIAM HARVEY AND THE CIRCULATION OF BLOOD (1628)

William Harvey, an English physician who studied with Fabrizio d'Acquapendente at the University of Padua, a leading medical school, wrote "De Motu Cordis," from which this passage comes, in Latin in 1628. This description of the heart as a muscular pump perhaps seems obvious to the modern reader. But before Harvey's work, people spoke about vague and immeasurable "vital spirits" and were unaware that the heart circulated blood through the lungs and the rest of the body. Through the observation of cold-blooded animals, a quantitative approach to the volume of blood, a simple experiment with ligatures tied around the arm, and a correct interpretation of the valves described by d'Acquapendente, Harvey freed medicine from the chains of Galenic authority.

Chapter XIV: Conclusion of the Demonstration of the Circulation
And now I may be allowed to give in brief my view of the circulation of the blood, and to propose it for general adoption.

Since all things, both argument and ocular demonstration, show that the blood passes through the lungs, and heart by the force of the ventricles, and is sent for distribution to all parts of the body, where it makes its way into the veins and porosities of the flesh, and then flows by the veins from the circumference on every side to the centre, from the lesser to the greater veins, and is by them finally discharged into the vena cava and right auricle of the heart, and this in such a quantity or in such a flux and reflux thither by the arteries, hither by the veins, as cannot possibly be supplied by the ingesta, and is much greater than can be required for mere purposes of nutrition; it is absolutely necessary to conclude that the blood in the animal body is impelled in a circle, and is in a state of ceaseless motion; that this is the act or function which the heart performs by means of its pulse; and that it is the sole and only end of the motion and contraction of the heart.

Source: *Scientific Papers: Physiology, Medicine, Surgery, Geology, with Introductions, Notes and Illustrations*, The Harvard Classics, vol. 38 (New York: P. F. Collier & Son, ca. 1910).

JAMES LIND'S SCURVY EXPERIMENT (1747)

James Lind, a physician who worked as a surgeon in the English navy, was preoccupied with scurvy, a debilitating disease that was prevalent among sailors. In one of the most famous experiments in the history of medicine, he took 12 sailors, all ill to a similar degree with scurvy, and managed them in the same way, with one exception. He varied only the experimental treatment, thus creating a "controlled trial." Citrus fruits cured the scurvy. Lind was both modest and perhaps not entirely aware of the importance of his finding. He wrote about his remarkable discovery in a slightly convoluted passage in the middle of a long book, so it would have been easy for most readers to miss.

The following are the experiments.

On the 20th May 1747, I selected twelve patients in the scurvy, on board the *Salisbury* at sea. Their cases were as similar as I could have them. They all in general had putrid gums, the spots and lassitude, with weakness of their knees. They lay together in one place, being a proper apartment for the sick in the fore-hold; and had one diet in common to all, viz., water gruel sweetened with sugar in the morning; fresh mutton broth often times for dinner; at other times light puddings, boiled biscuit with sugar etc.; and for supper barley and raisins, rice and currants, sago and wine, or the like. Two of these were ordered each a quart of cyder a day. Two others took twenty five drops of elixir vitriol three times a day upon an empty stomach, using a gargle of it for their mouths. Two others took two spoonfuls of vinegar three times a day upon an empty stomach, having their gruels and their other food sharpened with vinegar, as also the gargle for their mouth. Two of the worst patients, with the tendons in the ham quite rigid (a symptom none of the rest had) were put under a course of sea water. Of this they drank half a pint every day and sometimes more or less, as it operated, by way of gentle physic. Two others had each two oranges and one lemon given them every day. These they eat with greediness, at different times, upon an empty stomach. They continued but six days under this course, having consumed the quantity that could be spared. The two remaining patients took the bigness of a nutmeg three times a day of an electuary recommended by an hospital surgeon made of garlic, mustard seed, horseradish, balsam of Peru and gum myrrh, using for common drink, barley water boiled with tamarinds, by which, with the addition of cream of tartar, they were gently purged three or four times during the course.

The consequence was, that the most sudden and visible good effects were perceived from the use of oranges and lemons; one of those who had taken them being at the end of six days fit for duty. The spots were not indeed at that time quite off his body, nor his gums sound; but without any other medicine than a gargle for his mouth, he became quite healthy before we came into Plymouth, which was on the 16th of June. The other was the best recovered of any in his condition, and being now deemed pretty well, was appointed to attend the rest of the sick.

Next to the oranges, I though the cyder had the best effects. It was indeed not very sound. However, those who had taken it, were in a fairer way of recovery than the others at the end of the fortnight, which was the length of time all these different courses were continued, except the oranges. The putrefaction of their gums, but especially their lassitude and weakness, were somewhat abated, and their appetite increased by it.

As to the elixir of vitriol, I observed that the mouths of those who had used it by way of gargle, were in a much cleaner and better condition than many of the rest, especially those who used the vinegar; but perceived otherwise no good effects from its internal use upon the other symptoms. I indeed never had a great opinion of the efficacy of this medicine in the scurvy, since our longest cruise in the Salisbury, from the 10th of August to the 28th of October 1746; when we had but one patient in the scurvy, a marine, who, after recovering from a quotidian ague in the latter end of September, had taken the elixir vitriol by way of restorative for three weeks; and yet at length contracted the disease, while under a course of a medicine recommended for its prevention.

There was no remarkable alteration upon those who took the electuary and tamarind decoction, the sea-water, or vinegar, upon comparing their condition, at the end of the fortnight, with others who had taken nothing but a little lenitive electuary and cream of tartar occasionally, in order to keep their body lax, or some gentle remedies in the evening, for relief of the breast.

Source: James Lind, *A Treatise on the Scurvy*, 3rd edition (London: Printed for S. Crowder, 1772), 149–152.

EDWARD JENNER'S INOCULATION EXPERIMENT (1798)

Edward Jenner, a physician who studied in London but lived in a rural area of England, was familiar with the folk belief that those ill with cowpox (also known as Variolae vaccinae*), a mild illness, did not become ill with smallpox, a far more severe disease. In this detailed account of his work, he describes how he inoculated eight-year-old James Phipps with cowpox and then with "variolous" matter from a young woman ill with smallpox.*

The boy became slightly ill after the cowpox inoculation but not at all after the small-pox inoculation (soon to be called vaccination*). Jenner had succeeded in making Phipps immune to smallpox, and he had done so safely. As well as being a brilliant observer and daring experimenter, Jenner then became a tireless advocate for vaccination. Vaccinations against smallpox are one of the greatest triumphs in medicine.*

CASE XVI.—Sarah Nelmes, a dairymaid at a farmer's near this place, was infected with the cow-pox from her master's cows in May, 1796. She received the infection on a part of her hand which had been previously in a slight degree injured by a scratch from a thorn. A large pustulous sore and the usual symptoms accompanying the disease were produced in consequence. The pustule was so expressive of the true character of the cow-pox, as it commonly appears upon the hand, that I have given a representation of it in the annexed plate. [In original.] The two small pustules on the wrists arose also from the application of the virus to some minute abrasions of the cuticle, but the livid tint, if they ever had any, was not conspicuous at the time I saw the patient. The pustule on the forefinger shews the disease in an earlier stage. It did not actually appear on the hand of this young woman, but was taken from that of another, and is annexed for the purpose of representing the malady after it has newly appeared.

CASE XVII.—The more accurately to observe the progress of the infection I selected a healthy boy, about eight years old, for the purpose of inoculation for the cow-pox. The matter was taken from a sore on the hand of a dairymaid, who was infected by her master's cows, and it was inserted, on the 14th of May, 1796, into the arm of the boy by means of two superficial incisions, barely penetrating the cutis, each about half an inch long.

On the seventh day he complained of uneasiness in the axilla, and on the ninth he became a little chilly, lost his appetite, and had a slight headache. During the whole of this day he was perceptibly indisposed, and spent the night with some degree of restlessness, but on the day following he was perfectly well.

The appearance of the incisions in their progress to a state of maturation were much the same as when produced in a similar manner by variolous matter. The only difference which I perceived was in the state of the limpid fluid arising from the action of the virus, which assumed rather a darker hue, and in that of the efflorescence spreading round the incisions, which had more of an erysipelatous look than we commonly perceive when variolous matter has been made use of in the same manner; but the whole died away (leaving on the inoculated parts scabs and subsequent eschars) without giving me or my patient the least trouble.

In order to ascertain whether the boy, after feeling so slight an affection of the system from the cow-pox virus, was secure from the contagion of the smallpox, he was inoculated the 1st of July following with variolous matter, immediately taken from a pustule. Several slight punctures and incisions were made on both his arms, and the matter was carefully inserted, but no disease followed. The same appearances were observable on the arms as we commonly see when a patient has had variolous matter applied, after having either the cow-pox or smallpox. Several months afterwards he was again inoculated with variolous matter, but no sensible effect was produced on the constitution.

Here my researches were interrupted till the spring of the year 1798, when, from the wetness of the early part of the season, many of the farmers' horses in this neighbourhood were affected with sore heels, in consequence of which the cowpox broke out among several of our dairies, which afforded me an opportunity of making further observations upon this curious disease.

Source: Edward Jenner, *The Three Original Publications on Vaccination against Smallpox*, The Harvard Classics, vol. 38, part 4 (New York: P. F. Collier & Son, 1909–14).

Further Reading

Allen, Arthur. 2007. *Vaccine: The Controversial Story of Medicine's Greatest Lifesaver*. New York: W. W. Norton.

Blake, John B. 1952. "The Inoculation Controversy in Boston: 1721–1722." *New England Quarterly* 25 (4) (December): 489–506. doi:10.2307/362582.

Boylston, A., and A. E. Williams. 2008. "Zabdiel Boylston's Evaluation of Inoculation against Smallpox." *Journal of the Royal Society of Medicine* 101: 476–477. doi:10.1258/jrsm.2008.08k008.

Boylston, Art. 2012. "The Newgate Guinea Pigs." *London Historians* (September): 1–3.

Boylston, Arthur. 2012. "The Origins of Inoculation." *Journal of the Royal Society of Medicine* 105: 309–313.

Brown, T. H. 1988. "The African Connection: Cotton Mather and the Boston Smallpox Epidemic of 1721–1722." *Journal of the American Medical Association* 260 (15): 2,247–2,249. doi:10.1001/jama.260.15.2247.

Camac, C. N. B. 1959. *Classics of Medicine and Surgery*. New York: Dover Publications.

Frankenburg, Frances Rachel. 2009. *Vitamin Discoveries and Disasters: History, Science, and Controversies*. Santa Barbara, CA: Praeger/ABC-CLIO.

Gross, Cary P., and Kent A. Sepkowitz. 1998. "The Myth of the Medical Breakthrough: Smallpox, Vaccination, and Jenner Reconsidered." *International Journal of Infectious Diseases* 3 (1): 54–60. doi:10.1016/S1201-9712(98)90096-0.

Harvey, William. 1958. *Exercitatis anatomica de motu cordis et sanguinis in animalibus*. Springfield, IL: Charles C. Thomas.

Henderson, Donald A. 2009. *Smallpox: The Death of a Disease: The Inside Story of Eradicating a Worldwide Killer*. Amherst, NY: Prometheus Books.

Lind, James, C. P. Stewart, and Douglas Guthrie. 1953. *Lind's Treatise on Scurvy: A Bicentenary Volume Containing a Reprint of the First Edition of a Treatise of the Scurvy*. Edinburgh, Scotland: Edinburgh University Press.

Nuland, Sherwin B. 1988. *Doctors: The Biography of Medicine*. New York: Knopf.

Porter, Roy. 1997. *The Greatest Benefit to Mankind: A Medical History of Humanity*. New York: W. W. Norton.

Riedel, Stefan. 2005. "Edward Jenner and the History of Smallpox and Vaccination." *Proceedings (Baylor University Medical Center)* 18 (1) (January): 21–25.

Era 2: 19th Century

INTRODUCTION

The 1800s were marked by medical discoveries that made surgery easier, safer, and less painful. The discoveries also clarified the nature of nutrition and a number of common infections, including sexually transmitted diseases. Researchers worked on vaccines against lethal diseases, such as rabies, the bubonic plague, and cholera. Researchers did not think that the subjects of experiments had to understand or consent to the procedures.

One of the major advances was the discovery of surgical anesthesia. Experiments with ether, cocaine, chloroform, and nitrous oxide, some first performed by the experimenters on themselves, led to pain-free surgery. Cleanliness was also deemed important for safe surgery, but this concept was surprisingly difficult for doctors to comprehend. Oliver Wendell Holmes (1809–1894) in Boston and Ignaz Semmelweis (1818–1869) in Vienna tried to convince those who delivered babies to wash their hands, but both physicians were ignored or ridiculed. However, Joseph Lister (1827–1912) in Great Britain was more successful in promoting a clean operating room. Advances in hygiene combined with the use of anesthetics paved the way for surgical experiments.

Louis Pasteur (1822–1895) and Robert Koch (1843–1910), two great rivals and scientists, made discoveries that changed medicine. Pasteur identified the causes of animal illnesses, such as anthrax. Koch identified the cause of tuberculosis and formulated postulates that organized future experimentation. He explained that to be certain that a bacterium caused a specific illness, that bacterium always had to be present in a case of the illness and then be grown in a pure culture. When readministered to an animal, it must then cause the original disease and once again be found in that animal.

With the development of the microscope and the invention of stains by Koch, Paul Ehrlich (1854–1915), and Hans Christian Gram (1853–1938), microorganisms invisible to the naked eye could be seen for the first time, and physicians began to understand that these microorganisms caused illnesses. The laboratory thus became an inseparable part of medicine. Diagnosis was no longer just clinical, and the importance of cleanliness—a way of eliminating, or at least decreasing, the possibility of transmitting these microorganisms—finally became accepted. The earlier admonitions of Holmes and Semmelweis had been correct.

Medical researchers began to form hypotheses, weigh evidence, quantify findings, and understand the importance of replication of the experiment. The idea that medical experiments could be performed to increase our knowledge and expertise took hold.

Much of human experimentation in the 1800s was related to the development of vaccines. Vaccines can be developed in animals, but at some point, they have to be tested in humans. Toward the end of the previous century, in 1796, English doctor Edward Jenner (1749–1823) had successfully vaccinated his gardener's young son with cowpox, which led to the boy's immunity against the deadly smallpox—and the eventual elimination of the disease. Almost a century later, in 1885, Pasteur tried out a relatively untested treatment on a nine-year-old boy, Joseph Meister, who had been bitten by a rabid dog. The child survived, and Pasteur became an international hero. He named his treatment "vaccination" in honor of Jenner's earlier discovery and established the Institut Pasteur in Paris, where many went on to conduct important experiments, including Waldemar Haffkine (1860–1930), who studied there with one of Pasteur's students, Elie Metchnikoff (1845–1916), and who created vaccines for cholera and plague.

Other experiments were more exploratory and perhaps exploitative. In 1822, French Canadian fur trapper Alexis St. Martin (1802–1880) was shot in the stomach; William Beaumont (1785–1853), an American army surgeon, tended to his wounds. St. Martin survived, but he developed a fistula, an abnormal connection between his stomach and skin. The fistula did not heal, and Beaumont, seizing the opportunity, studied digestion by dropping food on bits of string into St. Martin's stomach through the fistula, pulling out the food and examining it to try to understand the digestive processes. Years of experiments followed. Beaumont paid St. Martin and housed him and his family for many years. Yet, St. Martin sometimes fled, and after his death, his relatives buried him as deeply as possible to protect him from further experimentation.

In the 1840s, in Alabama, J. Marion Sims (1813–1883) repeatedly operated on three black slave women who, after long labors, had developed fistulas between the vagina and bladder or vagina and bowel. Sims housed and supported these women, as Beaumont had done for St. Martin. For decades, Sims was celebrated as the father of gynecology, thanks in part to the surgical advances he made while experimenting on these women. He was elected president of the American Medical Association in 1876, and a statue of him was erected in New York. Some have criticized him because of these early anesthesia-free operations on three vulnerable women; others have noted that anesthesia was not available at the time and that he was operating on these women to help them.

During this century, many experiments were carried out to better understand how disease is transmitted. Contagious matter, such as pus or discharge, was transferred from patient to patient in attempts to grasp the nature of illness. Researchers studied venereal diseases, using blind or mentally retarded children, beggars, prostitutes, or the terminally ill, considering these individual as already damaged and therefore suitable for medical experimentation. The best-known of these experiments was carried out by German venereologist Albert Neisser (1855–1916), who discovered *gonococcus*, the bacterium that causes gonorrhea. Neisser infected prostitutes with syphilis while trying to invent a vaccine against the illness. The case led to the Prussian government later issuing a directive to researchers about the importance of consent. He was fined but continued his illustrious career. His Norwegian colleague and rival Gerhard Armauer Hansen (1841–1912) lost his job because of somewhat similar experimentation with leprosy.

Some individuals used themselves as subjects. Daniel Carrión (1857–1885), a Peruvian medical student, had been studying the illness verruga peruana for three years. This illness, endemic in Peru, is marked by large wart-like lesions. He asked a friend to inoculate him with blood from the wart of a young boy with that illness. He developed Oroya fever, a serious illness marked by fever, enlarged spleen and liver, and anemia, and died. He had proved the connection between these two illnesses. Oroya fever and verruga peruana are both caused by the bacterium *Bartonella bacilliformis*.

Researchers used themselves or family members in other types of experiments. Sigmund Freud (1856–1939), the neurologist better known for his creation of psychoanalysis, took cocaine and then measured its effect on his arm strength; he also subjected his daughter to psychoanalysis, then an experimental psychological procedure. Scottish physician and physiologist John Scott Haldane (1860–1936) breathed such noxious gases as carbon monoxide and chlorine to determine their effects; he also used his son in some experiments. American surgeon William Stewart Halsted (1852–1922), who had experimented on himself with cocaine to explore its analgesic properties, also performed quasi-experimental operations or procedures on his sister and mother. James Simpson (1811–1870), Carl Koller (1857–1944), and Horace Wells (1815–1936) all experimented on themselves with anesthetic agents.

As the 19th century drew to a close, medical experiments began to seem like magnificent achievements, thanks largely to Pasteur's development of a safe rabies vaccine. Illnesses were finally beginning to be understood, but very few cases could yet be safely or effectively treated. Such advances, which we now take for granted, would not come until the 20th century.

TIMELINE

1818	James Blundell (1791–1878) successfully transfuses blood from husband to wife after she bleeds heavily during childbirth.
1825–1833	William Beaumont (1785–1853) performs experiments on Alexis St. Martin (1802–1880), who had sustained a fistula in his stomach after a gunshot wound.
1845–1849	J. Marion Sims (1813–1883) performs experimental gynecological operations on black women and is later criticized, perhaps unfairly, for not using anesthesia.
1846	William Morton (1819–1868), a dentist, uses ether to anesthetize a patient at Massachusetts General Hospital.

1847	Sir James Simpson (1811–1870), a Scottish obstetrician, experiments on himself and two friends and discovers the anesthetic properties of chloroform.
1860–1936	Life of John Scott Haldane, who experiments on himself and others to make discoveries regarding breathing to improve safe working conditions for miners and divers.
1879	Gerhard Armauer Hansen (1841–1912), Norwegian physician and discoverer of the cause of leprosy, injects leprosy matter into two patients who are ill with a different type of leprosy and is censured for this.
1882–1884	Kanehiro Takaki (1849–1920), a Japanese naval physician, changes the usual diet on a Japanese training ship and lowers the incidence of beriberi.
1884	Carl Koller (1857–1944), an Austrian ophthalmologist, applies cocaine to his eye as well as a colleague's and proves its anesthetic properties.
1884	Sigmund Freud (1856–1939) suggests that his friend and fellow-physician Ernst von Fleischl-Marxow (1846–1891) try cocaine to see whether it will help with his opiate addiction.
1885	Louis Pasteur (1822–1895) vaccinates a nine-year-old boy against rabies using a vaccine that was not thoroughly tested, but it is nonetheless effective.
1892	Waldemar Haffkine (1860–1930) inoculates himself and friends with a vaccine against cholera and bubonic plague.
1892	Albert Neisser (1855–1916), German physician and discoverer of *gonococcus*, the organism that causes gonorrhea, begins his experiments with inoculations of syphilitic serum into subjects without their consent.
1892	Max von Pettenkofer (1818–1901) drinks a flask of cholera bacilli, to disprove the theory that cholera is a contagious disease, and develops mild diarrhea.
1897	Giuseppe Sanarelli (1864–1940) announces, mistakenly, that he has discovered the cause of yellow fever after injecting people with what he thinks is yellow fever toxin.
1898	Neisser publishes the results of his studies of syphilis injections into young women, which leads to outrage.

REFERENCE ENTRIES

ANESTHESIOLOGY

Anesthesiology is the physiologic and pharmacologic management of patients during surgery. The discovery of anesthetic drugs made surgery tolerable, and some of the drugs were discovered by researchers experimenting on themselves.

The use of drugs to relieve the pain and anxiety of surgery dates back to prehistory; seeds of the opium poppy have been found in the ruins of Swiss lakeside villages occupied in the 3rd millennium BCE, and the Egyptians were using opium extracted from those seeds around 1300 BCE. In the 1st century CE, Roman physicians used such drugs as mandragora bark, hyoscyamus seed, and extract of opium poppies to induce sleep or relieve pain. By the 13th century, other substances, such as mulberry, flax, hemlock, lapathum, ivy, and lettuce seed, were sometimes used as well.

The path to the synthesis and use of modern anesthetic agents was long. Valerius Cardus (1515–1544), a German botanist, pharmacist, and physician, synthesized ether (which he called sweet oil of vitriol) in 1540, but it was not used in anesthesia in any organized manner for the next 300 years. Joseph Priestley (1733–1804), the English philosopher and chemist, discovered nitrous oxide ("laughing gas") in 1772. English chemist Humphry Davy (1778–1829) experimented with it on animals and humans, including himself, and suggested it could be used in surgery. However, it remained for Hartford, Connecticut, dentist Horace Wells (1815–1848) to actually use it for that purpose in 1845.

In 1859, Albert Niemann (1834–1861), a young German chemist, isolated cocaine from the Peruvian coca leaf. Many noticed that it had local numbing effects. Neurologist and father of psychoanalysis Sigmund Freud (1856–1939), fascinated with cocaine, mainly because of its stimulant effects, talked about it with one of his colleagues, Carl Koller (1857–1944), a young ophthalmologist who was looking for a way to make cataract surgery less painful.

Inspired by his discussions with Freud, Koller applied cocaine to one eye of a frog but not the other and showed that the cocainized eye was indeed numb. In 1884, Koller tried the same experiment on himself and a colleague, cocainizing their own eyes. They found that they could press on their corneas and push pinheads into them painlessly. As a result, cataract surgery became less terrifying. Building on Koller's work, American surgeon William Halsted (1852–1922) pioneered the use of cocaine as a regional anesthetic agent, injecting it directly into the nerves instead of just applying it topically. (Both Freud and Halsted used cocaine themselves; Halsted became addicted.)

True surgical anesthesia began in 1842 when Georgia physician Crawford W. Long (1815–1878), who had participated in "ether frolics" as a medical student, used the gas on surgical patients. He did not, however, publish his findings, claiming he had been too busy practicing to write journal articles.

Horace Wells had his own tooth extracted painlessly under the influence of nitrous oxide. Emboldened by this success, he arranged for it to be used during another surgical extraction at the Massachusetts General Hospital (MGH), but it did not sufficiently anesthetize the patient, who cried out in pain. On October 16, 1846, Wells's partner, William Morton (1819–1868), an American medical student and dentist, was involved in the first successful operation using general anesthesia at MGH. Morton applied ether to a patient who had a large tumor on his neck, and the man lost consciousness. The surgeon, John Collins Warren (1778–1856), removed the tumor. The patient regained consciousness, and Warren famously announced, "Gentlemen, this is no humbug." The demonstration was a stunning success, and ether anesthesia became a surgical standard in the United States and Europe within months.

James Young Simpson (1811–1870), a Scottish obstetrician, however, was dissatisfied with ether's side effects, which included nausea, and experimented with many other agents. (Ether also had the disadvantage of being flammable.) After first experimenting with chloroform on himself and friends, he began to use the new drug with his patients, and it became popular in England. It was widely used in obstetric practice after Queen Victoria delivered her eighth child in 1853 with its assistance. Church officials objected to its use and said that relieving pain during childbirth violated the will of God.

Jack E. McCallum

BEAUMONT, WILLIAM, AND ALEXIS ST. MARTIN

The names of William Beaumont and Alexis St. Martin will forever be joined in the history of medicine. Beaumont saved St. Martin's life after he was shot in his stomach. The wound healed, but St. Martin developed a fistula. Beaumont took advantage of this development by binding St. Martin to himself through a contract and carrying out over 200 medical experiments on him over the next eight years.

A military physician and clinical physiologist, William Beaumont was born into a farming family in Lebanon, Connecticut, on November 21, 1785. As a young man, he refused his father's offer of an adjoining farm and moved to upstate New York, where he worked briefly as a teacher before beginning an apprenticeship with a physician in St. Albans, Vermont.

When the War of 1812 began, Beaumont, then 27 years of age, enlisted as a surgeon's mate. He participated in both the Battle of Niagara and the siege of Plattsburgh, where he took a particular interest in pleurisy and other pulmonary infections that plagued the American forces.

After the war, Beaumont entered private practice in Plattsburgh, New York, but he found civilian medicine boring. So, in 1820, he convinced his friend and army surgeon general Joseph Lovell to appoint him physician to the military base on Mackinac Island in the territory that later became Michigan.

While working on Mackinac Island in 1822, he was called on to treat a young fur trapper or voyageur, Alexis St. Martin (born in Canada in 1802), who had been shot in the stomach. Beaumont dressed the wound—expecting the trapper to die—but over the course of several months, St. Martin surprisingly recovered, although with a fistula, or passage, between his stomach and skin that never healed.

Beaumont saw the opportunity to study digestion in a way that had not been done before. He took St. Martin into his home and began a series of over 200 experiments on him over the next eight years. When Beaumont was transferred to Fort Niagara in 1825, he took St. Martin with him, employed him as an orderly and personal servant, and continued his experiments.

The experiments were uncomfortable and intrusive. St. Martin would lie down, and Beaumont would tie some food to a string, insert it into St. Martin's stomach through the fistula, and then retrieve it and document the resulting gastric movements and secretions. Beaumont showed for the first time that gastric secretions only occurred after the stomach was presented with food. He collected this "gastric liquor," measured it, and even tasted it. He showed that digestion was affected by emotions and general health and was due to chemical processes, not fermentation or mechanical activities of the stomach. Beaumont also witnessed peristalsis—the rhythmic contractions of the gastrointestinal tract, through the fistula.

The relationship between the two men was fraught. St. Martin was grateful that Beaumont had saved his life, but he tired of the experiments and disliked being displayed to others. Beaumont and St. Martin had signed a contract that was similar to labor contracts of the time. According to the contract, St. Martin had to comply with Beaumont's requests, while Beaumont had to support him. At one point, St. Martin, although a French Canadian, enlisted in the American army as an orderly, thus further formalizing their relationship, as Beaumont was an officer.

St. Martin eventually ran away back home to Canada. While in Canada, he married and fathered two children. Beaumont paid for St. Martin's whole family to move to live with him and his wife in Fort Crawford, on the upper Mississippi. Experiments resumed for the next two years. In 1831, St. Martin and his wife and four children returned to Canada. A year and a half later, St. Martin rejoined Beaumont in Washington, D.C., where Beaumont then lived. St. Martin once again returned to Canada in 1834, this time not to return.

Beaumont carried out his experiments on St. Martin in his own home, with little help or support from others. For most of them, he had little or no laboratory equipment. He published his results in the epochal book *Experiments and Observations on the Gastric Juice and the Physiology of Digestion* in 1833. That same year, he also wrote what has been called the first American document about the ethics of experimenting on humans, stating that "the experiment is to be discontinued when it causes distress to the subject" and that there must be voluntary consent.[1]

Beaumont left the army soon after his book was published and practiced medicine privately in St. Louis until his death in 1853. St. Martin lived with his fistula to age 83 and died in 1880. His family is said to have delayed the burial so that his body would decompose and then buried him so deeply that no one could ever experiment on him again.

Jack E. McCallum

Reference

1.   The quotation from Beaumont about ethical research can be found in George J. Annas and Michael A. Grodin, *The Nazi Doctors and the Nuremberg Code: Human Rights in Human Experimentation* (New York: Oxford University Press, 1992), 125.

BERIBERI EXPERIMENTS IN JAPAN

Long present in Southeast Asia, the illness beriberi became more common when mechanical grain milling was developed in the 1800s, leading to a decrease in the nutritional value of rice. One of the first people to carry out experiments to discover the cause of beriberi was a Japanese medical officer, Kanehiro Takaki.

Beriberi is a complex illness that results from a lack of thiamine. It has two forms: in "wet" beriberi, the person suffers from heart problems and swelling of the legs. In "dry" beriberi, the legs become painful and weak, and walking is difficult. If the person is alcoholic or has lost weight quickly, dry beriberi can sometimes also be accompanied by confusion and memory loss. Both forms of the disease are associated with diets that consist mostly of rice.

Beriberi had existed for centuries in Southeast Asia among people whose diet was mainly rice, but it became more widespread in the nineteenth century with the advent of mechanized grain milling. Until that point, rice was milled by hand to remove the indigestible husk. This kind of milling was done in small quantities on a daily basis and not all of the skin or pericarp was removed. Rice prepared this way retained moderate amounts of thiamine.

Around 1870, however, steel rollers for milling all types of grain were invented, and there were many immediate benefits. Using these rollers, the outer layers of grain were removed more thoroughly, easily, and efficiently than milling by hand. The mechanized mills also did a better job of removing dirt, insects, and some of the grain fats, making the grain less likely to rot or become rancid during storage. The milled grains therefore had a longer shelf life. Most people preferred the appearance, taste, and texture of machine-milled grains, and so this type of grain became associated with wealth and refinement. This new technology was widely and quickly adopted, but it came with a price: in the case of milled, or white, rice, even less thiamine remained than after hand milling, so as the new mills spread, so did beriberi.

Kanehiro Takaki (1849–1920) (sometimes Takaki Kanehiro) was a medical officer in the Japanese Imperial Navy and one of the earliest people to experiment with finding a nutritional link to beriberi. Beriberi, known as *kakké* ("leg disease" in Japanese), had existed in Japan for centuries, just as in the rest of Southeast Asia, and the Japanese navy, in particular, had been hard-hit: one-third of enlisted men between 1878 and 1882 developed it. The Japanese assumed that bacteria caused the illness, so they sent Takaki to St. Thomas's Medical Hospital in London for further medical education that might help him to address the problem. He mastered bacteriology in England, but he also learned that few men on English ships developed beriberi. Takaki thought that the relatively protein-rich diet was protective against the disease.

Takaki returned to Japan and convinced the authorities, as an experiment, to add protein to the diet supplied to the crew of a Japanese training ship. They added meat, milk, and vegetables to supplement the usually white rice–heavy fare. In 1882, this ship sailed from Japan to New Zealand and along the western coast of South America to Honolulu, and then returned to Japan in 1884. Beriberi was less common among the crew than was usual on trips of this sort. As a result of this experiment, Takaki concluded that lack of protein was the cause of beriberi. Although his theory was not quite correct, it did lead to diet changes that prevented beriberi. In addition, as the Japanese navy increased the variety of food to the diet of the seamen, the men's overall health improved.

Takaki was made a baron in recognition of his achievement. However, his experiment had little influence on the rest of the world or even other branches of the Japanese military.

Frances R. Frankenburg

FREUD, SIGMUND

Sigmund Freud, the neurologist better known for inventing psychoanalysis, was in his younger days a medical researcher of a different sort. He was one of the first Europeans to experiment with cocaine.

Sigmund Freud was born in Moravia in 1856 to a Jewish middle-class family. At the age of 17, he began to study medicine at the University of Vienna, and by the age of 26, he was a physician. Although this sober intellectual is better known now for his theories of the unconscious and the development of psychoanalysis, for a short time, he experimented with cocaine. His enthusiasm for it played an important part in an ophthalmologist's discovery of cocaine's anesthetic properties and in Freud's own perception of the importance of dreams—which led to another experiment of sorts.

In the spring of 1884, the 28-year-old Dr. Freud was concerned about the health of his friend Ernst von Fleischl-Marxow (1846–1891), another physician. While performing an autopsy, Fleischl-Marxow's right thumb became infected, and it subsequently had to be amputated. Following the surgery, he developed painful nerve growths, known as traumatic neuromas, at the site of the amputation. He began to use morphine to control the pain and became addicted to the drug.

At the same time, Freud was reading about the work of a German army physician, Dr. Theodor Aschenbrandt, who gave cocaine—provided by the German pharmaceutical company Merck—to soldiers. Aschenbrandt noticed that cocaine improved the soldiers' endurance. Freud also read reports from other physicians suggesting that cocaine cured morphine addiction. In April 1884, Freud encouraged Fleischl-Marxow to try cocaine both to build up his strength and to fight the morphine addiction.

Freud also bought some cocaine from Merck and began to experiment with it himself, taking it by mouth. It energized him and lifted his spirits. He performed laboratory experiments with a dynamometer (a device that measures power) to try to determine whether cocaine increased muscular strength or decreased reaction time. He reviewed the work of many scientists, most now forgotten, who had also experimented with cocaine, and he was most impressed by the descriptions of its mild stimulant and antidepressant effects. He recommended cocaine as a treatment for morphine or alcohol addiction. In the final paragraph of a review, he noted its possible use as a local anesthetic, but this seemed to be an afterthought, as he did not emphasize it or develop the idea.

In September 1884, one of his colleagues, ophthalmologist Carl Koller (1857–1944), with whom Freud had talked about cocaine, used the drug to first anesthetize the eyes of animals and then his own and his colleagues' eyes. As a result of these successful experiments, Koller developed painless cocaine-assisted cataract surgery and was celebrated internationally for his achievement.

In 1885, with a better understanding of the analgesic properties of cocaine, Freud tried to treat trigeminal neuralgia, a painful condition affecting a facial nerve, with injected cocaine but was unsuccessful, perhaps because of his lack of surgical expertise and skill. He continued to take cocaine by mouth, mainly as a stimulant when depressed or anxious, for the next few years.

Freud had hoped that the cocaine would help Fleischl-Marxow stop using morphine, but Fleischl-Marxow continued to use it—along with cocaine. He died in 1891, addicted to both drugs.

Meanwhile, Freud and a colleague, Wilhelm Fliess (1858–1928), an ear, nose, and throat surgeon, were collaborating in approaches to psychological problems. Fliess had a number of theories, one of which posited a connection between the nose and the genitals. Freud was fascinated by this theory. Freud himself had nasal surgery and often used cocaine to relieve his bothersome nasal congestion.

Freud asked Fliess to see one of his patients, Emma Eckstein, to whom he may have earlier recommended cocaine. Fliess recommended surgery to remove a bone from her nose to treat some of her psychological problems. The surgery went badly. This surgery could be considered to have been a therapeutic experiment that failed.

Perhaps bothered by this case, Freud had a complicated dream about cocaine and the nose. Freud reviewed his dream from multiple angles. He realized that the dream was not an accurate replication of any particular event, and he wondered about the reasons for the differences between the dream and his memory. He examined all of the differences and thought about the meanings of the words of the dream and each particular incident. By going over and over this dream—or, in other words, by "analyzing" it—he had found "the royal road to the unconscious." Each difference had psychological significance. This dream became the second chapter in one of his early masterpieces, *The Interpretation of Dreams*, published in 1900. By analyzing this cocaine-related dream, Freud had just created psychoanalysis. One of the first people that he subjected to the process was himself. He also analyzed his daughter, Anna (1895–1982), who grew up to become a psychoanalyst herself and created the field of child psychoanalysis.

Psychoanalysis is a painstaking process during which a person talks freely with an analyst for several days a week in an attempt to find patterns and causes of some feelings and behaviors. It is perhaps stretching the word "experiment" to label each analysis so, as the findings, such as they are, are difficult to replicate. The process is not scientific because the psychoanalytic concepts are impossible to measure or quantify. But Freud had invented a new form of psychological treatment that seemed scientific to him.

Freud's experiments with cocaine led indirectly to its use as a helpful anesthetic agent for surgical procedures but certainly not as a treatment for depression or anxiety. (We now know that cocaine is not an antidepressant, can worsen anxiety, and is addictive.) Perhaps his invention of psychoanalysis and his analysis of himself and his daughter could be considered psychological experiments, but despite their immense cultural influence, they have not been seen as scientific or as part of medicine.

Freud later developed cancer of his jaw and palate. He became unable to tolerate the pain, and in 1939, at his request, his doctor administered a lethal overdose of morphine.

Frances R. Frankenburg

HAFFKINE, WALDEMAR MORDECAI WOLFF

Waldemar Mordecai Wolff Haffkine developed and used vaccines against cholera and bubonic plague, which he tested on himself, prisoners, and many thousands of people in India.

Waldemar Mordecai Wolff Haffkine (1860–1930) was born in Odessa, at that time ruled by Russia. He studied at the department of natural sciences at the University of Odessa, where he came under the influence of microbiologist and future Nobel Prize–winner Elie Metchnikoff (1845–1916). In 1889, Metchnikoff, who was working with Louis Pasteur (1822–1895), a chemist and microbiologist, at the Pasteur Institute in Paris, offered Haffkine the only vacant position—that of librarian. By 1890, Haffkine had become assistant to the director of the institute, Émile Roux (1853–1933), the French bacteriologist who worked closely with Pasteur and had helped to develop the diphtheria vaccine.

At the time that Haffkine was beginning his career, one of the five great cholera pandemics of the 19th century was raging through Asia and Europe. Cholera is a devastating and often fatal diarrheal illness caused by the bacterium *Cholera vibrio*. Haffkine focused his research on creating a vaccine for it. He developed a strain of *Cholera vibrio* by passing it through the peritoneal cavity of guinea pigs, thus producing a culture of live cholera bacilli that had "fixed virulence"—meaning that the potency of this preparation would not change over time. This kind of culture was known as an "exalted" strain. He also produced an attenuated, or weakened, form of the bacterium by exposing it to blasts of hot air.

Haffkine inoculated guinea pigs, rabbits, and pigeons with the attenuated culture and then with the exalted strain. The animals did not become ill. In July 1892, building on these initial positive results, Haffkine inoculated himself with the weakened culture and then six days later with the exalted culture. He then inoculated three Russian friends. All survived, and Haffkine looked for a further opportunity to test his vaccine. His senior colleagues, including both Metchnikoff and Pasteur, were not interested, nor were authorities in Germany, France, or Russia. Haffkine's work was appreciated by others, however, and he was persuaded by Lord Dufferin (1826–1902), the former viceroy of India, to go to India, where cholera was killing hundreds of thousands.

He arrived in India in 1893 and was met with suspicion. On one occasion, a crowd of villagers threw stones at him and broke some of his equipment. To show them that his vaccine was safe, Haffkine asked an assistant to revaccinate him in front of the villagers. This demonstration went smoothly, and many present allowed themselves to also be vaccinated. He went on to vaccinate people in Calcutta, 20,000 laborers in the tea gardens of Assam, and inmates in the Gya (sometimes Gaya) Jail. As a result of these vaccinations, the mortality rate from cholera in the tea gardens dropped from between 22–45 percent to 2 percent. Haffkine had to stop his work, however, when he became ill with malaria in August 1895 and returned to France.

In December 1895, while lecturing in London, Haffkine reported that between April 1893 and the end of July 1895, he and his colleagues had inoculated over 42,000 people. In some cases, only the first injection had been given. Later statisticians examined his data and concluded that three of the eight trials reported by Haffkine showed that Haffkine's inoculation might have been effective. In March 1896, against his doctor's advice, Haffkine returned to India and performed another 30,000 vaccinations in seven months.

In October 1896, an epidemic of the deadly bubonic plague struck Bombay (now Mumbai), and the Indian government asked Haffkine for assistance. Also known as the Black Death, the plague is caused by the bacterium *Yersinia pestis* and is marked by large and painful lymph nodes, fever, and chills. It had been absent from India for many years but returned in 1896, probably brought in from Hong Kong. Haffkine embarked upon the development of a vaccine in a small laboratory in a corridor of Bombay's Grant Medical College. He used goat flesh as a medium for growing his cultures (beef or pork products being unacceptable to the Hindu and Muslim populations). Within three months, a form of the vaccine was ready for human trials, and on January 10, 1897, Haffkine tested it on himself. He developed a fever and malaise but recovered within two days.

In early 1897, bubonic plague struck the Byculla jail in Bombay, and some of the prisoners volunteered to be inoculated. Two of the 154 volunteers developed plague and survived. Of the 170 controls, 12 caught the plague, and 6 died. Although the numbers vary slightly in different accounts, the lesson was clear: vaccination against the plague was successful. At the end of 1897, plague broke out in the Umerkhadi (sometimes Umerkadi) Common Jail in Bombay, and 401 prisoners volunteered to be inoculated. The prisoners were lined up in the jail yard, and every other prisoner was inoculated. Of the 127 not inoculated, there were 10 cases of plague and 6 deaths. Of the 147 inoculated, there were 3 very mild cases of plague.

One of Haffkine's supporters was Sir Sultan Shah, Aga Khan III, KCIE (1877–1957), head of the Khoja Muslim community. The Aga Khan was vaccinated and paid for Haffkine's laboratory to be moved and established in his own lodge. He also encouraged the Muslim community to be inoculated.

In 1898, Haffkine organized a trial of the vaccine in the village of Undhera. Half of the population was vaccinated while the other half, the control group, was not. Six weeks later, he found that among the 71 inoculated, there were 8 cases of plague and 3 deaths; among the 64 controls, there were 27 cases and 26 deaths. In recognition of his work, Haffkine was appointed the director of the Plague Laboratory in Bombay.

In 1902, 19 Indian villagers who had been inoculated against plague from a single bottle of vaccine died of tetanus. An inquiry indicted Haffkine, and he was relieved of his position and returned to England. The report was unofficially known as the "Little Dreyfus Affair," referencing Haffkine's Judaism. (The Dreyfus affair involved the 1895 conviction of French army captain Alfred Dreyfus, who was Jewish, for allegedly betraying France to Germany. The unjust conviction was blamed on French anti-Semitism.) The Lister Institute of London reinvestigated the claim and overruled the verdict: it was discovered that an assistant had failed to sterilize a bottle cap.

By experimenting both on himself and many others, including prisoners, Haffkine had discovered moderately effective vaccines against two bacterial diseases that were responsible for killing millions of people—cholera and black plague. Not well-known in the Western world today, he is honored in India, where an institute—the Haffkine Institute in Mumbai—has been named after him. Work against infectious diseases continues there today.

Frances R. Frankenburg

HALDANE, JOHN SCOTT

John Scott Haldane was a Scottish physiologist and physician who experimented on himself to determine the safety of conditions in mines and the effects of various gases.

John Scott Haldane (1860–1936) was born in Edinburgh and studied at the University of Jena in Germany. He received his medical degree from Edinburgh University in 1884 but did not go into practice as a physician, being more interested in physiology. One of his first projects as a young doctor was to measure the excretion of certain substances in people ill with scarlet fever. Then he examined the excreta of smallpox victims and of himself. His career of self-experimentation had started.

Another early project, beginning his lifelong interest in respiration and social issues, was the study of the air in the slums of Dundee. He visited these neighborhoods and took samples of the air in small bottles, finding that homes and schoolrooms contained high concentrations of carbon dioxide, molds, hydrogen sulfide, and bacteria. He also studied sewer gases, which could cause explosions, and explored the sewers that ran under the Parliament buildings in London. He lowered himself into sewers to smell the gases and later invented the practice of lowering rodents into sewers to test air quality.

To more fully investigate and understand the effects of various gases on breathing, he built small airproof lead-lined chambers in which the concentration of these gases could be manipulated and measured. One such early chamber was in his own home in Oxford. He would often shut himself up to expose himself to different gases and monitor his responses, at times relying on his children to see if he was still breathing. He discovered that increasing concentrations of carbon dioxide led to rapid breathing and a sensation of panic, and that lower concentrations of oxygen led to unconsciousness. He often exposed himself to high concentrations of carbon monoxide, a poisonous gas produced by burning coal or other fuel, and then tested his physical endurance.

One of his major areas of research and concern was the safety of miners in southwest Britain. In the 19th century, Wales, Cornwall, and Devon were among the richest mining areas in the world, producing coal, tin, lead, copper, and iron. Mining was dangerous work, however, in part because of the occasionally poor air quality. Haldane often descended underground to examine the air and test it with small rodents and birds. Because of their rapid metabolism, small animals are more sensitive to changes in the air they breathe than humans.

The idea of using canaries in mines to measure air quality was Haldane's; if the bird died, the miners would know of the presence of toxic gases and have time to escape. These birds were used to protect miners until the 1980s, when a variety of chemical or electrical carbon monoxide detectors and sensors were developed. Indeed, the use of canaries in mines became so well-known that the expression "canary in the coal mine" has evolved to refer to something that serves as a warning or early indicator of danger.

Another mining problem was that coal dust explosions and fires led to accidents and deaths from injuries, burns, exposure to poisonous gases, or lack of oxygen. Haldane raced to mine disasters to sample the air and again climbed down into the mines. He took blood from dead miners; he performed autopsies on the miners and also on pit ponies, the horses that hauled coal underground.

This work was, of course, hazardous, and he would reassure his wife that he was safe by sending her telegrams. If the gases had affected him, he would sometimes become confused and send multiple telegrams, having forgotten the ones that he had already sent.

In 1905, the British navy asked Haldane to investigate decompression sickness, a problem that bedeviled divers working underwater. When divers breathe pressurized air, some of it dissolves into the tissues. If the diver comes up too quickly, nitrogen rediffuses out of the tissues as bubbles that can cause pain, depending on where they lodge. Sometimes the person bends over in agony; hence, the sickness became known as "the bends." Decompression sickness is also associated with work in caissons—large structures underwater on which bridges are placed—so it became known as caisson disease as well.

To investigate this problem, Haldane built a pressure chamber, which resembled a seven-foot-long boiler turned on its side. There were two six-inch-long windows and one entrance that looked like a manhole. He would go into the chamber for hours at a time, experimenting with different pressures, rates of "ascent," and gas compositions. He also put goats into the chamber because of their sensitivity to decompression sickness. He donned a diving suit himself and went underwater, which was all the more remarkable as he did not know how to swim.

At the time that he began his work, it was considered safe for divers to come up slowly at first, but then more rapidly. Haldane showed that divers had to come up very slowly for the entire duration of the ascent to avoid the bends, particularly as they neared the surface. In addition, the rate of ascent needed to be adjusted according to the length of time underwater. He devised dive tables to help people understand how fast they could safely come up. These tables, or versions of them, were used for decades.

In 1911, Haldane traveled to Pikes Peak in Colorado, 14,000 feet high, to study the effects of high altitudes on breathing, again using himself as a subject. During his time on Pikes Peak, he concluded that people acclimatize to high altitudes as their lung alveoli (air sacs) begin to secrete oxygen into the blood. This is no longer thought to be the case.

During World War I, Haldane's expertise was particularly useful. When the Germans used poison gases at Ypres, Haldane went to the front and identified the gases as chlorine and bromine. Haldane was already familiar with chlorine poisoning because, in his earlier work with sewers, he had encountered chlorine disinfecting agents, which released chlorine gas. At the front, he took blood samples and performed autopsies. After his return to Oxford, Haldane repeatedly sealed himself and a colleague in his airproof chamber—exposing the two of them to chlorine gas—to work out its toxicity and methods of protection against it. He had done similar work 20 years earlier with carbon monoxide. With the help of his son, by then a soldier, he was able to improve gas masks for the British forces.

In addition to his discoveries and inventions that led to safer mining, submarining, and more effective gas masks, Haldane made significant advances in the physiology of respiration.

As is clear from his work, Haldane believed in experimentation on himself and also that one should never subject animals to experiments before experimenting on oneself. He was not fanatical about this however. He did come up with the idea of the canary in the mine, and he did use goats in diving chambers. He would also sometimes experiment on his own son, who, in his own career, would carry on his father's work in respiration and self-experimentation.

In 1936, Haldane went to Persia to investigate cases of heat stroke in the oil refineries. He died later that year in Oxford, shortly after his return to England.

Frances R. Frankenburg

HALSTED, WILLIAM STEWART

William Stewart Halsted, one of the most important figures in the history of American surgery, experimented with cocaine as an anesthetic agent and devised regional, or local, anesthesia, a way of numbing a body part during surgery without interfering with consciousness. He experimented on two family members, invented new surgical procedures and techniques, and improved surgical education.

William Stewart Halsted (1852–1922) was born in New York City to a wealthy family, the oldest of four children. He had a privileged education, attending Phillips Academy in Andover, Massachusetts, and then Yale College. He obtained his medical degree from Columbia University in New York in 1877, though such a degree was not then what it is today. In the late 1800s, medical education and practice were quite backward throughout the United States, particularly when compared to Europe. In many American medical schools, students did not even have to be high school graduates. They were not expected to attend lectures, dissect cadavers, or examine patients.

Aware of the inadequacies of his medical education, Halsted traveled to Austria and Germany to further his studies. (He remained impressed with German medicine for the rest of his life.) In 1880, he returned to New York, where he became a successful physician. He was hardworking and ambitious and became adept at dissections and a master of anatomy. He also formed an important friendship with William Welch (1850–1934), a pathologist who would later help to create the Johns Hopkins School of Medicine.

Halsted was an adventurous and fearless surgeon with such self-confidence that he was willing to treat his own family members in ways that were innovative and practically unheard of at the time. In 1881, his sister bled heavily after delivering a baby, and he performed one of the first emergency blood transfusions, transfusing his own blood into her. Almost unbelievably, he operated on his own mother in 1882: she became ill, and he removed stones from her gallbladder—on her kitchen table in the middle of the night. This was one of the first times such a surgery had been performed in the United States.

Halsted's career course changed trajectory after he learned of the work done by ophthalmologist Carl Koller (1857–1944) in 1884, in which he used cocaine as a topical anesthetic agent for cataract surgery. Dentists and eye surgeons—those men who inflicted great pain on their patients—began to apply cocaine directly to teeth and eyes to numb them. Halsted took the next step and injected cocaine directly into the nerves that carried sensations from the area about to be operated on. This was the beginning of regional, or local, anesthesia. For example, he injected cocaine into an area in the face just under the eye. Cocaine applied here numbs the nerves carrying sensation from the upper jaw and makes dental extractions less painful.

Halsted would use cocaine deftly and successfully in multiple other procedures. Together with his New York medical students, he expanded the uses of the drug. Halsted's experimental work increased the number of operations, both dental and otherwise, that could be performed with local anesthesia. Halsted also showed that cocaine interfered with the transmission of sensation but not with the control of muscles. The patient who received an injection of cocaine was conscious, could follow any instructions of the surgical team, and felt no pain.

Halsted could not have known it at the time, but injected or snorted cocaine is different from cocaine consumed by mouth because of its quick onset of action. Halsted, with some of his colleagues and students, began to sniff cocaine powder. Many of these young doctors, including Halsted, became addicted—Halsted probably for the rest of his life. Later, in an attempt to overcome his cocaine use, he began to use morphine, which only resulted in his becoming addicted to both drugs.

Meanwhile, Halsted's friend Welch was becoming more involved with a new institution in Baltimore, Maryland: the Johns Hopkins Hospital and School of Medicine. Welch, too, had studied in Germany and was determined to create a medical school and hospital to rival German institutions. He recruited Halsted in 1886 to join him in the newly formed pathology laboratory. The other two physicians who made up the "Big Four" founding members of Johns Hopkins were William Osler (1849–1919) and Howard Kelly (1858–1943). Within a few years, most of the advances in American medicine were coming out of Baltimore.

In 1889, Halsted became temporary chief of the department of surgery; a year later, surgeon-in-chief; and then, two years later, professor of surgery. Halsted developed the (now outmoded) technique of radical mastectomy, in which the entire breast and surrounding tissue, including part of the armpit, were removed to treat breast cancer. Until Halsted's work, there was no treatment for or management of breast cancer. Women often did not seek medical attention until the cancer involved the whole breast, at which point doctors could do little to help. Using his formidable knowledge of anatomy and attention to detail, Halsted was able to safely remove the entire breast and associated tissue and at least make the woman more comfortable for some time.

Halsted introduced the use of rubber gloves in surgery, initially to help an operating room nurse who had developed dermatitis, probably due to her exposure to mercuric chloride, which was then used as an antiseptic agent. (He later married the nurse with the sensitive skin.) He improved hernia and thyroid surgeries and propagated the art and science of safe surgery by scrupulous aseptic technique, gentle handling of the tissues, and attention to stopping blood loss. A pioneer in medical education, he started the first formal surgical residency training program in the United States and developed the concept of surgical residencies in which residents took on more responsibility as they matured.

Halsted had immense self-confidence, which allowed him to experiment with new treatments and to operate on his sister and mother, possibly saving their lives. On the other hand, his self-experimentation with cocaine (and later morphine) imperiled his health and career. Despite his addictions, Halsted made major contributions to surgery, perhaps the most important of which was the establishment of experimental laboratories at Hopkins and his encouragement of students to experiment and find new ways of treating surgical problems.

Frances R. Frankenburg

HANSEN, GERHARD ARMAUER

Gerhard Armauer Hansen was the Norwegian codiscoverer (along with Albert Neisser of Germany) of the leprosy bacillus, the bacterium that causes leprosy. His experiments on leprosy patients without their consent led to his losing his position in a leprosy hospital.

Leprosy is a chronic infection caused by the bacterium *Mycobacterium leprae*, which leads to nodules, or granulomas. Because the bacterium grows best at cooler temperatures, it damages the exterior parts of the body, such as the nose and toes, but rarely the warmer internal organs. In the past, if leprosy only affected the skin, it was known as cutaneous, or nodular, leprosy. If it also led to patches of skin discoloration and damaged the peripheral nerves, leading to loss of sensation, it was known as maculo-anesthetic leprosy.

Although primarily thought of as a tropical illness, leprosy was common in Norway in the 1800s. In an attempt to find out whether the illness was contagious, researchers, including Daniel Cornelius Danielssen (1815–1894), a physician and leading leprosy researcher, inoculated themselves and others with material from leprous nodules, which sometimes led to skin ulcers but never to leprosy itself. The work of Gerhard Armauer Hansen (1841–1912) and Albert Neisser (1855–1916) finally established the infectious nature of the illness.

Hansen was born and educated in Norway. After he completed his medical training, he worked as a clinician in a research center at a hospital for leprosy patients. Danielssen was his mentor. In 1873, Hansen discovered rod-shaped microorganisms in nodules taken from these patients. He could not prove that these microorganisms caused the illness, however, because the leprosy bacillus is difficult to grow in culture or to transfer to animals. (The only other animal that develops leprosy is the armadillo.)

In 1879, in yet another attempt to show its contagiousness, Hansen injected matter from a patient with cutaneous leprosy into the arm of a man with maculo-anesthetic leprosy to see if he could transmit the cutaneous type of leprosy into a patient with the other type. No untoward consequences resulted from this experiment. He then injected similar matter into the eye of a female patient with maculo-anesthetic leprosy. The patient had not given consent in either experiment. The woman claimed that her eye was inflamed and painful for seven weeks after

Hansen's injection, and she initiated court proceedings against him. In 1880, the City of Bergen Law Courts found Hansen guilty, and he lost his position in the leprosy hospital. The scientific community, on the other hand, did not think that the sentence was warranted. Hansen continued his work with leprosy; indeed, leprosy is sometimes known as Hansen's disease.

Meanwhile, in 1879, Neisser visited Hansen, who gave him some specimens and unstained slide preparations. Neisser was a skilled microscopist who had studied with physician and microbiologist Robert Koch (1843–1910) and had access both to the superior fuchsin and gentian violet stains and a Zeiss microscope. He visualized the bacteria more clearly than Hansen was able to. (Bacteria are almost impossible to see unless they are stained. The stains, or dyes, highlight the organism's structures.) In 1880, Neisser announced that he had discovered the bacterium that caused leprosy. Conflict ensued between the two.

Later research has shown that leprosy is not highly infectious and that most people are not susceptible to developing the illness, thus explaining the failures (and safety) of the earlier person-to-person transmission experiments.

Frances R. Frankenburg

HOOKWORM

Hookworm infestation—which causes severe anemia—is common in places with warm and damp weather and poor sanitation. A parasitologist discovered how it was transmitted when he spilled some hookworm larvae onto his own hands, first by accident and then on purpose.

The hookworm, *Ankyloma dudodenale* or *Necator americanus*, is a parasite that can attach to the human intestine. Infestation is common in tropical climates and causes anemia. It was also common in Europe throughout the 1800s among miners and construction workers who worked in humid conditions. The disease it caused was therefore sometimes known as miners', or bricklayers', anemia. It was investigated by John Scott Haldane, who was better known for his experiments involving gases and respiration but who was also concerned about illnesses in Cornish miners. Hookworm eggs could be found in human feces, and it was assumed that transmission was via the fecal-oral route.

Arthur Looss (1861–1923) was a German zoologist and parasitologist who studied various parasitic illnesses in Egypt. In 1896, he accidentally spilled some larval cultures of hookworm onto his hand while dropping them into the mouths of guinea pigs. He saw that his skin became irritated, and he wondered if the parasites had passed through the skin. Later, after examining his feces for evidence of infestation with another parasite, he saw hookworm eggs. He repeated the cutaneous exposure to larval hookworm eggs, this time on purpose. He then examined a sample of his skin under a microscope and saw that the larvae had disappeared. They had penetrated into the skin. (Haldane had reported similar experiments with the transmission of hookworm, but with negative results.)

Looss repeated this experiment on a young boy whose leg was about to be amputated. An hour before the surgery, he applied hookworm larvae to the boy's leg. After amputation, he examined the leg and saw that most of the larvae had entered it through the hair follicles. Looss had shown that hookworms do not necessarily use the fecal-oral route to infect humans, but rather can infect humans through the skin. In 1904, Fritz Schaudinn (1871–1906), the great German zoologist who discovered *Treponema pallidum*, the causative agent of syphilis, and who had distinguished between the pathogenic and nonpathogenic forms of *Entamoeba* (a microorganism that lives in the human bowel), confirmed these findings.

Hookworms usually enter the body through the feet. Walking barefoot in areas contaminated with human fecal matter, either by unsanitary privies or the use of human waste as fertilizer, rapidly spreads the parasite. The hookworm larvae enter the skin of the foot and then the blood or lymphatic circulation and travel to the lungs. From the lungs, they either travel up to the throat themselves or are coughed up and then swallowed. Once in the human intestine, the larvae "hook" onto the small intestine and feed on the individual's blood. Persons infested with hookworms become sluggish and listless because of the iron-deficiency anemia. What was often seen as laziness and personality flaws in many people who lived in tropical areas is now thought to be a consequence of hookworm-caused anemia.

In 1931, hematologist William Castle (1897–1990) and pathologist Cornelius Rhoads (1898–1959) conducted a several-month-long study for the Rockefeller Anemia Commission as part of the Rockefeller Foundation's work in trying to combat hookworm in Puerto Rico. Most of the population in Puerto Rico was infested with hookworms. Castle emphasized the importance of replacing the lost iron with supplemental iron. Once that was done and the anemic population became healthier and stronger, medication to eliminate the worms became more effective, and it was easier to encourage the population to build better latrines and wear shoes.

Looss's discovery of the ability of the hookworm larvae to penetrate the skin explained how anemia could be so common and debilitating in some areas of the world and focused attention on proper disposal of feces and the importance of wearing shoes.

Frances R. Frankenburg

NEISSER, ALBERT

Albert Neisser was a German physician who discovered the bacterium *Neisseria gonorrhoeae*, which causes gonorrhea. His later experiments with syphilis were performed without the consent of his subjects and led to Prussian guidelines about human experimentation, in which such activity was forbidden.

Albert Neisser (1855–1916) was a German physician who studied microbiology. He had a special interest in venereal diseases, those diseases spread by sexual contact. At that time, the details regarding the transmission of these diseases were not entirely understood, and there was no particularly effective or safe treatment. While still a resident in the combined specialty of dermatology and venereology, Neisser made the discovery for which he is most famous.

Gonorrhea is a contagious disease that is usually spread through sexual contact. An infected woman can also spread the infection during childbirth, leading to ophthalmia (an eye infection) in the newborn child. Not all people with gonorrhea have symptoms though, and people without symptoms can still spread it. In 1879, at the age of 24, Neisser found the same microorganism present in over 20 adults with gonorrhea and in several infants and adults with ophthalmia. (The exact numbers vary in different accounts.) He stained the bacterium with methyl violet (sometimes described as methylene blue) and examined it with the newly devised Zeiss microscope and Abbé condenser (a lens that focuses light from the light source onto the specimen being examined). He described a new species of coccus (spherical bacterium) that appeared in pairs, which he identified as the cause of gonorrhea. His colleague Paul Ehrlich (1854–1915) named the new bacterium *gonococcus*. The microorganism is now known as *Neisseria gonorrhoeae*, "*Neiserria*" deriving, of course, from Neisser's own name.

He then turned his attention to the other main venereal disease, syphilis, a complicated illness with primary, secondary, latent, and tertiary forms caused by *Treponema pallidum*. In 1892, during tests of a vaccine against syphilis, he administered a subcutaneous (under the skin) injection of cell-free serum from syphilitic patients into four young females—one of whom had gonorrhea—hoping that this would serve as a kind of vaccination. They did not develop syphilis.

Emboldened by this success, he then injected syphilitic serum into the veins of four prostitutes between the ages of 17 and 20. All subsequently developed syphilis. These women had not given consent, and the public was outraged. Neisser claimed that the prostitutes had developed syphilis in another "normal" way. The case was sufficiently notorious that it reached the Prussian parliament and led to a 1900 directive regulating experimentation, forbidding experiments on individuals without their express consent. Most physicians of the time supported Neisser. (There is still no vaccine for syphilis, perhaps because *T. pallidum*, sometimes known as a stealth organism, does not elicit an immune response.)

Neisser also became involved in a conflict about the discovery of the cause of leprosy. In 1879—the same year that he identified *N. gonorrhoeae*—Neisser made advances in the staining of the bacillus that causes leprosy. That year he visited the Norwegian physician Gerhard Armauer Hansen (1841–1902) and took some tissue samples of Hansen's leprous patients back to Germany. Neisser successfully stained the bacteria with fuchsin and gentian violet and announced his findings in 1880, claiming to have discovered the pathogenesis of leprosy. Hansen had discovered the bacterium in 1873 but had never been able to culture the organism and prove its link to leprosy, so the two men now share credit for the discovery.

Frances R. Frankenburg

PASTEUR, LOUIS

The rabies vaccination that French scientist Louis Pasteur administered to nine-year-old Joseph Meister in 1885 is one of the most famous experiments in medical history. Rabies, although rare, is a terrifying and fatal disease that has always struck fear into people. Pasteur's ability to prevent what seemed likely to be a horrible death for the boy made medicine appear to be a lifesaving science in the 19th century. We now know that Pasteur was perhaps taking a greater risk with this experiment than was appreciated at the time.

Rabies is a viral disease that animals transmit to humans, usually through a bite or a scratch. In large parts of the world, the animal most often responsible for transmitting the virus to humans is a dog; in America, it's usually a bat. Once in the body, rabies travels along the nerves at a rate of one to two centimeters a day until it reaches the brain, where it causes inflammation. One to three months after the bite, the person becomes violently agitated, hydrophobic (afraid of water), and produces excessive saliva. In almost all cases, once the illness is diagnosed, the outcome is lethal. In a less common form of rabies, paralysis begins at the site of the bite and slowly progresses and worsens until the person becomes comatose.

Chemist and microbiologist Louis Pasteur (1822–1895) made a number of discoveries that influenced many areas of science and medicine, his work with rabies being his last major achievement. Much of his work, including that with rabies, was controversial, perhaps because of its newness.

Pasteur's first discoveries had to do with the handedness of some molecules or crystals. Molecules that are identical in structure but not superimposable—similar to a left hand and a right hand—possess chirality, or handedness. This is characteristic of organic, rather than inorganic, molecules. Most amino acids, for example, are left-handed, while most sugars are right-handed. Pasteur did some of the early work establishing this understanding of chirality, using the fact that the handedness of a molecule is reflected in the way in which it polarizes light.

Pasteur then became fascinated by the world of microorganisms. He proved that the transformation of grape juice to wine and dough to bread is due to fermentation that is carried out by a live organism: the single-celled fungus called yeast.

In the early 1860s, Pasteur disproved the then-popular theory of spontaneous generation: the idea that living organisms could arise from nonliving matter. For example, broth that had been boiled so that any living organisms were killed was known to become moldy. Many believed that it became moldy due to spontaneous generation. To test this theory, Pasteur boiled broth in a flask with a crooked neck. This neck, also known as a swan's neck, prevented the introduction of air into the flask. Nothing grew in the broth. Pasteur had proved that living microorganisms did not spontaneously arise from the broth but are present in the air, and it is those airborne microorganisms that cause the mold.

Later, in what may have been the first time that a microorganism was identified as the cause of a disease, Pasteur studied a disease that was devastating the French silk industry and showed that microorganisms were infecting silkworms.

These and other experiments allowed Pasteur—along with other scientists such as his rival, bacteriologist Robert Koch (1843–1910)—to develop the germ theory of illness. Pasteur and Koch showed that diseases such as anthrax, cholera, and rabies were indeed caused by microorganisms. The idea that specific microorganisms, so small that they could not be seen by the naked eye, could lead to illness in man and other animals was revolutionary.

Famously, Pasteur discovered that heat could kill microbes. This was a way of controlling unwanted microorganisms in the production of wine. The process, known today as pasteurization, was named after him and is now used to keep many other foods, such as milk and juices, safe from disease-causing bacteria.

In the 1870s, Pasteur developed a vaccine against chicken cholera, and in May 1881, he conquered the problem of anthrax in sheep by vaccinating half a herd and then exposing the entire herd to anthrax; only the vaccinated sheep survived. This was done in public in Pouilly-le-Fort, on the southern outskirts of Paris. In both cases, the vaccine, consisting of a live but weakened, or attenuated, culture of the microbes, led to a mild illness that protected the animal from a more severe form of the illness. This was similar to the observations that a mild case of smallpox or a case of cowpox prevented the person from developing a more severe form of smallpox. Pasteur called his methods "vaccinations" in honor of Edward Jenner's invention of the smallpox vaccine.

In 1880, Pasteur began to work on the problem of rabies. Optical microscopes, the technology of the time, allowed bacteria—but not the much smaller viruses—to be seen. Because rabies is caused by a virus, Pasteur was never able to see the microbe responsible for rabies. Nor was he able to grow cultures of it, as he had done with chicken cholera and anthrax. Nevertheless, he was convinced that a microbe caused the illness.

In 1879, French veterinarian Pierre-Victoire Galtier (1846–1908) reported that he had transmitted rabies from dogs to rabbits. Galtier noted the lengthy incubation period and suggested that a possible remedy could be put in place after a bite, but he did not proceed further than this prescient suggestion.

To determine how to prevent rabies, Pasteur first had to learn how to spread it. Rather than waiting for rabid animals to bite others, he inoculated healthy animals by injecting saliva or brain tissue from rabid animals into the healthy animals' brains. As Galtier had done, Pasteur passed the rabies virus from one animal to another: from dog to rabbit and then on to other rabbits. The incubation period became shorter, eventually less than eight days. At the same time, the material also became more virulent.

Pasteur's goal was to make a vaccine that was both weaker than the rabies virus, so that a person given the vaccine would not develop the illness, and also faster acting. If given to a person bitten by a rabid animal, the vaccine had to create antibodies before the slow-moving rabies virus could get into that person's central nervous system.

Pasteur tried his vaccine on dogs—the number of animals is not clear. In August 1884, he reported that he was passing rabies through large numbers of monkeys and that this process caused the virus to lose its virulence but maintain its ability to lead to immunity. He reported that after exposure to rabies, 2 out of 3 control dogs became ill, but not a single dog out of 23 vaccinated dogs developed the illness.

In a therapeutic experiment—and a transition to working with human subjects—Pasteur used a vaccine on two hospitalized people ill with probable rabies. One person recovered, but the other person died. These trials were not publicized.

His first trial involving a healthy person occurred after a nine-year-old Alsatian boy, Joseph Meister (1876–1940), was bitten 14 times on July 4, 1885, by a dog that was clearly rabid. His local physician had heard about Pasteur's promising work with rabies in dogs and told Meister's parents to take their son to Pasteur in Paris to ask him for his help.

Pasteur conferred with Alfred Vulpian (1826–1887) and Jacques-Joseph Grancher (1843–1907), two respected Parisian physicians, and then decided to vaccinate Meister. This was a terrifying step because the boy was still healthy and had not yet developed any symptoms of rabies. If he had developed and died from rabies, then his death could have been attributed to the original dog bite—or perhaps to rabies caused by the vaccine. His critics could have argued that the boy might never have even developed rabies because not everyone bitten by a rabid dog develops the illness. It was also possible that Meister could have had a bad reaction to the vaccine.

Emile Roux (1853–1933), a physician working with Pasteur, chose not to participate, fearing adverse consequences. Grancher, supervised by Pasteur, began the injections on July 6, 1885. Meister received 13 injections of dried spinal tissue of a rabid rabbit over the next 10 days. Each injection was stronger the previous one; that is, it came from fresher or younger spinal tissue. The boy did not develop rabies or any adverse reactions to the injections. Pasteur was celebrated internationally as the hero who had defeated rabies. In October 1885, Jean-Baptiste Jupille (1869–1923), a shepherd boy, was bitten repeatedly by a rabid dog as he tried to defend other boys. He was the second boy Pasteur treated, and he too survived.

Many physicians of the time soon raised questions about these experiments. They saw the vaccinations as foolhardy and improper, in part because Pasteur was not a physician (he was a chemist and microbiologist), and he had never worked with human illnesses prior to his work with rabies. Another issue that raised safety concerns was the fact that he changed his account of the material he had used for the vaccinations. At first, he had reported that the use of monkey spinal cords had been successful in work with dogs. But in a later description of the experiment on Meister, Pasteur said that he no longer was using monkey spinal cords. He said that he and Emile Roux had discovered that rabbit spinal cords, once aged and dried, were still able to transmit the virus, but in a less virulent form. The implication was that monkey spinal cords had been effective but that rabbit spinal cords were safer.

A later review of Pasteur's laboratory notebooks by the contemporary historian Gerald Geison suggests that his vaccination of dogs with monkey spinal cords was not successful after all. Beginning in May 1885, just two months before Meister's vaccination, Pasteur made the switch to using rabbit spinal cords to vaccinate dogs. This was likely not sufficient time to see if there were would be any adverse effects from these injections before he directed the treatment of Meister. What's more, he had never used the rabbit spinal cords on dogs that had been bitten by rabid animals, only healthy dogs. In other words, Geison argued, Pasteur had used a preparation on Meister that had not been thoroughly tested on animals.

Pasteur's vaccination was used on others, with mostly successful results. Some of the vaccinated people did become ill as a consequence of the inoculations. This illness was probably due to an autoimmune reaction to the nervous tissue in the vaccine and was manifested as an ascending paralysis in which paralysis began in the legs and moved up the body. Pasteur's coworkers covered up at least one vaccination-caused death.

Over time, postexposure rabies vaccinations have become safer, and now rabies immune globulin is used as well. People at high risk for developing rabies, such as spelunkers who are exposed to bats or laboratory workers exposed to live rabies virus, can receive effective preemptive vaccinations. The most important development in the control of rabies has been the widespread prophylactic vaccination of dogs.

None of the subsequent developments, however, have taken away from the drama of the vaccination of the young Joseph Meister. Because of this initial triumph, enough money flowed from all parts of the world to allow for the establishment of the Institut Pasteur in Paris in 1887 which continues to conduct biomedical research. Joseph Meister worked there as a guard for many years, and Pasteur is entombed there. In front of the institute is a statue of the shepherd boy being bitten by a rabid dog.

Frances R. Frankenburg

SANARELLI, GIUSEPPE

Giuseppe Sanarelli was an Italian physician who believed (incorrectly) that yellow fever was transmitted by *Bacillus icteroides*. In 1897, in Montevideo, Uruguay, he injected several people—without their consent—with a solution of a toxin from that bacterium and caused an international uproar.

Giuseppe Sanarelli (1864–1940), born in Monte San Savino, Italy, had studied at the prestigious Institut Pasteur in Paris, and in 1895, he was invited to head the new Instituto de Higiene Experimental at the University of Montevideo in Uruguay.

Yellow fever was prevalent in that area of South America, and in 1897, Sanarelli announced that he had found that a toxin excreted by the bacterium *Bacillus icteroides* was the cause of the disease. He injected an inactivated and filtered solution, containing the toxin—and not the actual bacillus—into some hospitalized patients who had not given consent. Two people received subcutaneous injections and became mildly ill. Three people received intravenous injections, and two of the three became very ill. Sanarelli performed liver and kidney biopsies on some of the subjects, looking for complications of yellow fever. Sanarelli said that the patients developed yellow fever, but that is almost certainly not the case. There were, fortunately, no deaths.

Some mistaken reports of this experiment mentioned that Sanarelli had injected the live bacterium into patients, causing yellow fever and three deaths. These reports, alarmed many of course. At a conference where Sanarelli's work was discussed, a physician described his experiment as ridiculous. Sir William Osler (1849–1919), the preeminent clinician of the time, said about this comment and about Sanarelli's work (possibly believing that three subjects had died), "To deliberately inject a poison of known high degree of virulency into a human being, unless you obtain that man's sanction, is not ridiculous, it is criminal."[1] This has become an oft-quoted warning about the dangers of research and the importance of obtaining consent.

Walter Reed (1851–1902) and James Carroll (1854–1907), researchers in Cuba working for the Yellow Fever Commission in Quemados, Cuba, investigated Sanarelli's claim about *Bacillus icteroides*. They examined patients with yellow fever but were unable to find the bacillus. By 1902, Sanarelli's theory had been discredited: his microorganism had been shown to cause not yellow fever but hog cholera. Yellow fever was later shown to be caused by a mosquito-borne virus.

An important consequence of Sanarelli's work was greater care with respect to consent. George Sternberg (1838–1915), director of the Yellow Fever Commission, knew of the controversy surrounding Sanarelli and was determined not to be so reckless in his own work with yellow fever. Indeed, one of the achievements of his commission was the requirement of informed consent from all of subjects

Frances R. Frankenburg

Reference

1.   Osler, "Discussion of G. M. Sternberg," 71.

SIMS, J. MARION

J. Marion Sims was the first surgeon to successfully operate within the peritoneal cavity (the space between the wall of the abdomen and the organs) and is generally considered the father of surgical gynecology. However, his work is controversial because his early work in surgical gynecology was done—without anesthesia—on slaves who may not have been able to give informed consent.

James Marion Sims (1813–1883) (known as J. Marion Sims) was born in the Lancaster district of South Carolina. He graduated from the South Carolina College at Charleston in 1832 and enrolled in the Charleston Medical School the following year. His performance at both institutions was, by his own admission, singularly undistinguished. He received his doctorate in 1835 from Jefferson Medical College of Philadelphia.

Sims began his career in his home county, but extending the lack of success he had begun in college, his practice faltered and he moved to Alabama. In his new home, he became skilled at repairing birth-related tears (also known as fistulas) between the vagina and bladder or the vagina and bowel. That success was partly due to his use of wire sutures, which he first created from the wire springs used to give suspenders elasticity before India rubber became available. The wires were easier to clean and less prone to infection than either the fiber or gut material in general use at the time.

Another reason for his surgical success was his access to subjects. Between 1845 and 1849, J. Marion Sims repeatedly operated on three black slave women who had fistulas. He housed and supported these women. He has been criticized because he did not use anesthetic agents when operating on the black women, but he did later when operating on white women. As well, because of their status as slaves, they were what is now called vulnerable subjects and perhaps not able to give voluntary consent to these procedures. (His apologists note that anesthesia had not been invented at the time that he started these operations, that women suffered terribly from these problems, that he might have helped the three women, and that not all surgeons used anesthesia even when available for the correction of the fistulas.)

Sims was an inveterate innovator. He was the first to operate successfully on an abscess of the liver, he managed to remove a lower jaw from an incision inside the mouth to avoid an external scar, and he devised an operation to drain an obstructed gallbladder (although he had been preceded in that by a few months by a surgeon in Indiana).

In 1853, he moved to New York City and founded the Women's Hospital of the State of New York and is credited with having started the specialty of gynecology in the United States. In 1861, he moved to Europe for health reasons, where he visited Napoleon III at St. Cloud and treated the Empress Eugénie. While in Paris, he demonstrated his surgical technique to French surgeons and started a successful referral practice with patients from across the continent seeking his help. He briefly returned to the United States in 1865 but went back to France when the war with Prussia started in 1870.

During the Franco-Prussian War, Sims accepted a position as surgeon in chief to the Anglo-American Ambulance Corps, a volunteer medical unit that initially served with the French and then with the Prussian army. His experience in France led to his landmark paper "The Careful Aseptic Invasion of the Peritoneal Cavity for the Arrest of Hemorrhage, the Suture of Intestinal Wounds, and the Cleansing of the Peritoneal Cavity, and for All Intraperitoneal Conditions," which he presented to the New York Academy of Medicine on October 6, 1881, and which is credited with initiating the practice of surgery of the abdominal cavity.

After the war, Sims divided his time between Europe and New York City and continued an active surgical practice in both. He died in New York City in 1883 and was honored with a statue in Bryant Park in that city.

Jack E. McCallum

VENEREAL DISEASE EXPERIMENTS

Throughout Europe and the United States, venereal diseases were studied in numerous experiments in the 1800s, many of them on patients without their consent, to determine the details of their transmission from person to person. A few physicians experimented on themselves. There was also an interest in syphilization, or inoculating people with weaker forms of syphilis, to protect against the disease.

Venereal diseases are those illnesses that are spread by sexual intercourse. The two most important are gonorrhea and syphilis. Men with gonorrhea usually have a brief, itchy genital discharge. In contrast, women may have no symptoms, although they can have a vaginal discharge and some can develop pelvic inflammatory disease, a serious condition that can lead to trouble becoming pregnant and or chronic pain. Pregnant women with gonorrhea can infect their children at birth; the babies typically develop severe eye infections, or gonococcal ophthalmia, which can lead to blindness. Sometimes people with gonorrhea also have eye or joint infections.

Syphilis has protean manifestations. For these reasons, it was referred to as the "great imitator" by William Osler (1849–1919), the distinguished clinician and one of the four founders of the Johns Hopkins Hospital. It was also known as "the pox" because of the skin lesions it produces. Syphilis has three active stages: primary (in which ulcers or chancres appear on the genitals); secondary (which is characterized by generalized rash, fever, and enlarged lymph nodes); and tertiary (during which neuropsychiatric problems appear, including psychosis, dementia, pain, and loss of physical control over a variety of bodily functions). A patient may experience a long period without symptoms, known as latent syphilis, between the secondary and tertiary stages.

In the 1800s, physicians were unsure of how to classify the venereal illnesses, nor did they know which stages of the illnesses were infectious, and whether there were systemic complications.

In 1767, John Hunter (1728–1793), a mid-18th-century Scottish physician, to test whether syphilis and gonorrhea were the same or different diseases, had inoculated a person—possibly himself—with pus from a person who, unbeknownst to him, probably had both illnesses. This misadventure led to much confusion about the difference between the two illnesses, until the 1800s, when Philippe Ricord (1800–1889), the great French venereologist, experimented on people with venereal illnesses, inoculating them with pus from their own lesions. Eventually, he established that syphilis and gonorrhea are indeed distinct infections. Ricord believed (incorrectly) that the lesions of secondary syphilis were not contagious. Several physicians documented cases of infection arising from exposure to people with secondary syphilis: one physician is said to have infected himself with pus from a lesion of secondary syphilis, and physicians in Prague and France deliberately inoculated others with matter from these lesions. But the experiments that drew the most attention, and notoriety, were those conducted by two physicians who reported their experiments to the French Academy of Medicine.

In 1859, French physicians Joseph-Alexandre Auzias-Turenne (1812–1870) and Camille-Melchior Gibert (1797–1866), rivals of Ricord, injected the contents of the syphilitic lesions of people with secondary syphilis into four patients at the Hôpital St.-Louis in Paris, all of whom developed syphilis. These four patients already had lupus, a chronic autoimmune disease that can damage many parts of the body. Auzias-Turenne and Gibert announced the results of their experiment at a meeting of the French Academy of Medicine—and were harshly criticized by their colleagues.

Most doctors argued that what Auzias-Turenne and Gibert had done was wrong and that their actions had embarrassed both the Academy of Medicine and French hospitals. Gibert said that he had hoped that the syphilitic infection and a mercury treatment that the patients were given might treat the lupus. No one, however, seems to have taken the therapeutic intent of the experiment seriously. The experiment did confirm the general belief that secondary syphilis was contagious. (Auzias-Turenne also incorrectly believed that one could acquire immunity from syphilis by being inoculated with weaker forms of the illness, and he promoted syphilization as a form of vaccination.)

Physicians were unsure of the relationship between gonorrheal urethritis, gonorrheal ophthalmia, and nongonorrheal ophthalmia. There was also confusion between gonorrhea and trachoma, a bacterial disease of the eye that leads to the formation of a "pannus" or membrane on the eye. Some physicians believed that inoculation of an eye afflicted by pannus with material from a person ill with gonorrhea could eliminate the pannus.

To study and parse these confusing infections, physicians performed a series of experiments, many of them odd and or ethically questionable. In 1855, a physician accidentally infected his own eye while treating an infant with an eye infection and then transferred pus from his eye into a patient's atrophic eye. The patient's eye developed a discharge that the physician inoculated into the urethra of a mentally retarded man who then developed gonorrhea. Discharge from this man's urethra was then put into the urethras of two other people, and then the discharge from one of these people was transferred into the nonfunctioning eye of yet another person who developed a discharge.

After German venereologist Albert Neisser (1855–1916) identified the gonococcus as the cause of gonorrhea in 1879, experimentation with gonorrhea perhaps increased, as the gonococcus bacterium could now be identified. In 1883, George Sternberg (1838–1915), America's leading microbiologist of the time, attempted to infect himself and two colleagues by inserting cotton soaked in gonococci into each other's urethras. (None became infected.)

In Austria, dermatologist Ernest Finger (1856–1939), along with colleagues in Vienna, infected six men who had recovered from gonorrhea with gonococci to see if they had developed immunity to the illness, but they had not. The Viennese doctors also infected seven dying and febrile men with gonococci to see if high temperatures protected them from infection. The findings were inconclusive.

In Italy, in 1894, Guido Bordoni-Uffreduzzi (1859–1943) cultured pus from the ankle of a young woman with gonorrhea and then inserted the matter into the urethra of a young man who subsequently developed gonorrhea.

Neisser also experimented with syphilis. In 1892, during tests of a vaccine against syphilis, he administered a subcutaneous (under the skin) injection of cell-free serum from syphilitic patients into four young females—one of whom had gonorrhea—hoping that this would serve as a kind of vaccination and prevent them from becoming ill. They did not develop syphilis. Emboldened by this success, he injected syphilitic serum into four prostitutes between the ages of 17 and 20. All subsequently became ill with syphilis. Unlike the experiments of Auzias-Turenne and Gibert, however, this experiment did lead to change. The public outrage at what Neisser had done is credited with the passage in 1900 of Prussian legislation regulating experimentation on humans.

In 1905, German zoologist Fritz Schaudinn (1871–1906) and German dermatologist Erich Hoffmann (1869–1959) identified the spirochete *Treponema pallidum* as the cause of syphilis. Just one year later, German bacteriologist August Paul von Wassermann (1866–1925) invented an immunological medical test to detect the presence of a certain antibody in a patient's serum. This test, now known as the Wassermann test, allowed the diagnosis of syphilis to be made in the laboratory. Thanks to the development of the Wassermann test, experiments of the type done by Hunter and Ricord no longer needed to be performed, and the identification of venereal diseases became more accurate and reliable. In general, human experiments similar to those described above became less common, perhaps both because of a better understanding of the infections and the legislative action taken by the Prussian government.

Frances R. Frankenburg

VON PETTENKOFER, MAX

Max von Pettenkofer was a respected German physician and a pioneer in public health who is famous for swallowing live cholera bacilli to prove that the great bacteriologist Robert Koch was wrong in emphasizing the microorganism as the sole cause of the illness. The experiment was brave but misleading.

Cholera is an infectious illness that causes a rapid onset of severe vomiting and diarrhea. It is often lethal because of the dehydration it causes. In the 1800s, there were five cholera pandemics in Asia and Europe. Some physicians thought—mistakenly—that cholera was caused by a miasma, or unhealthy smells or vapors. Bacteriologist Robert Koch (1843–1910) traveled to Egypt and India to study the disease, and in 1883 discovered the comma bacillus, or *Vibrio cholera*, that causes the illness. In London, physician and epidemiologist John Snow (1813–1858) then showed in 1855 that water contaminated by feces from cholera victims was the principal mode of transmission.

Meanwhile, Max von Pettenkofer (1818–1901), a German physician, believed that several factors usually had to combine for illness to occur and that the illness was not as simple as exposure to a microbe. From his review of 10 cholera outbreaks, he concluded that the following four conditions were needed: the organism itself, certain types of subsoil that allow the fermentation of organic material and then the release of the cholera germ, the correct seasonal conditions, and individual susceptibilities. Von Pettenkofer thought that the emphasis on the bacterium or clean water, to the exclusion of other factors, was mistaken. However, he did recognize the importance of clean water: indeed, he developed the first large city pure-water system in Munich.

In 1892, at the age of 74, he declared that cholera was not solely a contagious disease and that Koch was wrong. To prove his point, he obtained access to Koch's bacillus (in one account from the diarrhea of a man with cholera) and drank one milliliter of broth, containing 1 billion live cholera bacilli. Before drinking it, he took sodium bicarbonate (commonly known as baking soda) so that no one could say that his stomach acidity had killed the bacteria. He developed mild diarrhea but not full-blown cholera. Elie Metchnikoff (1845–1916)—who would later win a Nobel Prize for his work with immunology—and bacteriologist Rudolph Emmerich (1852–1914) repeated Von Pettenkofer's experiment with similar results. Von Pettenkofer declared that Koch was mistaken.

Von Pettenkofer was an intelligent scientist and physician, and his argument that disease is often multifactorial was reasonable. He had the courage to test his own theory—on himself. In retrospect, he was prescient in thinking that there must be, as we now call it, a host-microbe relationship that is important to the understanding of infectious diseases. But his experiment was misleading. Not all people exposed to the cholera bacteria will become ill, but the bacillus is the cause of the illness.

In his later years, he became depressed and committed suicide by shooting himself. In English-speaking countries, he is now remembered for his brave self-experiment, which led to the wrong conclusions. In Germany, he is honored for his contributions to public health.

Frances R. Frankenburg

DOCUMENTS

INHUMANE EXPERIMENTATION ON AFRICAN AMERICAN SLAVES (1855)

This excerpt from the autobiography of John Brown shows how inhumane human experimentation can be. Doctor Hamilton, who had a "great name," takes advantage of a vulnerable person, a slave, and experiments on him to make money, not advances in medicine. There is of course no question here of informed consent. The experiment is just one element of the ongoing exploitation of Brown. This episode, which seems more like torture than anything else, is not an isolated case. Harriet Washington describes in detail the history of experimentation on black Americans in Medical Apartheid: The Dark

History of Medical Experimentation on Black Americans from Colonial Times to the Present.

I had been fourteen years with Stevens, suffering all the time very much from his ill-treatment of me, when he fell ill. I do not know what his malady was. It must have been serious, for they called in to treat him one Doctor Hamilton, who lived in Jones County, and who had a great name. He cured Stevens, who was so pleased, that he told the Doctor to ask him any favour, and it should be granted. Now it so happened that this Doctor Hamilton had been trying a great number of experiments, for the purpose of finding out the best remedies for sun-stroke. I was, it seems, a strong and likely subject to be experimented upon, and the Doctor having fixed the thing in his mind, asked Stevens to lend me to him. This he did at once, never caring to inquire what was going to be done with me. I myself did not know. Even if I had been made aware of the nature of the trials I was about to undergo, I could not have helped myself. There was nothing for it but passive resignation, and I gave myself up in ignorance and in much fear.

Yet, it was not without curiosity I watched the progress of the preparations the Doctor caused to be made. he ordered a hole to be dug in the ground, three feet and a half deep by three feet long, and two feet and a half wide. Into this pit a quantity of dried red oak bark was cast, and fire set to it. It was allowed to burn until the pit became heated like an oven, when the embers were taken out. A plank was then put across the bottom of the pit, and on that a stool. Having tested, with a thermometer, the degree to which the pit was heated, the Doctor bade me strip, and get in; which I did, only my head being above the ground. He then gave me some medicine which he had prepared, and as soon as I was on the stool, a number of wet blankets were fastened over the hole, and scantlings laid across them. This was to keep in the heat. It soon began to tell upon me; but though I tried hard to keep up against its effects, in about half an hour I fainted. I was then lifted out and revived, the Doctor taking a note of the degree of heat when I left the pit. I used to be put in between daylight and dark, after I had done my day's work; for Stevens was not a man to lose more of the labour of his slaves than he could help. Three or four days afterwards, the experiment was repeated, and so on for five or six times, the Doctor allowing me a few days' rest between each trial. His object was to ascertain which of the medicines he administered to me on these occasions, enabled me to withstand the greatest degree of heat. He found that cayenne-pepper tea accomplished this object; and a very nice thing he made of it. As soon as he got back home, he advertised that he had discovered a remedy for sun-stroke. It consisted of pills, which were to be dissolved in a dose of cayenne-pepper tea, without which, he said, the pills would not produce any effect. Nor do I see how they should have done so, for they were only made of common flour. However, he succeeded in getting them into general use, and as he asked a good price, he soon realized a large fortune.

Having completed his series of experiment upon me, in the heated pit, and allowed me some days' rest, I was put on a diet, and then, during a period of about three weeks, he bled me every other day. At the end of that time he found

I was failing, so he left off, and I got a month's rest, to regain a little strength. At the expiration of that time, he set to work to ascertain how deep my black skin went. This he did by applying blisters to my hands, legs and feet, which bear the scars to this day. He continued until he drew up the dark skin from between the upper and the under one. He used to blister me at intervals of about two weeks. He also tried other experiments upon me, which I cannot dwell upon. Altogether, and from first to last, I was in his hands, under treatment, for about nine months, at the end of which period I had become so weak, that I was no longer able to work in the fields. I had never been allowed to knock off, I ought to say, during the whole of this time, though my bodily strength failed daily. Stevens always kept me employed: at hard work as long as I could do it, and at lighter labour, as my strength went away. At last, finding that the Doctor's experiments had so reduced me that I was useless in the field, he put me to his old trade of carpentering and joinery, which I took too very readily, and soon got a liking for.

Source: John Brown, (1855) *Slave Life in Georgia: A Narrative of the Life, Sufferings, and Escape of John Brown, a Fugitive Slave, Now in England*, ed. L. A. Chamerovzow (London: printed by editor).

LOUIS PASTEUR AND RABIES (1885)

Louis Pasteur, a French chemist and microbiologist, made a series of discoveries about microorganisms and found ways to protect animals from some illnesses. His work with rabies, perhaps his most famous, was controversial at the time because he was not a physician. A later historian has documented discrepancies between his original laboratory notebooks and his publications. Nonetheless, Pasteur did prevent a nine-year-old boy from developing rabies after being bitten by a rabid animal. Pasteur's physician colleagues injected the boy with a series of increasingly virulent inoculations of rabid rabbit marrow that made him immune to rabies. They went on to save a young shepherd who was bitten by a rabid dog while protecting others. Pasteur has been a medical hero ever since.

October 26, 1885.—*A Method for the Prevention of Rabies after the Bite of a Rabid Animal.*—The prophylaxis of rabies such as I exposed it in my own name and in the name of my fellow-workers in my preceding notes certainly constituted a real progress in the study of that disease. But the progress realised was more scientific than practical. In application it exposed to various accidents. Not more than fifteen or sixteen dogs in twenty could be made refractory to rabies with certainty.

It was advisable, on the other hand, to end the treatment with a last and very virulent inoculation, a control inoculation, in order both to confirm and to strengthen the refractory state. Furthermore, simple prudence required that one should keep the dogs in sight for a longer period than that of the incubation of the disease as produced by the direct and isolated inoculation of this last virus, so that it was occasionally necessary to wait three or four months before gaining the assurance of having produced a refractory state.

Such serious exigencies would considerably limit the scope of the method in practice.

Finally, it would have been difficult to put the method to emergency uses at a moment's notice, a condition required of it nevertheless, if we consider how casual and unforeseen are the bites of mad animals.

It was necessary, therefore, if possible, to discover a more rapid method, and one capable of giving, if I may so speak, a state of perfect security in the dog.

And it was impossible, too, before that desideratum was realised, to think of making any trial of the method on man.

After, I might say, innumerable experiments, I have at last found a method of prophylaxis both practical and rapid, and one which has proved successful in the dog with so much constancy in such a considerable number of cases already, that I feel confident of its general applicability to all animals and to man himself.

This new method rests essentially on the following facts: The rabbit, inoculated under the duramater, after trephining, with the spinal marrow of an ordinary mad dog, is always affected with rabies; it takes the disease after a length of incubation averaging about fifteen days.

If a second rabbit be inoculated from that first one, a third from the second, and so on, always by the same mode of inoculation, there is soon manifested in the succeeding rabbits a growing tendency towards a shorter incubation.

After a number of passages through rabbits, varying from the twentieth to the twenty-fifth, the incubation falls down to eight days, which remains the normal incubation time for the next twenty or twenty-five passages. Then it reached an incubation of seven days only, and recurring with striking regularity up to at least the 90th passage, which is the point we have reached at present, and there is barely as yet a slight tendency towards a shorter period of incubation than seven days.

The series was begun in November 1882, and has now lasted three years already. It has never once been interrupted, and never has it been necessary to have recourse to any other than the virus of rabbits of the same series which had previously died of rabies. Nothing is easier, therefore, than to have constantly at one's disposal, for considerable lengths of time, a virus of perfect purity and always identical with itself or as nearly so as possible. Therein lies practically the whole secret of the method.

The spinal marrows of the rabbits are virulent throughout the whole of their substance, with constancy of the virulence. If from those marrows we take portions a few centimetres long, using all possible precautions to keep them pure, and then suspend them in a dry atmosphere, their virulence diminishes slowly until at last it is all lost. The time that the virulence takes to disappear entirely varies somewhat with the thickness of the marrows, but most of all with the outside temperature. The lower the temperature, the longer is the virulence preserved. These points constitute the scientific part of the method.

After those preliminary explanations, here is the process for rendering dogs refractory to rabies in a relatively short time.

In a series of flasks, the air inside which is kept dry by dropping pieces of caustic potash into it, suspend every day a portion of fresh spinal marrow taken from a rabbit which has died of rabies of seven days' incubation. Every day also inject under the skin of the dog to be made refractory a full Pravaz hypodermic syringe of sterilised broth in which has previously been triturated a small piece of one of the drying marrows. Begin with a marrow old enough to make sure that it is not at all virulent. Previous experimentation will already have settled that point. On the succeeding days proceed in the same manner with fresher marrows, and use those of every second day, until finally we inoculate a last and very virulent one which has been drying only one or two days.

The dog has now become refractory to rabies, and will not take it anyhow inoculated, under the skin or on the surface of the brain.

Making use of this method, I had already rendered fifty dogs of all ages and of all races refractory to rabies, without having met with a single failure when, unawares, on Monday, July 6 last, three persons coming from Alsace presented themselves at my laboratory; they were—

Theodore Vone, a grocer from Meissengott, near Schelstadt, bitten on the arm on July 4 by his own dog, which had become mad.

Joseph Meister, nine years old, bitten also on July 4 at eight o'clock in the morning, and by the same dog. This child had been thrown down by the dog and had received numerous bites on the hand, the legs and thighs, some of them so deep that he could scarcely walk. The principal wounds had been cauterised with carbolic acid by Dr. Weber, of Villé, on July 4, at eight o'clock in the evening, twelve hours only after the accident.

The third person was the mother of little Joseph Meister, and had not been bitten.

The dog had been killed by his own master, and on opening his stomach it had been found stuffed with hay, straw, and chips of wood. The animal was certainly mad. Joseph Meister had been rescued from him all covered with saliva and blood. Mr. Vone had been severely contused on the arms, but he assured me that his shirt had not been traversed by the fangs of the dog. I told him there was nothing to fear, and that he could go home that same day, which he did. But I kept with me little Meister and his mother.

The weekly meeting of the Académie des Sciences was held on that same day, July 6. I saw there our colleague Dr. Vulpian, to whom I related what had occurred. Dr. Vulpian, joined by Dr. Grancher, professor at the School of Medicine, kindly consented to come at once and see the state and the number of the wounds of little Joseph Meister. He had been bitten in fourteen different places.

The advice of our learned colleague and of Dr. Grancher was, that owing to the depth and number of his wounds, Joseph Meister was exposed to almost certain death from hydrophobia. I then communicated to Drs. Vulpian and Grancher the new results I had obtained in my studies of rabies since the time of my lecture in Copenhagen a year before.

The child, being apparently doomed to inevitable death, I resolved, not without feelings of utmost anxiety, as may well be imagined, to apply to him the method of prophylaxis which had never failed me in dogs.

My set of fifty dogs, indeed, had not been bitten before they were made refractory to rabies; but that objection had no share in my preoccupations, for I had already, in the course of other experiments, rendered a large number of dogs refractory after they had been bitten.

I had that same year invited the members of the Commission on Rabies to witness that new and important progress.

On July 6, then, at eight o'clock in the evening, sixty hours after the bites of the 4th, and in the presence of Drs. Vulpian and Grancher, we inoculated into the right hypochondrium of little Meister, under a fold made in his skin, the half of a Pravaz hypodermic syringe containing the marrow of a rabbit which had died rabid on June 21 previous. Since that date the marrow had been kept in dry air, suspended in a bottle—fifteen days altogether.

On the following days the inoculations were renewed, always in the hypochondria and in the manner indicated in the following table:

July 7 at 9 A.M.	Marrow of	June 23 i.e.	14 days old
July 7 at 6 P.M.	"	June 25 i.e.	12 days old
July 8 at 9 A.M.	"	June 27 i.e.	11 days old
July 8 at 6 A.M.	"	June 29 i.e.	9 days old
July 9 at 11 A.M.	"	July 1 i.e.	8 days old
July 10 at 11 A.M.	"	July 3 i.e.	7 days old
July 11 at 11 A.M.	"	July 5 i.e.	6 days old
July 12 at 11 A.M.	"	July 7 i.e.	5 days old
July 13 at 11 A.M.	"	July 9 i.e.	4 days old
July 14 at 11 A.M.	"	July 11 i.e.	3 days old
July 15 at 11 A.M.	"	July 13 i.e.	2 days old
July 16 at 11 A.M.	"	July 15 i.e.	1 days old

The treatment, therefore, lasted ten days, and the total number of the inoculations was thirteen. I shall say later on that a smaller number of inoculations might have sufficed, but in this first case I had necessarily to act with peculiar circumspection.

Two fresh live rabbits were also inoculated on the brain with every one of the marrows used, in order to follow their degrees of virulence.

The observation of those rabbits brought out the following points: the marrows of July 6, 7, 8, 9, 10 were not virulent, for the rabbits inoculated with them did not become mad. The marrows of July 11, 12, 14, 15, 16 were all virulent, in ascending progression. The rabbits inoculated from the marrows of July 15 and 16 took rabies after seven days' incubation; those inoculated from the marrows of the 12th and 14th after eight days; those from July 11 after fifteen days.

I had, therefore, in the last days of the treatment, inoculated Joseph Meister with the most powerful rabies virus—namely, the virus of the ordinary mad dog, strengthened by a large number of passages through rabbits, a virus giving rabies to rabbits after seven days' incubation, to dogs after eight or ten days only. My action was justified by what I had observed in the fifty dogs of which I have spoken before.

When once the state of immunity has been reached, there is no danger attaching to the inoculation in any quantities of the most powerful virus. It has always appeared to me that the only consequence of such inoculations was to consolidate the refractory state.

Joseph Meister has, therefore, escaped from the hydrophobia which he might have developed in consequence of the bites he had received, and also from the hydrophobia, more powerful than the one resulting from ordinary canine madness, which I inoculated into him to test the immunity imparted by the treatment.

This last highly virulent inoculation has one more advantage: it limits the period of time during which fears may be entertained as to the results of the bites. If rabies could come on at all it would undoubtedly do so quicker after this most virulent inoculation than after the bites. As early as the middle of the month of August I looked forward with confidence to the future health of Joseph Meister. To-day, three months and three weeks after the accident, his health is still perfect.

What is the mode of action of the new method, just given, of the prophylaxis of rabies after bites? I do not purpose to deal fully with the question today, but shall content myself with a few preliminary remarks, which will help to explain the meaning of the experiments which I am still carrying on for the purpose of giving us a clear idea as to the best possible interpretation.

If we consider, on the one hand, the methods of progressive attenuation of mortal viruses and the prophylaxis which can be derived from them, and, on the other hand, the influence of atmospheric air on that attenuation, the first explanation which offers itself to the mind is that the continuous contact of the rabid marrows with dry air progressively diminishes their virulence until it is finally all lost.

It would hence appear that our prophylactic method rested on the use, first of all, of a virus without any appreciable degree of virulence, and then of viruses progressively virulent, from the lowest up to the highest.

I shall show later on that the facts do not agree with that hypothesis. I shall also give proof that the delays in the incubative periods of the rabies inoculated from day to day into fresh live rabbits, as just indicated, and for the purpose of testing the state of the virulence of our desiccated marrows, are due not to a diminution in the degree of virulence of those marrows, but to a diminution in the quantity of rabies virus contained in them.

Might it be, then, that the inoculation of a virus, the virulence of which should always remain identically the same, could bring on a state of refractoriness to rabies on condition that we proceeded in the use of it by very small but daily increasing quantities? That would be one way of interpreting the facts of the new method, and a way which I am occupied in verifying experimentally.

Yet one hypothesis suggests itself in explanation of the new method: a hypothesis which at first sight seems very strange, assuredly, but one nevertheless worthy of all consideration, for it is in keeping with certain known facts of the vital phenomena observed in several of the lower beings, and, in particular, in certain pathogenic microorganisms.

A large number of micro-organisms apparently give rise, in the media where they grow, to substances which have the property of opposing their own growth.

As early as the year 1880 I had initiated some researches having for their object to detect some such poison produced by the fowl-cholera microorganism and toxic to that same micro-organism. I have not been able, as yet, to demonstrate the presence of such a substance; but I am of opinion to-day that those studies ought to be taken up anew, and I shall not fail to do so myself, taking care to cultivate the micro-organism in an atmosphere of pure carbonic acid gas.

The microbe of swine-plague thrives in broths of very varying composition, but it is so rapidly stopped in its development, and the weight of it formed is so small, that it is occasionally barely possible to tell the presence of a crop of it by noticing the slender silky bands undulating in the nutrient medium. It looks as if at once had been produced a substance which had stopped the growth of the little being, whether sown in presence of air or *in vacuo*.

M. Raulin, once my assistant, and now a professor in the Faculty of Lyons, showed, in the very remarkable thesis which he presented in Paris on March 22, 1870, that the *Aspergillus niger* develops during growth a substance which stops, to some extent, the further production of that mould whenever the nutrient medium does not contain iron salts.

Might it be, then, that rabies virus was made up of two distinct substances, the one living and capable of multiplying in the nervous system, the other not living, but capable still, when in suitable proportions, of arresting the development of the first?

In an early communication I shall give the experimental and critical results arrived at with regard to this third hypothesis concerning the mode of action of the prophylactic method.

It is scarcely necessary in closing to remark that probably the most anxious question for the present is that of the time which may be allowed to elapse between the bite and the application of the treatment. That interval was, in the case of Joseph Meister, two days and a half, but it will certainly be considerably longer in a large number of cases.

On Tuesday last, October 20, obligingly assisted by MM. Vulpian and Grancher, I had to begin the treatment of a young man of fifteen who had been bitten six full days previously on both hands and in circumstances of peculiar gravity.

The Academy will not listen without some emotion to the story of the deed of bravery and of cool-mindedness done by the boy whose treatment I took in hand last Tuesday. Jean-Baptiste Jupille is a shepherd boy belonging to Villers-Farlay, in the department of Jura. Seeing a powerful dog with suspicious gait throwing himself upon a group of six of his comrades, all younger than himself, he seized his whip and rushed forward to meet the animal. The dog at once caught hold of Jupille by the left hand. Then followed a hand-to-hand fight, so to speak, the boy finally throwing down the animal and pinning him to the ground under his knee. Next, with his right hand he forced open the jaws of the beast, disengaged his left hand—all the while receiving new bites—and taking the thong of his whip he tied the muzzle of his enemy and with one of his wooden-shoes beat him dead.

I shall make it a point to acquaint the Academy with the results of this new trial.

Source: Renaud Suzor, *Hydrophobia: An Account of M. Pasteur's System* (London: Chatto & Windus, 1887), 88–101.

Further Reading

Allen, Arthur. 2007. *Vaccine: The Controversial Story of Medicine's Greatest Lifesaver*. New York: W. W. Norton.

Altman, Lawrence K. 1987. *Who Goes First?: The Story of Self-Experimentation in Medicine*. New York: Random House.

Annas, George J., and Michael A. Grodin. 1992. *The Nazi Doctors and the Nuremberg Code: Human Rights in Human Experimentation*. New York: Oxford University Press.

Benedek, Thomas G. 2005. "Gonorrhea and the Beginnings of Clinical Research Ethics." *Perspectives in Biology and Medicine* 48 (1) (Winter): 54–73.

Dracobly, Alex. 2003. "Ethics and Experimentation on Human Subjects in Mid-Nineteenth-Century France: The Story of the 1859 Syphilis Experiments." *Bulletin of the History of Medicine* 77 (2): 332–366. doi:10.1353/bhm.2003.0059.

Evans, Alfred S. 1973. "Pettenkofer Revisited: The Life and Contributions of Max von Pettenkofer (1818–1901)." *Yale Journal of Biology and Medicine* 46: 161–176.

Frankenburg, Frances Rachel. 2009. *Vitamin Discoveries and Disasters: History, Science, and Controversies*. Santa Barbara, CA: Praeger/ABC-CLIO.

Frankenburg, Frances R. 2014. *Brain-Robbers: How Alcohol, Cocaine, Nicotine, and Opiates Have Changed Human History*. Santa Barbara, CA: Praeger/ABC-CLIO.

Gawande, Atul. 2012. "Two Hundred Years of Surgery." *New England Journal of Medicine* 366 (18): 1,716–1,723.

Geison, Gerald L. 1995. *The Private Science of Louis Pasteur*. Princeton, NJ: Princeton University Press.

Gelfand, Toby. 2002. "11 January 1887, the Day Medicine Changed: Joseph Grancher's Defense of Pasteur's Treatment for Rabies." *Bulletin of the History of Medicine* 76: 698–718.

Goodman, Martin. 2007. *Suffer and Survive: The Extreme Life of J. S. Haldane*. London: Simon & Schuster.

Grzybowski, Sak A., J. Pawlikowski, and G. Iwanowicz-Palus. 2013. "Gerhard Henrik Armauer Hansen (1841–1912)—The 100th Anniversary of the Death of the Discoverer of *Mycobacterium leprae*." *Clinics in Dermatology* 31 (5) (September/October): 653–655.

Haffkine, Waldemar M. 1900. "On Preventive Inoculation." *Proceedings of the Royal Society of London* 65: 252–271.

Hawgood, Barbara J. 2007. "Waldemar Mordecai Haffkine, CIE (1860–1930): Prophylactic Vaccination against Cholera and Bubonic Plague in British India." *Journal of Medical Biography* 15: 9–19.

Ligon, B. L. 2005. "Albert Ludwig Sigesmund Neisser: Discoverer of the Cause of Gonorrhea." *Seminars in Pediatric Infectious Diseases* 16: 336–341.

Lutzker, Edythe, and Carol Jochnowitz. 1987. "Waldemar Haffkine: Pioneer of Cholera Vaccine." *American Society of Microbiology News* 53 (7): 366–369.

Nuland, Sherwin B. 1988. *Doctors: The Biography of Medicine*. New York: Knopf.

Osler, William. 1898. "Discussion of G. M. Sternberg, the Bacillus Icteroides (Sanarelli) and Bacillus X (Sternberg)." *Transactions of the Association of American Physicians* 13: 71.

Porter, Roy. 1997. *The Greatest Benefit to Mankind: A Medical History of Humanity*. New York: W. W. Norton.

Sartin, Jeffrey S. 2004. "J. Marion Sims, the Father of Gynecology: Hero or Villain?" *Southern Medical Journal* 97 (5): 427–429.

Vogelsang, T. M. 1963. "A Serious Sentence Passed against the Discoverer of the Leprosy Bacillus (Gerhard Armauer Hansen), in 1880." *Medical History* 7: 182–186.

Wall, L. L. 2006. "The Medical Ethics of Dr J Marion Sims: A Fresh Look at the Historical." *Journal of Medical Ethics* 32: 346–350.

Wasik, Bill, and Monica Murphy. 2012. *Rabid: A Cultural History of the World's Most Diabolical Virus*. New York: Viking.

Era 3: 20th Century to World War II

INTRODUCTION

In the early 20th century, human experimentation became more common as medicine became increasingly scientific and illnesses better understood. Scientists in the young fields of microbiology and nutrition debated about the causes of illness. A few causes, such as microorganisms, could be understood and manipulated. Nutrition advanced rapidly as specific nutritional deficiencies were linked to specific illnesses, in particular pellagra and beriberi. On the other hand, psychiatric illnesses still remained incomprehensible. Finally, the growing and seemingly benign interest in eugenics would turn malignant and begin to serve as justification for shocking acts of human experimentation—and genocide—in the years to come.

Human medical experiments in this era were often performed on convenient populations—with "convenient" being synonymous with "vulnerable." Experiments with pellagra, for instance, were carried out on prisoners and orphans and experiments with beriberi on inmates of an asylum. In the United States, in one of the most infamous and controversial studies in American medicine, physicians working for the U.S. Public Health Service began a 40-year longitudinal study of untreated or undertreated syphilis in poor black American men in Macon County, Alabama, without telling the men that they were participating in a study.

Some researchers had subjects who were desperate to participate in experiments. There was no cure for diabetes mellitus until Toronto researchers first administered insulin to patients who were grateful to receive an experimental therapy.

In the field of psychiatry, where effective treatments were still absent, neuropsychiatrist Julius Wagner-Jauregg (1857–1940) came up with an odd treatment for tertiary syphilis, the stage of syphilis associated with psychiatric symptoms. He infected these patients with malaria, and some got better. In the 1930s, experimental treatments for psychiatric illnesses, all based on serendipitous findings or mistakes, were also introduced. Manfred Sakel (1900–1957), a Viennese physician, accidentally overdosed some morphine addicts with insulin and then developed insulin coma as a new therapy for psychosis. Ladislas Meduna (1896–1964), a Hungarian neuropathologist, thought, incorrectly, that epilepsy and schizophrenia could not coexist; therefore, to treat schizophrenia, he induced seizures in some schizophrenia patients by injecting them with camphor. Ugo Cerletti (1877–1963) and Lucio Bini (1908–1964), two Italian physicians, modified Meduna's practice and applied an electric current across a mentally ill person's brain and cured him. Electrically induced seizures, despite the incorrect basis for their use, became a helpful treatment in psychiatry and are still used today, albeit in a modified form.

António Egas Moniz (1874–1955), a Portuguese neurologist, came up with perhaps the most radical treatment of all for serious medical illness—lobotomy, a surgical procedure in which nerve tracts traveling from the frontal lobe to other parts of the brain are severed. This procedure was enthusiastically adopted by the neurologist Walter Freeman (1895–1972) in the United States, and lobotomies were used for several decades. (They are not performed today, except in a modified form for patients with severe pain or obsessive-compulsive disorder.)

Eugenics, or the study of how to improve the population by improving the gene pool, seemed a benign field of research at first. But eugenics became the background for atrocious experimentation in Nazi Germany as doctors and politicians attempted to create a healthier and more Aryan nation by eliminating unwanted members of the population. Interestingly, concern about experimentation on the disadvantaged and the ill effects of medical practices had been expressed most clearly by guidelines and regulations issued in Germany in 1900 and 1933, but these regulations would be disregarded by the Nazi physicians.

As is often the case, wars influenced medicine and also experimentation. Following the brief Spanish-American War of 1898, the United States had become a colonial power, governing or controlling the previously Spanish colonies, Cuba, Puerto Rico, Guam, and the Philippines. The American presence in Cuba led to the early 20-century yellow fever experiments conducted by physician Walter Reed (1851–1902). American medical scientists also conducted cholera, beriberi, and amoebic dysentery experiments on inmates of the huge Bilibid Prison in the Philippine Islands.

During World War I, poison gas was a new and terrifying way of inflicting damage on the enemy. The Haldane father-and-son team in Great Britain explored the effects of poison gases on themselves so that they could identify the type used by the German army and devise better gas masks. After the war ended, Europe remained devastated. Viennese physicians worked with English doctors to address the problem of malnutrition in Viennese infants. This collaboration provided Harriette Chick (1875–1977) the opportunity to perform a series of experiments in Viennese foundlings, elucidating the cause, prevention, and treatment of rickets. These studies were similar to those done by Alfred Hess (1875–1933) in New York in his investigation of scurvy and rickets in orphanages. Rickets had been a poorly understood illness until its connection to sunlight and vitamin deficiency was shown.

The experimentation of this time yielded results that would lead to better medications and treatments. But the methods used by the researchers often reflected, from a 21st-century viewpoint, insensitivity to the autonomy or the well-being of the subjects.

TIMELINE

1900	The minister for religious, educational, and medical affairs in Prussia prohibits medical research on humans without consent.

1900–1901	Army surgeon-general George Sternberg (1838–1915) establishes the United States Army Yellow Fever Commission in Cuba and puts Walter Reed (1851–1902) in charge, who then proves that the anopheline mosquito is the vector of yellow fever. The subjects sign consent.
1901	John D Rockefeller Sr. (1839–1937) founds the Rockefeller Institute for Medical Research; in 1965, it becomes the Rockefeller University.
1905	William Fletcher (1874–1938) shows that patients in an asylum in Kuala Lumpur who eat polished rice are more likely to develop beriberi than those who eat unpolished rice.
1906	While developing a cholera vaccine, Richard Strong (1872–1948) gives prison inmates in the Philippines the bubonic plague by mistake.
1907	Henry Fraser and Thomas Stanton ask Javanese road builders, isolated in work camps, to choose which kind of rice to eat; those who eat white rice rather than parboiled rice are more likely to develop beriberi.
1909	Rockefeller creates the Rockefeller Sanitary Commission to eradicate hookworm in the South; it ends in 1914.
1912	Strong experiments with beriberi at Bilibid Prison, in the Philippines; inmates who sign consent are given cigarettes.
1913	Ernest Linwood Walker (1870–1952) and Andrew Walker Sellards (1884–1941) feed prisoners at Bilibid with *Entamoeba histolytica* cysts and find the cause of amoebic dysentery. The prisoners sign consent forms.
1913	Rockefeller establishes the Rockefeller Foundation that funds much medical research and continues the work of the Sanitary Commission.
1915	Joseph Goldberger (1874–1929) puts prisoners at the Rankin Prison Farm on a diet typical among the poor in the South and proves that pellagra is a nutritional illness.
1917	Julius Wagner-Jauregg (1857–1940) begins to treat neurosyphilis with malaria.
1918–1922	Leo Stanley (1886–1976) transplants testicular tissue from executed prisoners to elderly prisoners at San Quentin State Prison in an effort to stop the aging process.

1927	The Kaiser Wilhelm Institute for Anthropology, Human Heredity, and Eugenics is established in Berlin, partially funded by the Rockefeller Foundation.
1927	Manfred Sakel (1900–1957) begins to treat mental illness with insulin.
1929	Werner Forssmann (1904–1979) catheterizes his own heart; until this self-experiment, the procedure had been considered too dangerous to attempt.
1931	The German minister of interior requires consent from patients and subjects before procedures or experiments and only after they are fully informed of the nature of the treatment or research.
1931	A laboratory technician finds a letter from Cornelius "Dusty" Rhoads (1898–1959) in which Rhoads makes offensive comments about various ethnic groups; the letter tarnishes his otherwise exceptional career.
1932–1972	The Tuskegee Study of Untreated Syphilis lasts for four decades, during which black Americans with syphilis are not told that they have syphilis or that they are subjects of a study.
1922	Researchers at the University of Toronto inject insulin into diabetic patients and develop the first effective treatment for diabetes mellitus.
1927	William Castle (1897–1990) begins to use his own gastric juices to solve the riddle of pernicious anemia and distinguishes between intrinsic and extrinsic factors.
1934	Ladislas Meduna (1896–1964), a Hungarian physician, induces seizures in a mentally ill man, who subsequently improves.
1935	Egas Moniz (1874–1955) performs lobotomies in Portugal; he subsequently wins a Nobel Prize in Physiology or Medicine.
1936	Walter Freeman (1895–1972) begins to perform lobotomies in the United States and goes on to perform over 3,000 of these procedures.
1938	Ugo Cerletti (1877–1963) and Lucio Bini (1908–1964) treat a mentally ill man with electroconvulsive therapy; he improves.

REFERENCE ENTRIES

AMOEBIC DYSENTERY EXPERIMENTS AT BILIBID PRISON

In the early 1900s, Ernest Linwood Walker and Andrew Sellards investigated dysentery at Bilibid Prison in the Philippines. After describing their project to the prisoners and obtaining their written informed consent, they fed the prisoners different kinds of amoebic organisms to see which, if any, would make them sick. This work was notable for the early use of written informed consent and the contributions it made to the understanding of amoebic dysentery.

The human bowel is full of microorganisms living in a complicated web of relationships. Amoebae are one-celled protozoa that live in the crevices or crypts of the large intestine, where they feed on the abundant bacteria. Usually, they cause no illness in their host. In the active feeding stage of their life cycle, they are known as trophozoites. Sometimes these trophozoites encapsulate and form long-lived cysts that are excreted in the stool. If a person then ingests these cysts orally, the capsule of the cyst is digested in the small intestine, releasing trophozoites.

Amoebic dysentery, an intestinal infection caused by the organism *Entamoeba histolytica*, is common in the tropics and is spread through food or water contaminated with feces containing these amoebic cysts. Symptoms include severe and sometimes bloody diarrhea, abdominal pain, and weight loss. The cause of dysentery had been difficult to determine for several reasons. First, there are no animal models, and the incubation period can vary widely—from a few weeks to years. In addition, several types of amoebae live in the human intestines and can be difficult to distinguish from each other.

In 1903, the protozoologist Fritz Schaudinn (1871–1906) was the first to distinguish *Entamoeba histolytica* from its harmless counterpart *Entamoeba coli*. (*Entamoeba coli* should not be confused with the bacterium *Eschericia coli,* also known as *E. coli,* which is also an inhabitant of the human bowel. Most types of *Eschericia coli* are harmless, but some can cause diarrhea or more serious illnesses.) *E. histolytica* sometimes stops feeding on bacteria and instead penetrates into the intestinal mucosa and consumes red blood cells, kills the cells of the gut, and leads to inflammation of the gut, which in turn leads to the symptoms of dysentery. (Schaudinn himself died at the age of 34 from complications of a gastrointestinal amoebic abscess.)

The work that established the pathogenicity of *E. histolytica* was performed on prisoners in the Philippines by Ernest Linwood Walker (1870–1952) and Andrew Sellards (1884–1941). Walker was born in Maine and studied at Harvard. He worked as a bacteriologist for the Massachusetts Board of Health for 14 years while continuing to study medical parasitology and tropical medicine at Harvard, where he obtained a doctoral degree. Then he spent 4 years working at the bureau of science in the Philippine Islands. He was a protozoologist for three years and then chief of the biological laboratory.

In 1913, Walker and Andrew Sellards, a physician working at the Bilibid Prison, organized a number of experiments with the prisoners there. The advantage of the prisoners was—as is often the case with prisoners—their captivity. For example, their exposure to other organisms could be controlled, and it was easier to collect their feces than it would have been working with nonconfined subjects.

Walker and Sellards informed subjects about the nature of their experiments and told them that there was a risk of becoming ill with dysentery. The subjects signed consent forms that had been written in their own dialect. Walker and Sellards administered amoebic cysts in gelatin capsules to the subjects.

In one experiment, they fed 20 men *Entamoeba coli* organisms; 17 were infected, but none became ill. In another experiment, they fed 20 volunteers *E. histolytica* cysts, or trophozoites; 4 of the 18 who were infected with the parasite became ill.

The work of Walker and Sellards increased our understanding of dysentery and was groundbreaking in some ways. First, they definitively established that *E. histolytica* causes amoebic dysentery. They also showed that not all infected people became ill and that asymptomatic people could transmit the parasite to others through the fecal-oral route by passing cysts in their feces. Finally, they were some of the first researchers to have their subjects sign informed consent.

The issue of the subjects being prisoners has been problematic. Whether the prisoners understood what they were being asked to do, were promised something in return for their participation, or feared consequences if they refused to participate is not known.

Frances R. Frankenburg

BERIBERI EXPERIMENTS IN MALAYA

In Malaya in the early 1900s, British physicians investigated the cause of beriberi, a debilitating tropical illness. We now know that beriberi is caused by lack of thiamine, but this was difficult to prove. The physicians carried out experiments in large groups of people who were either in psychiatric hospitals or employed as road builders.

British investigators became interested in beriberi at the beginning of the 20th century because it was prevalent in Malaya, then a British-controlled territory (now Malaysia). It was not clear then if beriberi was an infectious illness or somehow related to diet.

William Fletcher (1874–1938), a British bacteriologist who had trained at the University of Cambridge, investigated beriberi in an experiment in a psychiatric hospital in Kuala Lumpur, Malaya. Psychiatric hospitals in those days were large institutions somewhat like prisons, in that the patients stayed for months or years and their diet was tightly controlled. In 1905, there was an outbreak of beriberi in this Kuala Lumpur hospital. Fletcher organized a trial to try to *disprove* the suggestion that parboiled rice was superior to white rice in preventing beriberi. (Parboiled rice has been partially boiled while still in its husk, thus allowing the antiberiberi vitamin, thiamine, to remain in the grain. White rice has been milled so that its husk, bran, and germ are removed.)

All of the patients were "lined up" and numbered. Patients were then assigned to one of two wards, depending on whether they had been given an even or odd number. One ward was supplied with white rice and one with parboiled rice. In all other ways, the patients were treated identically. Beriberi was more common in the white rice ward. This experiment led Fletcher to decide that beriberi was connected somehow with white rice and that it was *not* infectious, as many had thought. Yet he was unsure as to what the exact cause could be and what it was about the parboiled rice that might have prevented beriberi.

Two years later, in 1907, Scottish physician Henry Fraser and Canadian physician Thomas Stanton experimented with the diets of Javanese road builders living in two work camps in remote areas of Malaya. The laborers were healthy and located far from other populations—and were thus unlikely to be infected by any organisms that might cause beriberi. Until their work was finished, the laborers could not easily leave the camps. Fraser and Stanton informed the men that parboiled rice was suspected to be healthier than white rice. The laborers preferred the white rice. They were good subjects: healthy, isolated, informed, in a fashion—and trapped. Half of the men were given white rice—the better-tasting diet—and half were given parboiled rice, the rice thought to be healthier.

This experiment seems less exploitative than Fletcher's work with the mentally ill in Kuala Lumpur, in that the laborers were warned of the dangers of white rice. Fraser and Stanton found that laborers fed parboiled rice were indeed less likely to develop beriberi. In separate experiments, they also found that alcohol extracts of parboiled rice cured beriberi in chickens fed white rice. Fraser and Stanton suggested that the polished white rice lacked something necessary for metabolism of nerves.

More definitive work proving that beriberi was indeed a dietary disease was done by Dutch physician Christiaan Eijkman (1858–1930) in experiments with chickens, although he never quite realized the importance of his work. He established that chickens eating unpolished rice did not become ill, but he thought that there was a toxin involved and that a substance in unpolished rice, an anti-beriberi factor, somehow neutralized this toxin. Gerrit Grijns (1865–1944), another Dutch physician, continued Eijkman's work and showed that beriberi was not a toxic disease, as Eijkman had suggested, but a disease caused by the absence of a crucial substance in the outer layers of the rice grain.

American army physician Edward Vedder (1878–1952) successfully treated infants ill with beriberi with rice polish extract, and finally American chemist Robert Williams (1886–1965), in work with pigeons, identified the curative factor—vitamin B_1, or thiamine. The experiments with psychiatric patients and laborers had provided the critical information that guided later researchers in pinpointing both the dietary nature of the illness and its relatively simple treatment.

Frances R. Frankenburg

CARREL, ALEXIS

French surgeon, physiologist, and Nobel Prize–winner Alexis Carrel has been called the father of vascular surgery. He experimented with transplanting organs and was an innovator in the treatment of war wounds.

Alexis Carrel (1873–1944) was born in Sainte-Foy-lès-Lyon, a suburb of Lyons, France, the son of a textile merchant. Both his undergraduate and medical education were completed at the University of Lyons, which he joined as a faculty member after serving as a military surgeon to the Alpine Chasseurs. Carrel's interest in mysticism and his calls for a scientific study of the miracles at Lourdes led to conflict with the French medical establishment and resulted in his emigration to Montréal, Canada, and then to the United States, where he joined the faculty of the University of Chicago in 1904.

Carrel's father had died when Alexis was still a child, and his mother earned money doing embroidery. The young physician was fascinated with the delicate needlework and paid a professional embroiderer to teach him to sew. In 1902, he published a paper demonstrating that careful suturing made possible end-to-end anastomosis, or surgical connection of severed blood vessels. Prior to that time, the only treatment for a wounded artery had been ligation (or tying off) of the blood vessel, followed by the probable amputation of the involved limb.

He joined the Rockefeller Institute in New York in 1906, where he continued his work in vascular surgery. Most of his work was in animals, but he did perform some experimental work in humans. In one example, he joined an artery from a father to his infant who had had a severe intestinal bleed. His advances in vascular surgery earned him the 1912 Nobel Prize in Physiology or Medicine. His ability to repair blood vessels and his meticulous aseptic technique made organ transplantation seem possible for the first time. Carrel transplanted a kidney from one cat to another, but the problems of immunity and rejection prevented him from using the technique in humans.

When World War I broke out, Carrel volunteered for the French army and became a major. He worked with chemist Henry Drysdale Dakin to develop an antiseptic wound irrigation technique that saved hundreds of thousands of wounded limbs from infection and amputation. He summarized his experience in the book *Treatment of Infected Wounds*, which he wrote with Georges Debelly.

After the war, Carrel returned to the United States, where he resumed his studies of organ transplantation and tissue culture. He collaborated with aviator Charles Lindbergh (who was a skilled and innovated mechanic) to develop an extracorporeal perfusion pump that could be sterilized and used in open-heart surgery and organ transplantation. He and Lindbergh also shared an interest in eugenics and a conviction that Caucasians were superior to other races.

When World War II started, Carrel returned to France and became director of the Carrel Foundation for the Study of Human Problems under Philippe Pétain's Vichy government. That association led to accusations of collaboration with

France's Nazi occupiers, and it is likely that he would have been prosecuted after the war had he not died of heart disease in November 1944.

Jack E. McCallum

CASTLE, WILLIAM

Hematologist William Castle performed a unique type of self-experimentation and therapeutic experimentation that elucidated the physiology of vitamin B_{12} and led to a treatment for pernicious anemia. He used the contents of his own stomach to repair the bone marrow of ill patients.

William Bosworth Castle (1897–1990) was born in Cambridge, Massachusetts, and graduated from Harvard Medical School. He is best known for his investigations and experiments with pernicious anemia.

Pernicious anemia, first described by Thomas Addison (1793–1860) in England in the 1850s, is a rare autoimmune illness in which a person cannot absorb vitamin B_{12}, which is necessary for the production of red blood cells and neurological functioning. Symptoms include weakness, fatigue, rapid heartbeat, and neurological symptoms, including paresthesias (tingling or burning) and abnormal gait. Untreated, the illness is fatal.

Work done by American physicians George Hoyt Whipple (1878–1976), William Murphy (1892–1987), and George Minot (1885–1950) had shown that there was a dietary component to pernicious anemia and that patients with it could survive if they could eat 300 grams (about 10 ounces) of raw or lightly cooked liver every day, an unpleasantly large amount that was difficult to consume. (They received a Nobel Prize in Physiology or Medicine for this work in 1934.) Castle and his colleagues at the Thorndike Memorial Laboratory at Boston City Hospital also knew that patients with pernicious anemia had shrunken stomachs and produced stomach juice with little acid. Replacement of an ill person's stomach juices with those from a well person was ineffective in treating the disease.

In 1927, Castle put these findings together and concluded that there must be two factors present to prevent pernicious anemia: one present in healthy stomach juice, which he called *intrinsic factor*, and one present in some foods, which he called *extrinsic factor*. He suspected an interaction between these two factors. Large amounts of *extrinsic factor* found in liver were able to compensate for the ill person's lack of *intrinsic factor*.

Castle performed a series of experiments to demonstrate the existence of these two factors and the relationship between them. He ate hamburg steak and then extracted his own stomach contents. He poured the contents into the stomach of an anemic patient through a stomach tube. The patient improved. The timing was important. In other experiments, Castle had already shown that replacement of stomach juice alone had no effect. The stomach juice and steak had to be present together. Something had to happen between the factor in the stomach juice and the factor in the hamburg steak. The experiment worked well. The bone marrow of the patient began to make red blood cells. Castle's work showed, in a compelling manner, a clear connection between the stomach and the bone marrow.

Castle went on to perform the same experiment for another 60 patients. The patients were not told the origin of the substance in the flexible stomach tube. (One can imagine the hesitation that an ill patient—or anyone—would have in consuming his or her doctor's regurgitated meal.)

It is difficult to know how to classify this experiment. In a sense it was self-experimentation, in that Castle removed his own stomach contents. But Castle administered the results of his self-experiment to ill patients, particularly uninformed ill patients, in an attempt to treat their illness. Castle's experiment could not be done today because, among other reasons, of the element of deception or, at least, the withholding of information. Nor is it clear that this was exactly a therapeutic experiment, in that it was not used in actual practice. Castle and others were eventually able to prepare concentrated extracts of liver that patients found less odious to eat. They also discovered that injections of this extract worked even better than taking it by mouth.

It took another 20 years of work to define the nature of the substance in hamburg steak and liver that cured the anemia. This substance, Castle's extrinsic factor, turned out to be cobalamin, otherwise known as vitamin B_{12}. The intrinsic factor, as it continues to be known today, is a large protein that is secreted by the stomach. Vitamin B_{12} in the diet is usually bound to proteins. Stomach acids and enzymes break the B_{12} apart from the proteins, and then B_{12} is bound to other proteins. The protein-B_{12} compound travels to the duodenum, where the compounds are broken apart, and the B_{12} then binds with the intrinsic factor. It is this compound that is absorbed into the body.

Castle did other important work in medicine, but he is best known for this work that involved self-experimentation, laboratory investigation, and clinical observations.

Frances R. Frankenburg

ELGIN STATE HOSPITAL EXPERIMENTS

Experiments on mentally ill patients at the Elgin State Hospital in Illinois included radioactive injections and a series of nutritional experiments. These ethically questionable studies led to much of our current understanding about the importance of vitamins in the diet.

The Elgin State Hospital, also known as the Illinois Northern Hospital for the Insane, and today known as the Elgin Mental Health Center, was the location for a number of important but controversial human medical experiments in the early to mid-20th century.

Between 1931 and 1933, Elgin patients were injected with radium-266. There are two accounts given for the supposed purpose of the radium studies. One is that patients with schizophrenia were injected with radium to see if the element could treat the disorder. The other is that the patients were administered radium not for therapeutic reasons but for researchers to study how the body handles radioactivity. Little more is known about the radium injections.

Another set of experiments dealt with a seemingly more benign interest—nutrition. One of the leading nutritional researchers of the time was Max Kenneth Horwitt (1908–2000). Horwitt was born in New York City in 1908 and educated at Dartmouth and Yale. He was the founding director of the L. B. Mendel Research Laboratory at the Elgin State Hospital in Illinois and worked there from 1935 to 1968. He and his colleagues manipulated the diets of the long-term patients—those who stayed in the hospital for months to years—producing a number of important vitamin studies in the 1940s. These studies were performed with the knowledge and advice of the Food and Nutrition Board of the National Academy of Science and with input from the leading nutritional researchers of the time.

Because the patients lived at the hospital for so long, the researchers had a unique opportunity to study vitamin E. Vitamin E is stored in the body's fat, and to study the effects of its depletion in otherwise well-nourished people, it is necessary to perform the studies over several years. In one study, they fed subjects a diet deficient in vitamin E for five years. Vitamin E blood levels fell and the lifespan of red blood cells shortened, but there were no reports that the patients became ill in any way.

Other studies examined the effects of B-vitamin deficiency. The researchers fed subjects a diet deficient in vitamin B_2 (riboflavin) for several months, and many developed skin lesions. In a more disturbing experiment, the group fed schizophrenic and demented men diets deficient in vitamins B_1 (thiamine) and B_2 for over two years. The men became lethargic and lost interest in activities; some became violent. After vitamin B administration was resumed, the patients improved.

Hewitt and his colleagues also followed 36 male patients of the Elgin Hospital, who received diets low in vitamin B_1 for up to three years. During this time, the researchers took multiple blood samples to measure, for example, blood glucose, pyruvic acid, and lactic acid when the patients were fasting, resting, or exercising.

The Elgin projects continued for over 20 years, well until the 1960s, and much of what we know today about our nutritional needs for vitamins came from this research. Interestingly, in many of the publications arising from the experiments, careful acknowledgment is made of the hard work of the many scientists, technicians, physicians, and consultants, but no acknowledgment is made of the participation of the subjects, nor is there is a mention of consent, or even an indication of whether the subjects were informed that they were participating in a study.

Frances R. Frankenburg

EUGENICS

Eugenics, the effort to prevent, control, or eliminate disease thought to be due to genes, was intended to diminish suffering and to lead to a healthier population.

But the idea became associated with racism, forced sterilizations, and some of the cruelest experiments in history.

Eugenics in its modern form developed in the 19th century as a practical application of Charles Darwin's concept of natural selection. According to Darwin, some species of life-forms have a natural advantage over others due to inherited traits. Francis Galton (1822–1911) was a cousin of Darwin and shared some of his interests in the origin of life-forms and their development over time. Galton coined the term *eugenics* in 1883 from the Greek words meaning "good in birth" or "noble in heredity." He wanted to establish and develop a scientific field of inquiry dedicated to improving the human species.

Eugenics became popular in the United States after an increase in immigrants from southern Europe and the overcrowding of the nation's largest cities. Many politicians and writers sought an explanation and solution for the perceived cultural and physical inferiority of immigrants compared to white Protestant "natives." Some resented the "pollution" of their society by foreigners and looked to eugenics as a way to purify the national bloodline. Many eugenicists agreed with Galton's interest in reducing the number of (in Galton's words) "undesirables" and increasing the number of "desirables." Two forms of eugenics thus developed by the early 20th century: "negative" eugenics (to prevent undesirables from reproducing) and "positive" eugenics (to increase the presence of "desirables" in society).

Between 1900 and 1930, scientists across Europe, Latin America, the Russian Empire (and then Soviet Union), and the United States embraced eugenics as the solution for what was seen as an overpopulated and increasingly violent modern society. Both scientists and laymen convinced themselves that modern society should guide human evolution in the interest of world peace, public safety, and the "health of the race." For example, a university chair in racial hygiene was established in Munich, Germany, and held by Fritz Lenz, an eminent evolutionary biologist of his day. He supported the elimination of "inferior" people. Charles B. Davenport headed the American Station for Experimental Evolution, which was funded by the Carnegie Institution of Washington.

British, American, and German scientists established centers to research human heredity. The Kaiser Wilhelm Institute for Anthropology, Human Heredity, and Eugenics in Berlin, partially funded by the Rockefeller Foundation, was established in 1927 in Berlin, Germany, and gathered statistical data concerning human heredity found in medical records and oral family studies. Its first director was anthropologist Eugene Fischer, and its second director was Otmar von Verschuer, who was a mentor of Josef Mengele (1911–1979), the infamous Nazi doctor who performed experiments in the concentration camps.

Eugenicists associated ethnic and social differences with unalterable genetic traits, reflecting and reinforcing virulent ethnocentrism and racism. Criminality, prostitution, and other alleged signs of mental inferiority (often referred to as "feeblemindedness") stemmed from bad genes, scientists thought. Margaret Sanger (1879–1966), a major proponent of birth control in the 1920s, believed that the "unfit" and "undeniably feeble-minded" should not have children.

By the 1920s, new laws passed in American society reflected the influence of the eugenics movement. For example, the Immigration Act (1924) cut the quota of immigrants allowed to enter from such eastern and southern European nations as Italy, Poland, and Greece.

Some American scientists and social planners in the 1930s suggested sterilizing "undesirables" to stem the reproduction of supposedly genetically inferior people. Even as recently as the 1960s and 1970s, some doctors working for the federal government sterilized Native American women without their consent or knowledge at rural health clinics.

By 1930, more than 24 states had passed pro-sterilization laws. A revealing case of the influence of eugenics was *Buck v. Bell* (1927), in which the U.S. Supreme Court affirmed the constitutionality of sterilization laws. Justice Oliver Wendell Holmes delivered the majority opinion, in which he stated, referring to a family in which the grandmother and mother were allegedly "feeble-minded," that "three generations of imbeciles are enough." California, which experienced a heightened state of nativism between 1860 and 1940 due to its large population of Chinese and Japanese Americans, led the way in eugenics legislation and sterilization campaigns. By 1933, the state had forcibly sterilized more people in the name of eugenics than all other states combined.

Criticism of the social policies and the scientific basis of eugenics research increased during the 1930s. Scientists and social scientists, ranging from biologists to anthropologists, began to view social deviancy as a product of a poor environment rather than being due to inherited genetic traits. In 1930, the Catholic Church officially came out against eugenics and birth control. British and American biologists attempted to rescue the field of eugenics in the 1940s. They rejected the social prejudice that accompanied the scientific theory and instead emphasized its connection to the study of genetics. Genetics as a scientific school of inquiry grew rapidly from the reorientation of eugenics research during this time.

Germany continued to propound the eugenics movement, however. Manifested in the Nazi Party's attempt to eliminate world Jewry through the "final solution," eugenics embodied the core of German social scientific research until 1945. The Nazis put eugenics into practice throughout German society, forcing mentally challenged and "damaged" individuals, as well as homosexuals and other perceived social deviants, to undergo sterilization to maintain the purity of the fatherland. Mengele, for example, carried out cruel, inhumane, and immoral experiments on twins. With the horror of the Holocaust revealed, eugenics acquired a repugnant connotation during the post–World War II period that it is unlikely ever to lose.

Jason Newman

FORSSMANN, WERNER

In 1929, Werner Forssmann was the first person to catheterize the human heart, a procedure seen as so dangerous at the time that he had to do it on himself, in secret, and by deceiving his coadventurer. After this feat of courage and dexterity, he worked in obscurity as a urologist for some decades, until he was awarded the Nobel Prize in 1956.

Werner Forssmann (1904–1979) graduated from the University of Berlin medical school in 1929. At that time, physicians did not think that it was possible to safely insert any tubes into the human heart. Forssmann, however, had been impressed by a drawing of French physiologists passing a thin tube through the jugular vein of a horse into its heart to measure the pressure in the heart's chambers, and he saw other potential uses of this procedure.

In addition to recording pressures, Forssmann foresaw that a tube inserted into the human heart could take blood samples and also directly deliver medication. Instead of inserting a tube through the neck, as in the horse experiment, he decided that the antecubital vein in the arm (the vein in front of the elbow) would be more acceptable for human catheterizations.

The advantages of catheterization, however, were not so obvious to Forssmann's supervisor, who refused to allow Forssmann to try it. So, in 1929, Forssmann decided to proceed in secret. He befriended a nurse who had access to ureteral catheters, which were long and thin enough to be threaded into the heart, and she agreed to be the first person to undergo this experimental procedure. She obtained the catheter and operating room and prepared for the catheter's insertion. Forssmann inserted the catheter into his own left arm instead. Once the catheter was threaded up to his shoulder, he told the nurse what he had done, and together they walked down a flight of stairs to the radiology room so that he could continue the insertion under fluoroscopic guidance. He pushed the catheter into his right atrium. He repeated the procedure another five times over the next four weeks and then published an article describing the catheterization.

Later, he was the first person to inject radiopaque material through the catheter directly into the heart. He experimented first on rabbits, but they died during the procedure. He experienced greater success with catheterizations of the hearts of dogs. Then, he tried the experiment on himself, inserting a catheter into his heart using his femoral vein, a large vein in the groin, and then injecting sodium iodide into his own heart. The resulting pictures were not very clear, but they were the first images of a radiopaque substance injected into a living human heart. He catheterized his own heart another nine times.

In 1932, Forssmann joined the Nazi Party at the urging of a colleague. However, when offered human subjects for experimentation by Karl Gebhardt (who was later tried and executed at the Doctors' Trial in Nuremberg), Forssmann rejected the opportunity, feeling that it was wrong. Instead, he served as a physician in the German army and was captured by the Russians. He escaped and was then taken prisoner by the Americans. Eventually released, he resumed his medical career, but his career foundered because of his membership in the Nazi Party.

Physicians André Cournand (1895–1988) and Dickinson Richards (1895–1973), working together at Columbia University, used Forssmann's technique to catheterize patients and then further developed it so that they could take blood samples from the right atrium and pulmonary vein. This technique allowed them to describe with more exactness than had hitherto been possible the relationships between blood flow, blood pressure, and oxygenation in the pulmonary circulation.

In 1956, while working as a urologist, not as a researcher or a cardiologist, in a small town in Germany, Forssmann was astonished to be awarded the Nobel Prize in Physiology or Medicine for his work on catheterization, along with Cournand and Richards.

Frances R. Frankenburg

GERMAN MEDICAL RESEARCH ETHICS

One of the arguments the Nazi physicians used to justify their cruel, unethical, and often lethal experiments on humans was that there were no internationally accepted medical research guidelines. But pre–World War II Germany had more advanced research ethics than other countries of the time.

The Nazi physicians had many excuses for their horrific human medical experiments, arguing that no code of research ethics existed and that they were therefore breaking no laws. Of course, a code of ethics is not needed to condemn the sadism of their experiments and their intent to murder their subjects. But they were incorrect in stating that there were no codes of ethics. In fact, there were two earlier published German codes of research guidelines related to human experimentation.

German physician Albert Neisser's (1855–1916) inoculation of syphilis into people without their consent in the late 1800s was sufficiently notorious that it was discussed in the Prussian parliament. A panel composed of leading German clinicians, including pathologist Rudolf Virchow (1821–1902), reviewed the case, as did lawyers. Based on these reviews, in 1900, the minister for religious, educational, and medical affairs issued a directive to all hospitals and clinics, sometimes known as the Berlin Code, stating that medical interventions other than for diagnosis and treatment were forbidden under all circumstances if the subject was a minor, not competent, or had not given clear consent after having the procedure, including any adverse consequences, explained to him or her. The fulfilment of these requirements had to be carefully documented. All research interventions could be performed only by the medical director of the facility or with his or her authorization. The directive was not legally binding, but it was the first example of a modern government issuing regulations concerning medical experimentation; it applied to most of the northern part of the German Reich and most of the German population.

Three decades later, in 1930, there was once again a flurry of public concern about medical activities (if not actual experimentation) after 72 children died in Lübeck from tuberculosis when they received a contaminated Bacillus Calmette–Guérin vaccine (a vaccine for tuberculosis). As a result, in 1931, the Reich minister of the interior issued a circular titled "Guidelines for New Therapy and Human Experimentation." It was an elaboration of the guidelines included in the 1900 directive. The patient was to make his or her own decisions after the procedure had been clearly described. A written report was required for each clinical trial. Once again, the medical director of each institution was responsible for all clinical research. The regulations differed from the earlier ones in that they did allow experimentation on children if the risk was minimal. Experiments on dying persons were considered impermissible. Finally, the minister recommended that all physicians should be educated about these issues. These guidelines were now binding law.

Medical research ethics in pre–World War II Germany may have been more codified or advanced than in other countries, but, tragically, the guidelines were not followed by the later Nazi physicians.

Frances R. Frankenburg

GOLDBERGER, JOSEPH

Joseph Goldberger performed experiments on himself, his family and colleagues, and prisoners to prove the nutritional basis of pellagra, an illness that affected poor people.

Pellagra is a disease caused by a deficiency of niacin in the diet. It is known as the "illness of the four Ds": dermatitis, diarrhea, dementia, and death. The skin lesions begin as an erythematous rash, which then becomes rough and scaly. The lesions are symmetrical and found over the hands, face, neck, elbows, and knees. A variety of neurological problems, not just dementia, can develop. Patients complain of dizziness, weakness, depression, and paresthesias. They can become confused. If severe, pellagra can be fatal. Pellagra affected poor people in parts of Europe, Africa, and the southern United States.

Joseph Goldberger (1874–1929) carried out many of the experiments that established the cause of pellagra. He was born in Hungary and came to the United States at the age of seven. He graduated from Bellevue Hospital Medical College, joined the United States Public Health Service (PHS), and worked with infectious illnesses, including yellow fever, dengue, typhus, hookworm, and diphtheria. He traveled to Mexico and Cuba to study yellow fever and became ill with this terrible disease. He developed dengue in Brownsville, Texas, in 1907. Three years later, he fell ill with typhus in Mexico City.

Goldberger was asked to investigate pellagra, then thought to be an infectious illness and a serious problem in the South. For example, in the Georgia State Sanitarium in Milledgeville, Georgia, pellagra was the most common cause of death by 1909, overtaking tuberculosis. Pellagra was diagnosed in other parts of the country also, particularly in poor areas. In 1914, Goldberger went to the South and quickly became convinced that pellagra was not like the other infectious illnesses he had encountered. Nurses and physicians treating it rarely became ill themselves; he noted that they had a better diet than the patients.

Goldberger arranged for improved diets to be given to children in two orphanages in Jackson, Mississippi, and to patients at the Georgia State Sanitarium, and the incidence of pellagra decreased. This was an experiment of sorts and an early example of successful dietary intervention for the prevention of disease.

Goldberger continued his investigations of pellagra by arranging for an experiment at the Rankin State Prison Farm near Jackson. Although Mississippi was the state worst hit by pellagra, there were no reports of pellagra in any of Mississippi's prisons. Indeed, the prisoners seemed to have a better diet than other poor or institutionalized Southerners. Goldberger chose to do an experiment on the Rankin Farm prisoners, in part because he had a good working relationship with Earl Brewer, the governor of Mississippi.

Brewer and Goldberger told about 80 Rankin inmates that if they volunteered to eat a traditional Southern diet for about six months, and therefore run the risk of developing pellagra, they would get full pardons. Brewer and Goldberger selected 12 volunteers. Of this group, 7 were convicted murderers serving life terms. Two were wealthy brothers, serving time for embezzlement after their bank had failed. The brothers were friends of the governor.

In April 1915, the convict volunteers were moved to a scrupulously clean building separated from the other prisoners. Their diet was limited. Breakfast consisted of biscuits, fried mush, grits, brown gravy, cane syrup, and coffee. Lunch included cornbread, collards, sweet potatoes, grits, and syrup. Supper was similar to lunch. The usual Rankin prison diet was better than what the volunteers or research subjects received, in that it contained meat of some sort at all meals, buttermilk, peas, and beans.

Prisoners on the experimental diet became ill and weak within two weeks. Plus, they hated the diet. Yet this was standard fare for the Southern poor at that time. By the fifth month of the study, in September of 1915, six of the volunteers had developed dermatitis and other vague symptoms. Other physicians confirmed that in five of these prisoners these changes were consistent with the diagnosis of pellagra. The experiment had succeeded in establishing the nutritional basis of the disease.

Goldberger had induced pellagra by feeding otherwise healthy men a diet lacking meat, fresh milk, and vegetables. This experiment was criticized at the time from every angle. Its secrecy was deplored. Some thought that the prisoners were being treated too harshly, and others claimed they were being treated too leniently. Governor Brewer was accused of arranging the whole experiment to "spring" his two friends from prison. Skeptical physicians pointed out that the convicts might have been weakened by the poor diet, making them more susceptible to the real cause of pellagra, which was probably infectious.

Goldberger carried out more experiments to determine whether infection or diet caused pellagra. He arranged "filth parties" to test the contagion theory of pellagra. He attempted to transmit the illness to healthy volunteers by administering secretions or actual excreta of pellagrins (people suffering from pellagra) or injections of pellagrous blood. The volunteers included other physicians, himself, and his wife. The experiments went on for two months, and although some of the volunteers developed unpleasant side effects, such as diarrhea and pain at the site of blood injections, no one developed pellagra.

Goldberger was a member of every experimental group. He swallowed sodium bicarbonate (baking soda) with the capsules so that no one could say that his stomach acid had killed the putative infectious agent.

The inclusion of his wife among the "volunteers" was unusual, and Goldberger was one of the few physicians to have his wife be a subject in experiments. In an account that she wrote years later, she explained she had insisted on being a volunteer. The men would not let her swallow the pills but instead allowed injections into her abdomen of the blood of a woman dying from pellagra. The injection of seven cubic centimeters of blood into her stomach was so upsetting that one nurse who watched fled from the room crying. It is not clear why the experimenters gave her an injection instead of a pill. Did they think it more proper to inject a woman with the blood of another woman? Why was swallowing a pill thought to be worse than receiving an injection? The injection was in fact more dangerous than swallowing, but somehow the investigators found it less objectionable.

The filth parties showed that pellagra was probably not an infectious illness. These so-called parties and the Rankin prison studies would probably have had trouble being approved today because of the risks to the subjects. Because of Goldberger's past experience with infectious disease, however, he must have seen this risk of illness as just part of the quotidian nature of his work. Goldberger's experiments had clearly shown that pellagra was caused by the poor diet common in the South.

An animal model of pellagra was found in dogs; this allowed more experimentation and the determination that a diet lacking the vitamin niacin causes pellagra.

Many researchers contributed to working out the cause and cure of pellagra, but perhaps because of the variety and, at times, disgusting nature of his experiments, Goldberger usually gets the credit.

Frances R. Frankenburg

HALDANE, JOHN BURDON SANDERSON

As a young boy, John Burdon Sanderson Haldane, the son of physiologist John Scott Haldane, helped his father with his experiments and also at times was a subject of his experimentation. In his own career, the younger Haldane later experimented on himself and his colleagues. He was a brilliant man who made substantial contributions to the disciplines of mathematics, biology, and genetics.

John "Jack" Burdon Sanderson Haldane (1892–1964) was born in Oxford, England, and later studied at Oxford University. As a young boy, he went with his father, the well-known physiologist and researcher John Scott Haldane (1860–1936), into a mine that was filled with firedamp, more technically known as methane gas. His father asked him to recite the famous "Friends, Romans, Countrymen" speech of Marc Antony from Shakespeare's *Julius Caesar* until his legs buckled and he collapsed. Once on the ground, Jack recovered, thus showing that methane gas was lighter than air. The Haldanes' finding meant that miners could escape fire-damp by crawling on the ground of tunnels in the mines. When he was 13 and his father was experimenting with caisson disease (also known as "the bends"), Jack dove underwater. His diving suit was too large, but he had the presence of mind to adjust the valves to keep the air pressure in the suit high enough to keep the water out.

During World War I, when he was fighting in the trenches, he also worked with his father to improve the gas mask to better protect soldiers against the toxic gases, such as chlorine and bromine, that the Germans had started to use. Like his father, he was fascinated by the physiology of respiration. His father had shown that elevated carbon dioxide levels increased respiration. To find out whether that was due to an increased acidity in the blood resulting from carbonic acid, Haldane drank various acidic compounds, including diluted hydrochloric acid. At other times, he exposed himself to high concentrations of carbon dioxide. He also subjected himself to low atmospheric pressures in decompression chambers.

In 1939, the submarine HMS *Thetis* of the British Royal Navy sank off Liverpool; 99 men died. Haldane was asked to investigate. He conducted a series of experiments, one in which he and four colleagues sealed themselves into a small steel chamber and investigated whether a gradual rise in carbon dioxide would have the same effect as a rapid rise. During some of these experiments, Haldane vomited and had severe headaches; some of his colleagues were incapacitated. Nevertheless, he continued his investigations, increasing the risk by exposing himself to the increased pressure and cold that submariners would experience. As a result, one of his colleagues ruptured a lung, six colleagues and Haldane lost consciousness at varying times, and one colleague had a seizure. During these experiments, Haldane also suffered from the bends and sustained a spinal injury that would cause him pain for the rest of his life.

Haldane recruited a number of people to participate in similar experiments. Among these were Elizabeth Jermyn, his secretary; Dr. Juan Negrín, the former prime minister of Spain, also a physician and physiologist; and Helen Spurway, whom he later married.

A man of prodigious intelligence and interests, Haldane made contributions to the science of enzymes by doing work that led to a formula known as the Briggs-Haldane equation. He wrote books for children and popular books about science. He brought his mathematical genius to bear on many problems in biology and genetics and made significant contributions to evolutionary theory, writing about such topics as mutation rates, gene frequencies, genetic linkage, and population genetics.

In his later years, he became more concerned about the ethics of experimenting on animals and believed, as did his father, that one should experiment on oneself first, if possible, before subjecting animals to medical experiments.

Haldane was also an irascible man who had little patience for convention. He left England in 1956 and moved to Calcutta (now Kolkata), where he briefly worked at the Indian Statistical Institute. After quarreling with his colleagues there, he moved to Orissa (now Odisha). True to his principles, he requested at the time of his death that his body be used for medical studies. This request was not granted.

Frances R. Frankenburg

INSULIN

Until the 1920s, there was no effective treatment for diabetes. In 1922, a group of researchers in Toronto—Frederick Banting, Charles Best, James Collip, and J.J.R. Macleod—isolated insulin from beef pancreas. Two Toronto General Hospital clinicians then injected this insulin into a 14-year-old boy. This successful therapeutic experiment meant that diabetes became a treatable illness.

Diabetes mellitus type 1 is an autoimmune disease in which the beta cells of the pancreas no longer produce insulin, the hormone that allows sugar to enter cells of the body. Without insulin, sugar levels in the blood become elevated, the person loses weight, and organs throughout the body are damaged. The functions and structures of the pancreas were not well understood until the 19th century. French physiologist Claude Bernard (1813–1878) showed that the pancreas produces enzymes that are delivered to the gastrointestinal tract through the pancreatic duct and aid in digestion, and a German medical student, Paul Langerhans (1847–1888), discovered the presence of clusters, or islands, of clear cells within the pancreas. He did not understand their function but noted that these cells seemed different from those in the rest of the pancreas.

In 1889, Lithuanian German physician Oskar Minkowski (1858–1931) and German physician Joseph von Mering (1849–1908) removed the pancreas from a dog. The dog survived this difficult operation, but it developed diabetes as a result. Minkowski and von Mering demonstrated that there was indeed a connection between the pancreas and diabetes, but they were not able to elucidate the nature of that connection. Ligation (tying off) of the pancreatic duct—through which the pancreatic products presumably flowed—did not lead to diabetes. The pancreas was thus proved to have at least two products: one that prevented diabetes and one involved in digestion that was secreted through the pancreatic duct. Later, researchers began to suspect that the clusters of clear cells—later called, after the medical student, islets of Langerhans—were involved in the regulation of sugar levels in the body and might be the key to understanding diabetes.

In 1916, Romanian physiologist Nicolae Paulescu (1869–1931) prepared pancreatic extracts using saline that lowered the blood sugar of dogs. He published his findings in 1921, but as he wrote in French and lived in Romania, few people outside France or Romania were aware of his work. He did not test his extracts on humans. Other researchers used pancreatic extracts to lower blood sugar in animals, but the extracts always led to toxic reactions. The solution to the problem of diabetes seemed to lie in the product of the clear cells of the pancreas, but pancreatic extracts were considered too dangerous to try on humans because of their harmful constituents.

Meanwhile, Frederick Banting (1891–1941) was a young Canadian surgeon living in Toronto, trying to forge a medical career after distinguished service in the trenches in World War I. He read a paper by physician Moses Barron (1884–1972) about the ligation of the pancreatic duct and had the idea that if he ligated the pancreatic ducts of dogs that this would lead to the death of the pancreatic cells that synthesized the digestive enzymes. This in turn would make the recovery of the antidiabetes product of the pancreas—what we now call insulin—easier by protecting the antidiabetic substance from digestion by the pancreatic enzymes.

Banting convinced J.J.R. Macleod (1876–1935), an older and well-established Scottish physiologist who was the director of the University of Toronto physiology lab at the time, to give him some research space. A young medical student named Charles Best (1899–1978) was recruited to help Banting with the work. Banting and Best were young, enthusiastic, hardworking, and unencumbered by other responsibilities or the understanding of how difficult their job would be.

In May of 1921, Banting and Best began their experiments, at first with dogs. They ligated the dogs' pancreatic ducts and, after a few weeks, removed the pancreas (now without the digestive enzymes) and prepared a pancreatic extract. Then they removed the entire pancreas from other dogs, thus making the dogs diabetic. They administered the pancreatic extract to the newly diabetic dogs and sometimes succeeded in lowering the dogs' blood sugar. These experiments were difficult and time-consuming. In November 1921, they began to use the pancreases of fetal calves because the pancreases of these fetuses were richer in islets than in the cells that produced the digestive enzymes.

Macleod asked chemist James Bertram Collip (1892–1965) to help them purify the pancreatic extract. Banting and Best used Collip's improved extracts on rabbits. (This was another important advance because they no longer had to "de-pancreatize" dogs.) Collip had produced a pure extract that lowered the sugar in diabetic dogs and healthy rabbits without leading to the same toxic reactions that had hindered the work of other researchers.

Collip's extracts seemed safe enough to be tried on humans. According to some accounts, Banting and Best injected the extract (shortly to be named insulin) into themselves, with no adverse effects other than some dizziness. They were not allowed to inject it into patients, as they were not authorized to provide patient care. Then, on January 11, 1922, an intern at Toronto General Hospital working with Walter Campbell, head of the diabetes service, injected 7.5 cubic centimeters of insulin into each buttock of a 14-year-old diabetic boy, Leonard Thompson. Thompson was so malnourished from his untreated diabetes mellitus that he barely weighed 65 pounds. He was lethargic and being kept alive only by following the treatment of the time—a very restricted diet. Following the injection, Thompson's blood sugar decreased a little, but he developed a sterile abscess in his buttocks, suggesting that the extract was not yet pure enough.

Collip continued to work with pancreatic extracts and finally discovered that if he dissolved the extract in a solution of 90 percent alcohol, the "active principle" precipitated out of the solution into a powder. Campbell repeated the injection on

January 23, 1922. Thompson began to feel better and to gain weight. Thompson had been the subject of a therapeutic experiment that proved to be successful. In February, the team treated six more diabetic patients. Although some difficulty in preparing insulin in adequate amounts continued, the researchers had successfully shown that animal-derived insulin could lower the blood sugar of diabetic humans.

Banting and Best were lucky in that they had not been fully aware of the failures other scientists experienced doing similar work. If they had known of the problems the others had encountered, they might have been discouraged from making their own attempts. They also were aided by the use of new technology to measure blood glucose in small amounts. They chose their animal subjects well, using dogs and rabbits as test animals and dogs and calves for pancreatic extracts. The insulin in these animals is similar to that in humans, allowing an easy transfer from experimental laboratory work to the clinic.

Banting's original ideas of ligating the pancreatic ducts and using fetal calf pancreas, as it later turned out, were not needed. But these ideas gave Banting the conviction that he could do something that others could not and the confidence to proceed and to persevere. The researchers, clinicians, and patients were also lucky that the first injections worked well—but not too well. Insulin injections carry with them the risk of lowering the blood sugar too much, and thus, in extreme cases, can lead to death.

The Nobel Prize Committee awarded the Nobel Prize in Physiology or Medicine in 1923 to Banting and Macleod for the discovery of insulin. The selection of these two was controversial because Best's and Collip's contributions were not recognized, and some others thought that Paulescu should have received the prize for his earlier work. Banting immediately shared his prize money with Best; Macleod shared his with Collip.

Frances R. Frankenburg

INSULIN COMA THERAPY

In 1927, psychiatrist Manfred Sakel caused a coma in a psychotic patient by injecting him with insulin and thus causing low blood sugar. The patient's psychotic symptoms disappeared, and insulin coma became, for a number of years, a widely used treatment in psychiatry.

Manfred Sakel (1900–1957) graduated from the University of Vienna medical school in 1925 and trained as a psychiatrist. He then worked as an internist at a facility treating drug addicts in Berlin. In 1927, while treating a diabetic morphine addict, he gave her the newly discovered insulin, lowering her blood sugar so much that she became comatose. When she recovered, she had lost her craving for morphine.

Perhaps inspired by this result, he began to treat nondiabetic addicts with insulin, including one man who had a psychotic disorder as well an addiction. In this case, when the patient recovered from the coma, he was no longer psychotic. In some accounts, these events are described as accidental and caused by Sakel's misjudgment of the insulin dose. In others, they are described as purposeful experiments based on his biological theories of psychosis. (Other psychiatrists had used insulin before Sakel did, but almost always with glucose, as a way of increasing appetite in patients with anorexia or severe depression. Occasionally the person's sugar became too low and he or she became comatose, but this was not the intended result.)

Whether Sakel's work was experimental or serendipitous, he was, in any event, the first to recognize improvement in psychosis after insulin-induced hypoglycemia (low blood sugar) and the first to promote insulin coma as a treatment for schizophrenia—an illness with no effective treatment at that time.

It was not clear, though, whether the coma was necessary for the improvement to occur. Sakel's insulin treatment was elaborate. He prescribed a complicated series of insulin injections that lowered the person's blood sugar for two to three hours. At low levels of blood sugar, the person became unconscious and sometimes had a seizure. Nurses revived the patient with sweetened orange juice or, if the person was still comatose, glucose through a feeding tube. The safety of the treatments depended on excellent nursing care.

Insulin therapy became widely practiced until the 1950s. Because insulin coma therapy was occasionally accompanied by a seizure, it was sometimes known as insulin shock therapy. Perhaps the effectiveness of the insulin treatments was due to the quality of the medical attention received by these patients.

Eventually, other ways of causing seizures, such as metrazol or electroconvulsive therapy (ECT), and new psychotropic medications replaced insulin treatment. For a few years, psychiatric institutions offered all three forms of "shock" therapy—metrazol, insulin, and ECT—and some patients were treated with a combination of the three.

Frances R. Frankenburg

LOBOTOMY

Lobotomy, or prefrontal leucotomy, is a type of neurosurgery in which the fibers connecting the frontal lobes, or prefrontal cortex, with other parts of the brain, are cut. Early animal experiments led to therapeutic experiments in agitated patients who became calmer after the procedure. For several decades, lobotomies were widely used in patients for whom no other treatment seemed helpful. Lobotomies are now a byword for cruelty and psychiatric incompetence.

Beginning in the 1800s, there were some indications that surgery on the brain, formerly thought to be dangerous, could be safe. For example, people who suffered brain injuries sometimes survived their wounds. In one famous case in 1848, Phineas Gage, a 25-year-old railroad foreman, was tamping black powder into a blast hole when the powder ignited and sent a three-foot-long metal rod straight through his head. He remained conscious, and a physician removed the rod from

Gage's skull and brain. Gage recovered but became withdrawn, short-tempered, and "childlike." In this natural experiment, or experiment of nature, it seemed that damage to his frontal lobes had led to changes in his personality and impulse control.

In 1888, the Swiss psychiatrist Gottlieb Burckhardt (1836–1907) initiated the first systematic attempt at modern human psychosurgery. He was the director of a small Swiss asylum, where some of his patients were desperately ill. Beginning in December 1888, he operated on six patients, removing sections of their cerebral cortex, hoping to modify their behavior. Two patients experienced no change, two became quieter, one experienced convulsions and died a few days after the operation, and one improved. The response from his medical peers was hostile, and he did no further operations. As far as we know, there were no similar operations for the next 40 years.

In the early 1900s, progress was being made in neurology and surgery. Researchers were intrigued by the fact that the frontal lobes occupied a larger part of the human brain than they did in the brains of other animals. Injuries suffered by soldiers in World War I and neurosurgeries performed to remove tumors or seizure foci showed that this part of the brain could withstand a surprising amount of surgery.

John Fulton (1899–1960), a leading American neurophysiologist, had created the first primate research laboratory in the United States. In 1933, he and psychologist Carlyle Jacobson, in one famous set of experiments, removed half of the frontal lobes of two chimpanzees and noted that one of them, Becky, became calmer. (The other chimpanzee, less often written about, Lucy, became more easily frustrated after the surgery.)

António Egas Moniz (1874–1955), a neurologist at the University of Lisbon, who was well known for his advances in cerebral angiography, saw Fulton present his work at a conference in 1935. Whether Fulton's chimpanzee work influenced Moniz's subsequent work has been debated, but in any event, Moniz decided to perform a similar (but not identical) operation on mentally ill people to "separate" their emotions from their thoughts while retaining their intelligence.

In Portugal, in 1935, Moniz and his colleague Almeida Lima drilled holes in the skull of a patient and injected the connecting fibers of the brain with alcohol to destroy them. Later, Moniz used a tool called a leucotome to remove cores of white matter, the connecting fibers of the brain, under general anesthesia. Moniz claimed that his patients became calmer after the surgery. This procedure was known as a prefrontal lobotomy and led to the field of psychosurgery.

A year later, neurologist Walter Freeman (1895–1972) and James Watts (1904–1994), a neurosurgeon and protégé of John Fulton, began to perform lobotomies in the United States. For the first few years, Fulton encouraged Freeman and Watts in their work. Their therapeutic experiments had some scientific backing from Fulton's animal experiments. In turn, it was easier for Fulton to obtain support for his animal research by pointing to the clinical work that it had inspired.

For over a decade, lobotomies were widely performed in the United States. They were thought to be most useful for those suffering from agitated depression and at first were carried out in private hospitals. They were also of some—although limited—use in the treatment of people with schizophrenia and were carried out on many patients in state hospitals and the newly established Veterans Administration hospitals. Many hospitals reported that previously out-of-control patients improved with lobotomies and that a few were able to go home and resume their previous lives.

In 1946, copying the work of Italian neurosurgeon Amarro Fiamberti, Freeman decided to approach the prefrontal cortex through the eye sockets instead of going through the top or side of the skull. He practiced on cadavers, and by using an ice pick and hammer, he entered the brain by breaking through the thin layer of bone above the eyeball. Freeman performed transorbital lobotomies on patients using a leucotome that resembled an ice pick. After going through the top of the eye socket under the eyelid and entering the brain, Freeman rotated the tool to cut through the brain fibers and then repeated this on the other side. The transorbital lobotomy took 10 minutes or less.

This procedure was done by first rendering the patient unconscious with electroconvulsive shock. No anesthetist was needed. Freeman also claimed that the procedure was so simple and safe that it could be done by nonsurgeons. As most mental hospitals did not have operating rooms or surgeons on staff, this new method made the procedure easier to arrange. Eventually, Freeman performed transorbital lobotomies as outpatient procedures in his office, in addition to doing them in mental hospitals and teaching other doctors how to do them. Freeman became a sort of evangelist and traveled around the country performing and promoting these procedures. Freeman did follow-up visits on his patients and convinced himself (and others at the time) that these procedures were, for the most part, helpful and safe.

Freeman described successful procedures on physicians (including psychiatrists), a violinist, and an engineer and claimed that all of these professionals were able to perform their challenging jobs after the procedure. Freeman repeated his travels around the country to see how his patients were doing. He maintained files with information about them, their jobs, and their friends and family members so that he could find them. He sent them Christmas cards to maintain contact. Much of his reporting about his patients was personal, though, and no independent assessments were carried out.

Watts and Fulton were uneasy about Freeman's transition to transorbital lobotomies. Watts refused to have anything to do with these procedures, and in 1947, Fulton wrote to Freeman: "What are these terrible things I hear about you doing lobotomies in your office with an icepick? . . . Why not use a shot gun? It would be quicker!"[1]

In the United States between 1936 and 1951, about 20,000 patients were lobotomized, with Freeman himself performing between 3,500 and 5,000 of the procedures. Freeman, and other doctors who performed lobotomies, believed that the procedures relieved suffering caused by schizophrenia, depression, and other problems. Descriptions of people suffering from agitated depression with psychotic symptoms, or severe and terrifying hallucinations and delusions who improved after the procedure, make it clear that lobotomies—in a sense therapeutic experiments as there was no clear proof of their usefulness—were not necessarily cruel or reckless.

Lobotomies have been harshly criticized. Some lobotomies may have been done too quickly or at the behest of family members upset by a relative's behavior, which may not necessarily have been due to a psychiatric illness. Many people suffered hemorrhages or seizures following the lobotomy. Others had a loss of spontaneity, self-control, and self-awareness after the procedure. Some people became easier to "manage" at home or in the hospital, but at the cost of loss of spontaneity and initiative.

In 1949, Egas Moniz was awarded the Nobel Prize in Physiology or Medicine for "his discovery of the therapeutic value of leucotomy in certain psychoses." With the discovery of chlorpromazine and other antipsychotic medications in the 1950s, lobotomies became less popular. Some specifically targeted forms of psychosurgery are still performed for severe pain, intractable depression, or obsessive compulsive disorder, but lobotomies in general are now regarded as an embarrassing episode in the history of psychiatry.

Frances R. Frankenburg

Reference

1.   Pressman, *Last Resort*, 342.

MALARIATHERAPY

The venereal illness syphilis has many manifestations, one of which, neurosyphilis, is associated with neurological problems and psychosis. In the early 20th century, Julius Wagner-Jauregg, a Viennese neuropsychiatrist, experimented with malaria as a treatment for neurosyphilis. Malariatherapy became an accepted if unproven treatment for the illness, and Wagner-Jauregg received a Nobel Prize in Physiology or Medicine in 1927 for this work. Wagner-Jauregg's work was used by later experimenters who were interested in malaria itself.

Syphilis, a venereal illness caused by the spirochete *Treponema pallidum*, has a primary, secondary, latent, and tertiary phase. The tertiary phase—known as neurosyphilis or general paresis (weakness) of the insane—can develop anywhere from 5 to 20 years after the initial infection. Complications in this final phase can include psychosis, dementia, pain, cardiovascular problems, and loss of control over a variety of bodily functions.

Syphilis became increasingly common in Europe and North America in the 19th century, and by the early 20th century, as many as 20 percent of patients in American and European asylums were there because of the psychosis and dementia caused by tertiary neurosyphilis.

Physicians since the time of Hippocrates (ca. 460–ca. 370 BCE) had noticed that fever seemed to lead to an improvement in some illnesses. Julius Wagner-Jauregg

(1857–1940), a Viennese neuropsychiatrist, along with other physicians, began to treat psychotic patients by inducing fever. Wagner-Jauregg initially used typhus vaccines and injections of tuberculin. (Tuberculin is a protein derived from tuberculosis cultures, thought (incorrectly) by German physician and microbiologist Robert Koch (1843–1910) to be an effective treatment for tuberculosis. It is now used in smaller doses to test for exposure to tuberculosis). Wagner-Jauregg saw that tuberculin induced fevers in patients and that the patients who responded the best—in terms of becoming less psychotic—were those who had both the most severe reaction to the tuberculin and the ones who were ill with neurosyphilis. However, the symptoms of neurosyphilis often returned, and he looked for a more effective treatment. Wagner-Jauregg had noticed that patients with neurosyphilis seemed to improve the most when they had an actual infection, not just a fever induced by a foreign substance. So, in 1917, Wagner-Jauregg began to experiment with malaria as a treatment for neurosyphilis because this infection is associated with episodic high fevers.

Malaria did not occur naturally in Austria, but an Austrian soldier had returned from the Balkans ill with benign tertian malaria caused by *Plasmodium vivax*. In 1917, Wagner-Jauregg took blood from this soldier and injected or rubbed it into the skin of syphilitic patients. The patients developed high fevers that lasted 5 or 6 hours and recurred every 48 hours. They went through this two-day cycle several times and then were given quinine to treat the malaria and neosalvarsan to treat the syphilis. (Neosalvarsan, the drug then used to treat syphilis, by itself was not very effective against neurosyphilis but used nonetheless.) He reported some success in six of the first nine patients he treated. In fact, three patients recovered completely, returned home, and were able to work.

By using *Plasmodium vivax* he caused a mild form of malaria that was easily treated with quinine. In the absence of anopheline mosquitoes—the usual vectors of malaria—Wagner-Jauregg needed to maintain his supply of the parasite. He would sometimes inject blood from a syphilitic patient who had been given malaria into another syphilitic patient so that the supply of malarial blood would be replenished. In one incident, however, he inadvertently used *Plasmodium falciparum*, a species of the parasite that causes a more severe form of the disease, and three patients died.

Malariatherapy was accepted quickly and with enthusiasm as an effective treatment for the hitherto difficult-to-treat neurosyphilis. Contemporary psychiatrists, patients, and their families were convinced of its value. Other methods of heating patients continued to be tried, such as hot baths, placement in heated cabinets, and so on, but none seemed as safe or as effective as malariatherapy.

This experiment brought hope to patients and doctors. Perhaps the complications and intricacies of this treatment had a therapeutic effect, or at least added to it. However, the injection of one individual's blood into another person was dangerous because it could transmit other illnesses or lead to a transfusion reaction. The injection of blood was therefore replaced by the use of infected mosquitoes. Colonies of anopheline mosquitoes were established so that malariatherapy could be used even in places without a natural supply of them.

Malaria was used to treat neurosyphilis throughout Europe and the United States until the early 1950s, when the use of penicillin, more effective than neosalvarsan in treating neurosyphilis, became widespread. Whether malariatherapy was effective is difficult to determine, in part because it was reserved for less seriously ill patients who were more likely to tolerate infection with malaria, and partly because neurosyphilis typically varies in severity over time. When malariatherapy was introduced, the concept of controlled clinical trials that might have addressed the question of effectiveness had not yet become a standard of experimental therapeutics. Moreover, the mechanisms by which malariatherapy might have been useful, if it indeed was, remain unclear. One theory is that *T. pallidum* is sensitive to heat. Other theories are that perhaps malaria increases the antigenic properties of *T. pallidum* or in some other way increases the body's immune response to it.

Wagner-Jauregg was a complicated man. Although he was not Jewish himself, his first wife was Jewish, and he had many Jewish friends. However, he was known for telling anti-Semitic jokes and became increasingly anti-Semitic as he developed sympathy for the growing Nazi movement in Austria. He was protective of his ill patients, yet also supported the idea of sterilizing them. He was nominated for the Nobel Prize for his work with neurosyphilis. But a member of the Nobel Prize committee could not agree that a physician who inoculated people with malaria deserved a Nobel Prize. After this person retired from the committee, the Nobel Prize in Physiology or Medicine was awarded to Wagner-Jauregg in 1927 for his work on malariatherapy.

Wagner-Jauregg's work fostered more research into malaria. In 1925, a mosquito colony, or insectary, was established in a large psychiatric hospital in Horton, England, and became the center of malariatherapy in the United Kingdom. The laboratory maintained seven separate strains of malaria in the blood of psychiatric patients because the *Plasmodium* parasite could not be kept alive in culture. A number of discoveries about malaria resulted from the experiences gained in the Horton laboratory.

During the World War II effort to conquer malaria, many experts continued Wagner-Jauregg's practice of giving malaria to neurosyphilis patients or, indeed, to any patients with serious psychiatric illnesses, as a way of maintaining the *Plasmodia* strains. In the United States, malariologists used psychiatric patients at the Florida State Hospital in Tallahassee, the South Carolina State Hospital in Columbia, Manhattan State Hospital in New York, and St. Elizabeth Hospital (sometimes known as St. Elizabeths or St. Elizabeth's Hospital) in Washington, D.C., for the same purpose. The effects on the patients are difficult to judge because so much of the work was secret. The secrecy was due both to some unease about using psychiatric patients as hosts for malaria and the importance of keeping medical advances from the enemy. While most of these patients would never have become ill from malaria without this work, it is possible that some patients with neurosyphilis did benefit. Other patients, who may not have had neurosyphilis or may not have benefited from malaria, did receive extra attention and care that the malaria research brought to these often underfunded and overcrowded hospitals.

G. Robert Coatney (1902–1990), a parasitologist, had been working at a National Institutes of Health (NIH) laboratory at the South Carolina State Hospital, where he learned about the use of malaria in treating neurosyphilis. During World War II, he moved to Washington, D.C., and developed the NIH's antimalarial clinical testing programs there at St. Elizabeth Hospital. Coatney and his colleagues experimented with new antimalarial drugs in patients undergoing malarial treatment for neurosyphilis. The patient was infected with malaria and then administered the new drugs after they had been febrile for a suitable time. One strain of *P. vivax* became known, after the supposed location of the patients in whom it was grown, as the St. Elizabeth strain. Recent work suggests, however, that the person with this strain of malaria had actually been a patient at the South Carolina State Hospital.

Frances R. Frankenburg

RHOADS, CORNELIUS

Cornelius Rhoads was a distinguished scientist who made significant advances in hematology. His career was almost derailed by a letter he wrote about killing Puerto Ricans and experimenting with transplantation of cancer cells.

Cornelius Packard "Dusty" Rhoads (1898–1959) was born in Massachusetts and obtained his medical degree from Harvard Medical School in 1924. In 1931, Rhoads went to Puerto Rico to investigate hookworm and tropical sprue with hematologist William Castle (1897–1990), both working for the Rockefeller Foundation. That same year, a lab technician found a letter on his desk in which Rhoads described Puerto Ricans as "the dirtiest, laziest, most degenerate and thievish race of men ever to inhabit this sphere. . . . What the Island needs is not public health work but a tidal wave or something to totally exterminate the population. . . . I have done my best to further the process of extermination by killing off eight and transplanting cancer in several more."[1]

The letter was publicized and caused an uproar. Rhoads said that this letter was intended as a "parody," and others have seen it as typical medical gallows humor. He wrote a letter of apology. Several investigations, including one headed by Puerto Rican attorney general Ramon Quinones and one performed by the Rockefeller Foundation, cleared him of any misdoings, but Rhoads, who had already left Puerto Rico, never returned.

He went on to serve as the chief of the medical department of the American army's chemical warfare division during World War II. A wartime incident involving chemical warfare led, unexpectedly, to medical discoveries in the fight against cancer, in which Rhoads took part.

On December 3, 1943, German bombers hit American ships in the harbor of Bari in Italy. One ship, the *John Harvey*, exploded; it contained munitions and airplane bombs with mustard gas, and many people died. Autopsies showed that the victims had depletion of their bone marrow due to the mustard gas exposure. Such a finding was not entirely new: mustard gas had been used in World War I and was known to cause resulting bone marrow depression. The *John Harvey* incident was kept secret at the time, as the Allies did not want their readiness to use mustard gas known. While looking for antidotes for mustard gas, Alfred Goodman and Louis Gilman, two Yale pharmacologists, realized that the bone marrow toxicity of mustard gas or its derivatives could be of use in the treatment of bone marrow cancers. Rhoads played a major role in the development of nitrogen mustards as chemotherapeutic agents.

After the war, Rhoads became director of Memorial Hospital in New York and directed research into the use of mustard gas derivatives and other molecules in the treatment of malignancies. He was awarded many honors for his research.

Despite Rhoads's accolades and accomplishments, the letter he wrote in Puerto Rico cast a lasting shadow on his career. Many in Puerto Rico never accepted Rhoads's explanation or apology and considered the investigation to have been a whitewash. To this day, they continue to see his letter as racist and as evidence of his true beliefs and actions. In 1979, an anonymous donor established the Cornelius P. Rhoads Memorial Award to be presented by the American Association of Cancer Research to a young investigator each year. In 2003, Rhoads's name was removed from the award after protests about his earlier letter.

Frances R. Frankenburg

Reference

1.   Starr, "Ethics," 573.

ROCKEFELLER, JOHN D.

The enormously wealthy cofounder of Standard Oil, John D. Rockefeller Sr., was also a philanthropist who established a number of institutes and foundations that supported human experimentation—not always without controversy.

John D. Rockefeller Sr. (1839–1937), cofounder of Standard Oil, was reported to be the richest man in the world during his lifetime. He began giving money to charities as a teenager, and his donations increased in size as his wealth grew. As a young man, he was a major donor to Baptist causes. Later, the focus of Rockefeller's charitable giving changed as a result of a suggestion from his adviser, Frederick Taylor Gates (1853–1929). Gates had read *Principles and Practices of Medicine*, the authoritative book on medicine written in 1891 by William Osler (1849–1919), the great clinician. He described it as the most interesting book he had ever read, but he noted the absence of cures and realized how little was known about medicine. Gates wrote a memorandum to Rockefeller in which he mentioned the absence of any American researchers who could compare to chemist and microbiologist Louis Pasteur (1822–1895) or bacteriologist Robert Koch (1843–1910) in Europe. At the time, Rockefeller did not particularly believe in scientific medicine, trusting in homeopathy instead. However, Gates was persuasive and convinced Rockefeller to set up an institution for medical research that would have benefits for others and also for Rockefeller himself. The institution would improve his image, stained by the exposures of his unethical business practices by the muckraker Ida Tarbell (1857–1944), and it would deal with the problem of leaving too much money to his heirs. It might also lead to tax relief.

In 1901, Rockefeller founded the Rockefeller Institute for Medical Research, the first American institution whose sole purpose was experimental medicine. (The institute became the Rockefeller University in 1965.) Then, in 1909, he created the Rockefeller Sanitary Commission to eradicate hookworm in the South. In 1913, he established the Rockefeller Foundation that continued the work of the commission (which ended in 1914). The foundation went on to endow many medical research institutions and educational centers around the world, including the London School of Hygiene and Tropical Medicine, the Johns Hopkins and Harvard Schools of Public Health, and the School of Hygiene at the University of Toronto.

Unfortunately, the foundation has also been associated with some research abuses. In 1929, it funded German eugenics programs and supported the establishment of the Kaiser Wilhelm Institute of Anthropology, Human Heredity, and Eugenics in Berlin. This institute included the laboratory of Otmar Freiherr von Verschuer, where Josef Mengele (1911–1979), the notorious Nazi physician, had worked as a researcher before he began his inhumane experimentation at Auschwitz. The foundation also supported the Vanderbilt radioiron studies, in which radioisotopes were administered to schoolboys and pregnant women, which have been criticized for their lack of consent.

In the 21st century, the Rockefeller Foundation continues to be a major granting agency that funds projects that aim at improving the well-being of people worldwide.

Frances R. Frankenburg

SAN QUENTIN STATE PRISON EXPERIMENTS

Between 1918 and 1927, prisoners at San Quentin State Prison in California were subjected to many experiments, including testicular implants and vasectomies, by the chief surgeon, Leo Stanley, who was looking for a way to stop the aging process.

The desire to stop or reverse the aging process is a perennial one. During the 19th and 20th centuries, some physicians had the idea that male aging could be slowed by injecting men with testicular tissue from animals or other humans. One such doctor was Charles-Édouard Brown-Séquard (1817–1894), a distinguished physiologist and neurologist from Mauritius, who made many important contributions to endocrinology. At the age of 70, dismayed by the evidence of his own aging, he injected pulverized dog or guinea pig testes into himself over a period of about three weeks and claimed that it increased his physical and mental powers.

Later, French surgeon Serge Abrahamovitch Voronoff (1866–1951) would do somewhat similar experiments on himself and others. Voronoff, who had studied with Alexis Carrel (1873–1944), a Nobel Prize–winning surgeon and physiologist, grafted monkey testicular tissue onto human testicles in the 1920s and 1930s. He also followed the example of Brown-Séquard by injecting himself with ground-up dog and guinea pig testicles, and he experimented with transplanting chimpanzee and baboon testicular tissue into a human's scrotum. He believed that his grafting surgery could rejuvenate people, and his "monkey gland" grafts became popular among the wealthy in the 1920s.

Leo Stanley (1886–1976) was chief surgeon at the San Quentin Prison between 1913 and 1951 (except for the period of World War II when he was a medical officer in the U.S. Navy). He was innovative, for example, in being the first West Coast physician to use spinal anesthesia. He also performed plastic surgery on some inmates, hoping that they would have better lives if they had an improved physical appearance. The San Quentin convicts, in some ways, received better medical care than convicts in other prisons.

Stanley was also interested in reproductive issues, and he carried over this interest to his work at the prison. Eugenics, the effort to prevent, control, or eliminate disease thought to be due to genes, was a respectable idea in the United States in the 1920s, particularly in California. Sterilizations of men and women commonly took place in mental hospitals and prisons. Stanley supported the idea of eugenics and argued that "sterilization . . . will do much to stamp out crime." It was no surprise then that he encouraged many of the inmates to have vasectomies and told those who volunteered that he would speak on their behalf at parole board hearings.

At the same time, he believed that transplanting testicles from younger men into older men could rejuvenate them. To test this theory, he removed the testicles of about 30 executed prisoners and implanted them into older prisoners. He published reports of this work in the *Journal of the American Medical Association*. (He also tried to implant the testicles of animals into prisoners, but without success.)

Further confusing the situation, some researchers believed that vasectomy increased the blood supply to the testicles. Irish poet William Butler Yeats and Sigmund Freud were both vasectomized hoping that they would become more vigorous as a result of the surgery. Stanley himself was vasectomized. Stanley also wondered if exhibitionism and child abuse, sometimes associated with dementia, could be due to the loss of male hormones. The thinking was that old men, rejuvenated by testicular implants or vasectomies, might behave better.

Voronoff has been ridiculed by the scientific community, but at least in terms of ethics, his experiments were on wealthy men who chose the surgery. Similarly, Brown-Séquard experimented on himself, thus freely choosing the injections. Stanley's work, on the other hand, was much more troubling: he felt free to experiment on a vulnerable population, and, as far as we know, never obtained informed consent, had a control group, or conducted follow-ups.

Frances R. Frankenburg

SEIZURE THERAPY

In 1934, Ladislas Meduna induced seizures in a young man who had refused to eat for four years. Four years later, Ugo Cerletti and Lucio Bini sent an electric current through a subject's head. In both cases, the patient improved, and the use of seizures—particularly in the form of electroconvulsive therapy—became widely accepted as medical treatment. These were some of the most successful experiments in the history of psychiatry.

Until the early to mid-1900s there were no effective treatments for severe psychiatric illnesses. The first successful treatments were induced seizures. Seizures are caused by an episode of unusually excessive and coordinated electrical activity in the brain, leading to an alteration of consciousness or convulsions.

Ladislas Meduna (1896–1964) was a Hungarian neurologist and neuropathologist who believed that there was an antagonism of sorts between epilepsy, an illness marked by recurrent seizures, and schizophrenia, and that these two illnesses could not coexist. In 1934, he tested this belief by inducing seizures in a 33-year-old man who had been catatonic for 4 years, during which time he needed to be tube-fed. (Catatonia is a psychiatric syndrome marked by peculiar activities and often a refusal to eat.) Meduna injected the patient with camphor, and after 45 minutes, the patient had a seizure lasting 60 seconds. After the seizure ended, the patient showed no change in symptoms. Meduna repeated the injection a few more times, and the patient recovered from his psychiatric illness. He was able to return home and resume work.

Meduna also induced seizures using metrazol. His techniques were adopted by others but never became popular because the injections were painful and the wait between the injection and seizure was terrifying and unpredictable. Nonetheless, some patients improved; their psychiatric symptoms lessened or disappeared entirely. This was the beginning of convulsive therapy for psychosis and catatonia.

Two Italian psychiatrists, Ugo Cerletti (1877–1963) and Lucio Bini (1908–1964), took the next step. Cerletti had studied with the leading psychiatrists and neurologists of the day: Alois Alzheimer, Emil Kraepelin, Pierre Marie, and Franz Nissl. He was familiar with psychiatrist Manfred Sakel's (1900–1957) insulin coma therapy (sometimes used for psychosis) and Meduna's metrazol shock therapy. Bini had a particular talent and interest in machinery and the induction of seizures. Both psychiatrists were interested in the effects of seizures, and together they began to induce seizures in dogs by using electric currents from mouth to rectum. Not surprisingly, the mortality rate was quite high, as it was already well-known that electric shocks could be lethal. (Since the 1880s, electrocution had sometimes been used to execute criminals.) However, when the two researchers applied the current through the dog's head alone, the dog did not die. Cerletti and Bini realized that electric currents were relatively safe when applied only to the head. (Electric shocks become lethal when they pass through the chest and cause cardiac arrhythmias.) Still, the idea of deliberately passing electric currents through humans remained terrifying.

To further investigate the effects of electrically induced seizures, Cerletti went to an abattoir, where electric shocks were used in the slaughter of pigs. He saw that the electric shocks administered to pigs' heads did not actually kill them. Instead, the shock immediately rendered the pig unconsciousness, which made it easier for the butcher to then cut the pig's throat. Cerletti and Bini practiced applying electric currents across the heads of pigs. They adjusted the strength and duration of the current until they could assure themselves of its safety. They became convinced that if they could pass an electric shock across a human's head, they could safely produce a seizure that could be as therapeutic as the seizures produced by insulin or metrazol, but easier to induce.

Cerletti and Bini needed a subject on whom to try their new procedure. In 1938, the police found an incoherent and seemingly homeless person wandering around the Rome train station. The police took this man to the hospital where Cerletti and Bini worked, and the researchers decided to use him as a subject. Some of their colleagues gathered to witness the procedure. There are several accounts of what happened next. According to Cerletti, he and Bini administered a 70-volt electric shock for two-tenths of a second across the subject's head. He began to sing. Then he sat up and said, "Not a second. Deadly." All of the observers were nervous, and some disapproved.

Cerletti quickly administered another shock, this time with 110 volts for half a second. The patient had a grand mal seizure, recovered, and then spoke lucidly. The researchers administered more shocks over the next few days, and the patient made a full recovery. It also turned out that he was not homeless. He was a farmer in the countryside near Milan and had been treated successfully with metrazol the year before in Milan. He had recently traveled from Milan to Rome. This was the beginning of electroconvulsive therapy (ECT).

The experiment also illustrated that both ways of inducing seizures (chemical and electrical) were effective, but not long-lasting. Indeed, the patient from Milan became ill again two years later. Whether insulin shock therapy worked as well as electricity, metrazol, or camphor was never quite clear.

Over time, the procedure for ECT has been modified. Now the patient receives short-acting anesthesia and is unaware either of the passage of a brief electric current through his or her head or the subsequent seizure. Muscle-paralyzing agents are used to prevent any physical response or convulsion. ECT is the safest and quickest treatment for severe depression and catatonia, although it does cause some memory loss, which is usually temporary. The mechanism by which it works is still not known. Meduna's theory that epilepsy and schizophrenia do not coexist has since been shown to be incorrect.

Frances R. Frankenburg

STRONG, RICHARD PEARSON

Americans became drawn into beriberi research in the early 20th century because of their colonization of the Philippines. In what was one of the first human medical experiments to involve written signed consent, physician Richard Pearson Strong organized a nutritional trial involving prisoners in the Bilibid Prison in Manila. This relatively advanced approach to consent came as a consequence of a terrible and fatal accident in which prisoners were accidentally exposed to bubonic plague as part of a cholera vaccine test.

Richard Pearson Strong (1872–1948), an American physician, graduated from the first medical class at Johns Hopkins in 1897, a class imbued with the importance of experimental work. To further his education, he went to Germany to study at the Berlin Institute for Infectious Diseases. He became director of the biological laboratory of the Philippine Bureau of Science and inoculated many subjects, including himself, with experimental vaccines. Because Manila experienced cholera epidemics, he was interested in vaccines against that illness.

In 1906, he was responsible for a medical experiment on prisoners that went horribly wrong. Strong inoculated 24 prisoners at the large Bilibid Prison with what he thought was cholera vaccine—not to protect the prisoners from cholera, but to assess the side effects associated with this particular vaccine. No one explained to the Filipino prisoners the purpose of the experiment or asked their permission. Somehow, this cholera vaccine had been contaminated by active bubonic plague. All of the subjects became ill, and 13 of the 24 prisoners died from bubonic plague. The resulting investigation was unable to determine how exactly the error had had happened. The investigators did not find Strong criminally negligent but did raise questions about his use of prisoners. They noted how difficult it would have been for prisoners to refuse to cooperate. No official action was taken against Strong.

Strong continued his work with Bilibid prisoners but never worked with cholera vaccine or bubonic plague again. Instead, he performed nutritional experiments with the prisoners to see whether he could advance the field of beriberi research. Beriberi is a complex illness that had existed for centuries in Southeast Asia among people whose diet was mainly rice. It results—as we now know—from lack of thiamine and has two forms: In "wet" beriberi, the person suffers from heart problems and swelling of the legs. In "dry" beriberi, the legs become painful and weak, and walking is difficult. If the person is alcoholic or has lost weight quickly, dry beriberi can sometimes also be accompanied by confusion and memory loss.

Beriberi became more common with the advent of mechanized grain milling around 1870, which stripped the whole-grain rice of essential nutrients, including thiamine. A number of earlier researchers had determined that beriberi was not an infectious disease and had correctly connected it to diet. To confirm this theory, Strong decided to compare the effects of feeding prisoners a diet of white rice with or without rice polishings. (Rice polishings are the outer layers of rice that are rubbed off during the milling of rice; they contain many nutrients, including thiamine.)

In 1912, 29 Bilibid prisoners, all sentenced to death, agreed to participate in his new study. The prisoners who participated in this trial signed documents, written in their own dialects, that explained the experiment and its voluntary nature. In return for their participation, they were offered cigarettes and cigars. For about three months, some men were fed mostly polished white rice. The other men were fed polished white rice with the addition of rice polishings. One man in the polished white rice group died. His autopsy showed acute beriberi. Eight other men in that same group developed beriberi, but no one who was fed polished rice with rice polishings added became ill.

This was an important study in the history of human experimentation for two reasons. First, the prisoners gave written consent. (The problem of prisoners being able to give fully voluntary consent remained unaddressed however.) Strong's care in documenting their consent was probably due to the previous disastrous cholera vaccine study. Second, the study showed once again that beriberi was related to nutrition rather than to bacteria.

In 1917, Strong returned to the United States and became professor of tropical medicine at Harvard University.

Frances R. Frankenburg

STUDIES OF RICKETS AND SCURVY

Nutritional studies are difficult to do because they usually need to be carried out over long periods of time. As well, experimental diets are often monotonous or unpalatable. In the early 1900s, one solution to these problems was to study institutionalized infants on strictly controlled diets, who, because of their rapid growth and small body mass, can develop deficiency disorders quickly. Supervision of the diets of infants is also much easier than it is for adults. Experimentation on institutionalized infants by Harriette Chick and Alfred Hess was helpful in elucidating the causes of two vitamin-deficiency illnesses: rickets (from lack of vitamin D) and scurvy (from lack of vitamin C).

Harriette Chick (1875–1977) was an English scientist who, early in her career, was involved in experiments with plague transmission. As a young woman, she experimented on herself by letting a particular species of flea bite her to show that this species could indeed bite humans and thus transmit bubonic plague. In later laboratory work on proteins, she studied the method of action of disinfectants, showing the irreversibility of the coagulation of proteins. Her interests then turned to nutrition, and in 1922, she led a team from London's Lister Institute of Preventive Medicine to post–World War I Vienna to address the problems of childhood malnutrition, one of which was rickets. Rickets is caused by a deficiency of vitamin D, a strange vitamin that can be obtained by eating foods rich in vitamin D or by being exposed to sunshine. The bones of children with rickets do not form well, and, as a result, children with rickets have skeletal abnormalities and are usually quite short. Some researchers believed that this illness was due to poor hygiene, others that it was a nutritional deficiency. Exposure to sunlight seemed to prevent it.

Chick worked with Viennese pediatricians at the University Kinderklinik, a hospital with about 100 infants. She and colleagues established research units housing about 60 of those infants. Some developed rickets despite good hygiene and general care. Chick's team experimented with various treatment methods: some of the ill children were placed in the sun, some were exposed to a mercury vapor quartz light, and some had their diets supplemented with cod liver oil. Each of these treatments was effective in treating rickets. Chick did not generate the hypotheses that she tested, but she was the first to test them in a methodical and well-controlled manner in large numbers of infants and to show that the curative effects of light and cod liver oil (later shown to contain vitamin D) were the same.

Alfred Hess (1875–1933) was an American pediatrician also interested in, among many other topics, nutritional-deficiency diseases in children. Some of his work was done on orphans at the New York Home for Hebrew Infants and involved the investigation of scurvy, a disease caused by vitamin C deficiency. The symptoms of scurvy include lethargy, gum disease, muscle aches, poor wound healing, and easy bleeding. In a series of studies, he and his colleagues studied infants after orange juice had been withheld from their diet. The orange juice had been eliminated because it was thought that if milk was pasteurized at a lower degree (to 145°F instead of the previous 160°F), milk would retain its vitamin C content, and the children wouldn't need the addition of juice. However, this was not so, and some children given moderately pasteurized milk and no orange juice developed scurvy.

Hess and his colleagues were particularly interested in the petechiae—small bleeding spots—that occur with scurvy. Thinking that the problem might be the coagulability of their blood, Hess needed to test samples of the infants' blood. To get sufficient quantities, he took blood from the jugular vein (the prominent vein at the side of the neck) of the infants. Later, assuming (correctly) that the problem could be due to capillary (or small blood vessel) wall weakness, Hess and his colleagues tested capillary wall strength by using an inflated blood pressure cuff to stop the return of venous blood, leading to petechiae as blood seeped through the capillaries. Hess was criticized for using orphans for these studies, but he was exonerated by his peers.

As far as can be seen, no infants were seriously harmed by these experiments, and infants in control groups who did develop scurvy or rickets were always eventually treated. The work of Chick and Hess clarified the nature of these illnesses. Nonetheless, the idea of studying disadvantaged young children is disconcerting. The researchers did not mention consent in their papers.

Frances R. Frankenburg

TUSKEGEE STUDY OF UNTREATED SYPHILIS

One of the most controversial studies in the history of American medicine is the Tuskegee Study of Untreated Syphilis (TSUS), which lasted from 1932 to 1972. In this study, 400 black Americans with syphilis were followed for up to four decades without being told that they had the illness and with little treatment being provided. Effective treatment was blocked. In this observational study, inadequate treatment was the experiment.

Syphilis is a sexually transmitted illness caused by the bacterium *Treponema pallidum*. It has several phases: in the primary stage, a chancre (a type of skin ulcer) appears; in the secondary stage, there is a rash on the palms and soles. Latent syphilis has no symptoms, but in almost a third of those with latent syphilis, tertiary syphilis, which damages the heart and nervous system, can develop.

The origins of the Tuskegee Study of Untreated Syphilis (TSUS) were benign. Sears president Julius Rosenwald established the Julius Rosenwald Fund (also known as the Julius Rosenwald Foundation) for the "well being of mankind," in 1917. The fund supported many causes, including those to do with the health of black Americans. In 1929, the fund, along with the United States Public Health Service (PHS), was studying the prevalence of syphilis in six counties in the American South. The study was a demonstration project with the ultimate aim of showing that treatment could be provided to these patients.

Shortly thereafter, because of the Great Depression, the fund was no longer able to support the study. In 1932, the PHS decided to continue it on its own but changed the focus to study untreated syphilis for a brief period. Macon County, Alabama, was chosen as the site for the study because of the prevalence of syphilis in the area. Most of the inhabitants were cotton-growing sharecroppers who were black and poor. The study was named after the Tuskegee Institute, a prestigious medical institution founded by Booker T. Washington and located in the Alabama town of the same name.

One of the goals of the TSUS was to compare untreated syphilis in black Americans and Norwegians. In a comparable long-term study in Oslo, 2,000 Norwegian men and women with untreated syphilis were followed from 1890 until 1910. The Tuskegee study wanted to test the theory that syphilis had a different course in black people than it did in white people and that complications in black people were more likely to be cardiovascular than neurological. Another goal, which was not widely known, was to collect blood from the subjects to allow for the evaluation and standardization of diagnostic blood tests for syphilis. The key difference between the TSUS and the Oslo study, however, was that the Norwegians with syphilis did not receive treatment because their physicians correctly understood that the various treatments then available were ineffective, whereas by the time of the TSUS, treatment, although difficult to administer and tolerate, was available but intentionally withheld.

In 1910, Paul Ehrlich (1854–1915), a physician and scientist who worked in the fields of hematology, immunology, and chemotherapy, developed an arsenic-based medication, the first synthetic chemotherapeutic agent, called arsphenamine (salvarsan), also known as the "magic bullet," which was effective against syphilis. Two years later, he developed a slightly less toxic form of the drug, neoarsphenamine (neosalvarsan). Once these arsenical drugs were available, Norwegians with syphilis (including those participants in the study) were treated with them, and the Oslo study ended.

The Tuskegee study recruited 399 black men between the ages of 25 and 60 who had latent syphilis and 201 men without the illness to serve as the control group. The diagnosis was made by the Wassermann test, a blood test that detects the presence of antibodies to *Treponema*. According to some accounts, men with acute syphilis or syphilis for fewer than five years were not included. A few men with newly diagnosed syphilis were later added to the study.

The men were not told that they would be part of a study, nor that they had syphilis. Rather, they were told that they had "bad blood" and that they would be getting treatment for it. PHS doctors performed physical exams every few years and in some cases lumbar punctures. In a lumbar puncture, the physician inserts a needle between two lumbar vertebrae (the bones in the part of the backbone between the ribs and pelvis) to remove a sample of cerebrospinal fluid, the fluid that surrounds the spinal cord and brain. It is a safe and relatively minor procedure, but it is unpleasant and can result in a headache lasting a few hours or days. Physicians did provide some treatment for the men with syphilis at the beginning of the study, but it consisted of inadequate courses of mercurial ointment and neoarsphenamine, mostly as an enticement to convince the men to participate and also, perhaps, to prevent infection of their partners. Later, they were treated with "spring tonics" or aspirin. The 201 controls were also told that they were ill and given aspirin.

The study continued as the doctors realized the opportunity they had to study "untreated" syphilis over a number of years. The word "untreated" is inaccurate, as the men were provided with some, albeit inadequate, treatment, but it was used in the description of the study in publications arising from TSUS. The PHS physicians also realized that they might make their most interesting findings by examining their "untreated" subjects at autopsy. The subjects were thus promised $50 to help with funeral expenses on condition that an autopsy was performed.

In 1943, a little more than 10 years after the TSUS began, penicillin became available to treat syphilis. It was more effective, easier to administer, and less toxic than salvarsan or neosalvarsan. It was not, however, provided to the men in the study. Some subjects did get penicillin from physicians not connected with the TSUS, but many did not.

One of the key people who worked with the study for 40 years was a black nurse, Eunice Rivers Laurie (1899–1986), who had trained at the John Andrews hospital at the Tuskegee Institute. She was respected by both the subjects and staff and was the first author on one of the medical journal articles connected with the TSUS. She was perhaps the only person who was involved in the study from beginning to end. She knew the subjects well and spent much time with them; for example, she drove them to their hospital appointments and demanded that the PHS physicians respect the subjects. She thought that the men benefited from the study in that they received medical attention that they would not otherwise have received.

The true nature of the study was known in the local medical community. Physicians in Macon County (among them some black physicians), the Alabama Health Department, the Tuskegee Institute, local hospitals, and the Veterans Administration hospital in the area supported the study. The physicians were asked not to treat the syphilis of the TSUS subjects and they agreed. At the beginning of American involvement in World War II, the army drafted some of the younger men in the study. Per army protocol, these men should have been tested for syphilis and treated. However, the study personnel intervened, sending a list of 256 subjects to the draft board, and asked the board that should these men be drafted that they not be treated with penicillin; the board cooperated. How many of these subjects were still drafted is not clear.

The study was no secret in the medical community at large either. Thirteen reports about it, most describing the subjects as "untreated," were published between 1936 and 1973. Indeed, the American Medical Association and the National Medical Association (an association of black physicians) supported the TSUS.

In 1969, an ad hoc committee of the National Communicable Disease Center—now known as the Centers for Disease Control and Prevention (CDC)—reviewed the study in a three-hour meeting. The reviewers were impressed by the TSUS's length and uniqueness, and they discussed the possibility of treating the subjects. Several members said that treatment should be provided to those with active disease, while other members said it would not be helpful, presumably because of the length of the time that the subjects had been ill. The question of treatment was not further pursued, nor was the deceptive nature of the study discussed. The committee did agree, however, that such a study could never be done again. A reasonable step, at this juncture, would have been to tell each subject the nature of his disease and to arrange consultation and treatment if indicated. But no one suggested this, and the committee allowed the study to continue.

Peter Buxtun (sometimes spelled Buxton), a venereal disease investigator for the PHS, found out about the study while working at the PHS and protested. His protests were ignored for seven years. He finally told Jean Heller, a journalist, and the story she wrote about it appeared on the front page of the *New York Times* on July 26, 1972. Medical professionals saw nothing wrong with the study, but the public did. Responding to the negative publicity, the Department of Health and Welfare formed a nine-member panel that ended the study in 1972.

From a scientific point of view, the study was poorly designed. Indeed, there was never even a written protocol. The division of the subjects into two groups—the infected and the controls—was not clear, because if people from the control group became infected with syphilis, they were simply moved into the infected group. There is doubt as to the correctness of the diagnosis in some cases. It's also thought that some of the control subjects who became infected were treated, at least after 1939, although this is difficult to determine with certainty. As noted, many of the people in the infected group were treated to some extent, so they were really not "untreated," just partially treated.

What was the effect of not providing those with syphilis with a full course of treatment? That is impossible to determine because so many did receive treatment of some sort. By 1946, 25 percent of those with syphilis had died, but only 14 percent of the controls had died. In papers written about the TSUS, the increased mortality and morbidity in the "untreated" group were openly acknowledged. Another possible effect is that the patients might have infected their partners and caused babies to be born with congenital syphilis.

There was little justification for not treating people with syphilis with a full course of treatment in 1932. By this point, arsphenamine, or neoarsphenamine, had been available for approximately two decades, and medical opinion—although not unanimous—supported their use for either acute or latent syphilis in conjunction with a heavy metal, such as bismuth or mercury. The arsenical compounds and heavy metals were toxic and difficult to administer. Not all patients finished the course of treatment because it was so unpleasant. Some have argued that this treatment was so difficult and Macon County was so poor that many subjects would not have received or complied with it anyway. However, the fact that the study personnel made efforts to stop their subjects from getting treatment suggests that many physicians of the time would indeed have treated the men and that they would have cooperated with the treatment. The Oslo study had ended with the availability of arsenical drugs, suggesting that Norwegian physicians believed that these agents worked.

Any possibility that treatment was too difficult disappeared when penicillin became available at midcentury. Apologists for the study have argued that penicillin at that time was not available in great supply, and there was some uncertainty about its value in treating latent syphilis. But the TSUS requested that army boards not treat their subjects with penicillin, suggesting that they thought that penicillin was available and possibly helpful.

If the PHS genuinely believed—as the apologists for the study claim—that treatment for syphilis, especially latent syphilis, was not effective, then they could have followed the subjects with syphilis, treated or not, and compared them to men without syphilis and informed all subjects of the nature of the study. It seems clear that the PHS doctors did distinguish between treated and untreated syphilis—that was the important point of the study—because treatment worked. Otherwise there would have been no interest in an observational study of the untreated.

It bears repeating that the men were never informed that they were in a study or that they had syphilis, and they were told that they were getting treatment. The physicians deceived the subjects about treatment in a number of ways. For example, they wanted to perform lumbar punctures on the subjects. The physicians sent a letter to the subjects requesting them to agree to a "special examination." They did not say that they were asking permission to do a lumbar puncture; instead, they used the phrases "special examination" and "free treatment" interchangeably, as though the lumbar puncture was itself a free treatment. The low-dose treatments received at the beginning of the study were designed to get the cooperation of the subjects, not to truly treat their syphilis in any effective way. In other words, the basis for this study was deception and withholding of treatment that the researchers knew the subjects wanted and that could have been helpful.

The TSUS has now become a byword for racism and has exacerbated the distrust felt by many blacks toward white doctors and toward the idea of medical research or experimentation. The involvement of black health care professionals and the Tuskegee Institute is another tragic and complicated part of this experiment.

As a reaction to the TSUS, in 1974, the United States Congress passed the National Research Act, mandating the establishment of institutional review boards whenever facilities received federal grants. The act also established the National Commission for the Protection of Human Subjects of Biomedical and Behavioral Research. In 1979, this commission produced the Belmont Report, emphasizing that the foundations for ethical human experimentations are the *respect for persons*—requiring informed consent, the respect of privacy, and sensitivity to the existence of some vulnerable populations; *beneficence*—not harming the subject; and *justice*—ensuring the equitable sharing of burdens and benefits of research. The Tuskegee study had not honored any of these principles.

One of the many lessons of the TSUS is that perspectives on medical experimentation evolve. Enthusiasts carrying out a study to answer a question they and their colleagues found interesting were unable to appreciate how wrong the study would seem to later generations. The lack of education and poverty of the Tuskegee men made them vulnerable. But at the time of the study, they seemed like an ideal research population—captive by nature of these very characteristics. Their lack of mobility and trust in Nurse Rivers (as she was known to the subjects) and "government people" made a deceptive longitudinal study relatively easy to organize and to continue.

Litigation was inevitable. Lawyers suing on behalf of the subjects faced many legal difficulties, such as how to sue the government for misbehavior with respect to medical experimentation, the statute of limitations, and sorting out liabilities between state and federal agencies. The legal action was settled in 1974, with money being paid out to the survivors and medical care being provided for the survivors and their families.

Frances R. Frankenburg

YELLOW FEVER COMMISSION

In the wake of the Spanish-American War, physician Walter Reed headed a commission investigating yellow fever. Reed and his colleagues proved that the mosquito transmitted the illness, and this knowledge made prevention easier. During this work, Reed used written consent forms, perhaps for the first time.

Yellow fever is an acute hemorrhagic illness caused by the yellow fever virus, which is transmitted from one ill human to another by a bite of a mosquito, *Aedes aegypti*. In some cases of the illness, the liver is affected so badly that the person becomes jaundiced (hence the name yellow fever). There can also be such severe bleeding in the gastrointestinal tract that the infected person vomits blood. Because the vomitus appears black, the disease was then known to the Spanish-speaking world as *vómito negro*, or black vomit. The mortality rate ranges from 3 percent to 50 percent.

The disease is predominantly a tropical or warm weather illness and is now found mostly in jungles in South America and Africa. In the past, epidemics occurred in the United States, usually in coastal areas in the South, but yellow fever did reach inland to cause the Mississippi, or Memphis, epidemic of 1878 and as far north as Philadelphia, Portsmouth, and Halifax. Yellow fever also devastated Napoleon's troops fighting in Haiti from 1791 to 1804. France sold Louisiana to the United States in 1803 partly because it was unwilling to lose more troops to this American disease. Malaria and yellow fever contributed to the French failure to build the Panama Canal in the 1880s.

After the Spanish-American War of 1898, the United States temporarily controlled Cuba. The island was beset by infectious diseases, and during the brief war, the U.S. Army lost more men to malaria, typhoid, and yellow fever than it did to actual combat. The army was anxious to stop losing men to these illnesses during the postwar occupation and also to prevent yellow fever from spreading north from Cuba.

George Miller Sternberg (1838–1915), a bacteriologist and the U.S. Army surgeon general between 1893 and 1902, and Leonard Wood (1860–1927), a physician and military governor of Cuba between 1899 and 1902, believed that the removal of garbage and sewage from the streets of Havana would control yellow fever. Similar measures had been successful in eliminating typhoid fever. Havana streets were cleaned, but yellow fever did not disappear. So Sternberg appointed Walter Reed (1851–1902) as head of a commission to investigate it.

Walter Reed was a graduate of the University of Virginia School of Medicine and the Bellevue Hospital Medical College and had joined the United States Army Medical Corps in 1875. He had been assigned to positions in Arizona, Nebraska, and Alabama. When he was assigned to Fort McHenry in Baltimore, he took the opportunity to work with William Welch (1850–1934), a pathologist at Johns Hopkins, and studied typhoid fever, the hog cholera bacillus, smallpox, and malaria. In 1898, Reed was appointed as head of the War Department's Typhoid Board, with the job of studying the disease and making recommendations for controlling it. It was this work that drew Sternberg's attention, and Reed led the United States Army Yellow Fever Commission of 1900 to 1901, the fourth such commission. Reed's colleagues were three other U.S. Army physicians with experience in bacteriology: James Carroll, an English-born Canadian (1854–1907); Aristides Agramonte, a Cuban (1868–1931); and Jesse Lazear, an American (1866–1900).

Beginning in the 1800s, researchers had suggested that mosquitoes were involved in the transmission of yellow fever. The role of mosquitoes in transmitting other illnesses was also beginning to be appreciated. Scottish physician Sir Patrick Manson (1844–1922) had shown in 1877 that the mosquito could transmit filariasis, a parasitic illness in which there is swelling or tissue thickening throughout the body. In India, in 1898, British physician Ronald Ross (1857–1932) showed that *Plasmodium*, the parasite that causes malaria, could be transmitted by mosquitoes. (Ross received a Nobel Prize for this discovery.) But the transmission of yellow fever by mosquitoes was difficult to prove because, as it turned out, only one type of mosquito carries it. Carlos Finlay (1833–1915), a Cuban physician, had suggested in 1881 that the *Aedes aegypti* mosquito was the vector. He spent 20 years trying to prove it but was never able to do so.

The newly appointed commission gathered together in Havana in June of 1900. The team first investigated the theory of Italian physician Giuseppe Sanarelli (1864–1940) that *Bacillus icteroides* transmitted the illness. They failed to find the bacterium in blood or intestinal flora of patients with yellow fever and so disproved Sanarelli's theory.

They then turned to Finlay's theory. Because of the lack of animal models, the men agreed that they would have to experiment on humans and that they would begin with themselves. Agramonte was not eligible because he had been born in Cuba and might have been exposed to yellow fever and become immune. They took *Aedes aegypti* mosquito eggs harvested by Finlay and raised mosquitoes from them.

While Reed was away in Washington, Carroll and Lazear exposed themselves and nine volunteers to infected mosquitoes. At first, none showed any symptoms. But then Carroll and another volunteer, Private William Dean, became ill with yellow fever. Both recovered. Lazear noted that in these cases the mosquitoes had bitten an infected person very early in the illness and that there had been a period of at least 10 days before the mosquito bit the next person. After two separate exposures, perhaps accidental (this is not clear), Lazear became ill with yellow fever. He died on September 25, 1900. Lazear's death and the illnesses of Carroll and Dean were suggestive, but not proof, that mosquitoes had transmitted the illness. In none of these cases had the men avoided other mosquitoes or people ill with yellow fever. Reed returned from Washington to Cuba to organize some more careful experiments.

Reed and his colleagues decided to test the then-prevailing theory that yellow fever was spread by contact with an ill person or fomites (contaminated objects). Despite evidence to the contrary from the earlier experiments of Stubbins Ffirth (1774–1820), a medical student who had exposed himself to yellow fever fomites, and the many observations that nurses and doctors working closely with patients with yellow fever did not become ill, the theory remained popular.

Reed obtained support from military and civilian authorities, including the Spanish consul to Cuba. With funding from Leonard Wood, he established what he called Camp Lazear in the countryside, far from Havana, to make accidental exposures to yellow fever less likely. The camp consisted of two sheds for the experiments and seven tents for the volunteers. On November 20, 1900, the experiments began with 18 American subjects, mostly military, and 15 Spanish immigrants. The Spanish immigrants were asked to sign a written document outlining the risks of contracting yellow fever and the fact that there was no treatment for the illness. They were promised $100 for participating and an extra $100 if they became ill. They were also told that there was a good chance that they might become ill with yellow fever even if they did not participate in the experiment. They agreed to remain at Camp Lazear for the duration of the experiments. There may have been consent forms for the American participants, but none remain.

In one shed, the Infected Clothing Building, the furnishings included trunks and boxes of freshly soiled linens used by people ill with yellow fever at local hospitals. The stench of this material was at times overpowering. In three trials lasting 20 days at a time, subjects slept in sheets filthy with vomit, urine, and feces. One subject slept on a towel soaked in the blood of a man who had died from yellow fever. None of the seven volunteers developed the illness.

In the other shed, the Infected Mosquito Building, another set of complicated experiments was undertaken to further explore the mosquito theory. Men were exposed to mosquitoes at varying times after the mosquitoes had become infected. The subjects assigned to this shed thought that they were luckier because the shed was clean, the furnishings were steam sterilized, and there was good ventilation. However, within one week, four cases of yellow fever developed.

In subsequent experiments subjects were injected subcutaneously with blood from patients ill with yellow fever. Four of the volunteers became ill.

The conclusion was clear. Cleanliness and sanitation, although important in the control of other illnesses, had little to do with controlling yellow fever. Mosquitoes transmitted the illness by transferring infected blood from an ill person to a healthy person. The confusing element of the relationship—the time between the original mosquito bite and the transmission of the illness—was clarified. The delay between exposure to ill people and the development of illness had been described by an epidemiologist, Henry Rose Carter (1852–1925), in his observations of the natural course of yellow fever, but he had not blamed the mosquito. Finlay, who knew that the mosquito was involved, had never quite understood the timing.

Reed's mosquito experiments showed that, first, the mosquito had to bite an infected person while that person was in the early stages of the illness. Then, there had to be an incubation period of 10 to 14 days before the mosquito could transmit the illness. The mosquito could bite and infect multiple people for up to 71 days after the initial bite. After a person was bitten by an infected mosquito, there was a period of a few days before the person became ill.

In February 1901, Reed returned to Washington, and Carroll finished the experiments. In August 1901, he inoculated at least three subjects at Las Animas Hospital using blood injections. He filtered the blood first, which would have eliminated any bacteria. One subject became ill. Because the filtered blood was still infectious, it seemed likely that the microbe involved was a virus and not a bacterium.

Jesse Lazear, the 14 volunteers who became ill with yellow fever, and Walter Reed himself have all been regarded as medical heroes. The combination of self-experimentation, the death of Lazear, the ingenuity of the experiments, and the repeated exposure to mosquito bites and to disgusting matter caught the attention of the public. The method of yellow fever transmission was now clear, so there was no longer any need to fear catching the illness from yellow fever patients; plus, the transmission of the illness could now be stopped. American military medicine had made a huge advance. The key to yellow fever control was mosquito control.

Reed has been lionized for his work. A Broadway play, a Hollywood film, and a painting in a series of "Pioneers of American Medicine" memorialized his work.

A large military hospital in Washington, D.C., is named after him. However, it is important to put Reed's role in perspective: he had no theories of his own and had not risked his own life by exposing himself to mosquitoes. He was in Washington at the time of the first bites (for unclear reasons). He was older than the other members of the commission and perhaps more cautious because of that. But what he had done was organize well-thought-out experiments with volunteers and rapidly establish the vector and incubation times involved. He collaborated effectively with multiple authorities—both civilian and military—and with Spanish immigrants.

One of Reed's greatest accomplishments may have been his early—perhaps the earliest—use of written informed consent. In the consent form, many of the principles that apply to experimentation today are evident: the respect for autonomy, the emphasis on voluntariness, the outlining of risks and benefits, and compensation. The insistence that the volunteer be over the age of 25 is different from consents of today, as is the part forbidding the subject to leave the camp during the experiment. Perhaps this latter point can be understood as not wanting to put the subject and others at risk should the subject leave while ill.

More experiments followed after the Reed Yellow Fever Commission left Havana. Major William Gorgas (1854–1920), a physician and the chief sanitary officer of Havana, and Cuban physician Juan Guiteras (1852–1925) began to inoculate volunteers at Las Animas Hospital in Havana, hoping that an infection by a mosquito that had bitten a person with a mild case of yellow fever would lead to immunity. Reed, who had left Cuba by then, advised against this experiment. In the spring of 1901, the army offered volunteers $100 to participate in this study.

Clara Maass (1876–1901), a young nurse from New Jersey, was the only woman and the only American of 19 volunteers. She was bitten several times. She was bitten on August 14, 1901, became extremely ill, and died on August 24, at the age of 25. Two Spanish subjects also died. The deaths shocked many, and further experimentation was stopped.

Frances R. Frankenburg

DOCUMENTS

WILLIAM OSLER AND THE IMPORTANCE OF INFORMED CONSENT (1907)

William Osler, the preeminent clinician of his time and one of the "Big Four" founding physicians of the Johns Hopkins Hospital, was not himself a researcher, but he respected research and experimentation. Indeed, one of the missions of Johns Hopkins has always been "to foster independent and original research." Osler celebrated the work of Walter Reed, who had studied at Johns Hopkins University Hospital Pathology Laboratory, and had discovered that the mosquito transmitted yellow fever. Reed carefully obtained consent from subjects in his experiments. Osler insisted on "safety and full consent" when physicians experimented. With those conditions in place, Osler thought that human experimentation was one of the "brightest [pictures] in the history of human effort."

To each one of us life is an experiment in Nature's laboratory, and she tests and tries us in a thousand ways, using and improving us if we serve her turn, ruthlessly dispensing with us if we do not. Disease is an experiment, and the earthly machine is a culture medium, a test tube and a retort—the external agents, the medium and the reaction constituting the factors. We constantly experiment with ourselves in food and drink, and the expression so often on our lips, "Does it agree with you?" signifies how tentative are many of our daily actions. The treatment of disease has always been experimental, and started indeed in those haphazard endeavors of friends and relatives to try something to help the sufferer. Each dose of medicine given is an experiment, as it is impossible to predict in every instance what the result may be. Thousands of five-grain doses of iodide of potassium may be given without ill effect, and then conditions are met with in which the patient reacts with an outbreak of purpura, or a fatal result may follow. A deviation from what we had regarded as a settled rule, a break in a sequence thought to be invariable, emphasizes the impossibility of framing general rules for the body of the same rigid applicability as in physics and mechanics. The limits of justifiable experimentation upon our fellow creatures are well and clearly defined. The final test of every new procedure, medical or surgical, must be made on man, but never before it has been tried on animals. There are those who look upon this as unlawful, but in no other way is progress possible, nor could we have had many of our most useful but very powerful drugs if animal experimentation had been forbidden. For man absolute safety and full consent are the conditions which make such tests allowable. We have no right to use patients entrusted to our care for the purpose of experimentation unless direct benefit to the individual is likely to follow. Once this limit is transgressed, the sacred cord which binds physician and patient snaps instantly. Risk to the individual may be taken with his consent and full knowledge of the circumstances, as has been done in scores of cases, and we cannot honor too highly the bravery of such men as the soldiers who voluntarily submitted to the experiments on yellow fever in Cuba under the direction of Reed and Carroll. The history of our profession is starred with the heroism of its members who have sacrificed health and sometimes life itself in endeavors to benefit their fellow creatures. Enthusiasm for science has, in a few instances, led to regrettable transgressions of the rule I have mentioned, but these are mere specks which in no wise blur the brightness of the picture—one of the brightest in the history of human effort—which portrays the incalculable benefits to man from the introduction of experimentation into the art of medicine.

Source: William Osler, "The Evolution of the Idea of Experiment in Medicine," in *Transactions of the Congress of American Physicians and Surgeons, Seventh Triennial Session* (New Haven, CT: Published by the Congress, 1907), 7–8

ALBERT LEFFINGWELL AND THE CRUELTY OF VIVISECTION (1916)

Physician Albert Leffingwell was a vivisection reformer. In the late 1800s and early 1900s, the word "vivisection" referred to experimentation on both animals and humans. For over three decades, Leffingwell protested experimentation on animals and humans when it was carried out in secrecy and with cruelty. Leffingwell sparred with W. W. Keen, a leading surgeon, who claimed that vivisection was usually properly done and was necessary for progress in medicine. In this dramatic passage, Leffingwell writes about a physician who took advantage of a vulnerable patient who had already been severely injured. This physician went on to become a professor and a dean of a medical faculty. The description of the suffering of this young girl constitutes a powerful plea for physicians to act with more decency.

Chapter XVIII
The Final Phase: Experimentation on Man
. . .

I. The Case of Mary Rafferty

An instance of human vivisection which ended by the death of the victim, occurred some years ago in the Good Samaritan Hospital in Cincinnati. It would be difficult to suggest a name for a hospital more suggestive of kindly consideration for the sick and unfortunate: and to this charitable institution, there came one day a poor Irish servant girl by the name of Mary Rafferty.

She was not strong, either mentally or physically. Some years before, when a child, she had fallen into an open fire, and in some way had severely burned her scalp. In the scar tissue an eroding ulcer—possibly of the nature of cancer,—had appeared; and it had progressed so far that the covering of the brain substance had been laid bare. No cure could be expected; but with care and attention she might have possibly have lived for several months. We are told that she made no complain of headache or dizziness; that she seemed "cheerful in manner," and that "she smiled easily and frequently,"—doubtless with the confidence of a child who without apprehension of evil, feels it is among friends. The accident, however, had made her good "material"; she offered opportunity for experimentation of a kind hitherto make only upon animals. "It is obvious," says the vivisector, "that it is exceedingly desirable to ascertain how far the results of experiments on the brain of animals may be employed to elucidate the functions of the human brain."

At the outset the experiments seem to have been somewhat cautiously made. Nobody knew exactly what would be the result. The experiments began by inserting into Mary Rafferty's brain, thus exposed by disease, needle electrodes of various lengths, and connecting them a battery. As a result, her arm was thrown out, the fingers extended, but in the brain substance no pain was felt. Presently, as the experimenter grew bolder, other phenomena appeared. The vivisector shall tell the story in his own words:

"The needle was now withdrawn from the left lobe, and passed in the same way into the (brain) substance of the right. . . . When the needle entered the brain substance, SHE COMPLAINED OF ACUTE PAIN IN THE NECK, IN ORDER TO DEVELOP MORE DECIDED REACTIONS, the strength of the current was increased by drawing out the wooden cylinder one inch. When communication was made with the needles, HER COUNTENANCE EXHIBITED GREAT DISTRESS, and she began to cry. Very soon, the left hand was extended as if in the act of taking hold of some object in front of her; the arm presently was agitated with colic spasms; her eyes became fixed with pupils widely dilated; lips were blue, and SHE FROTHED AT THE MOUTH; HER BREATH-ING BECAME STERTOROUS; SHE LOST CONSCIOUSNESS AND WAS VIOLENTLY CONVULSED. The convulsion lasted five minutes, and was succeeded by coma. She returned to consciousness in twenty minutes from the beginning of the attack."

The experiment was a success. Upon the body of the poor servant girl, the distinguished vivisector had produced the "violent epileptiform convulsion" which Fritsch and Hitzig and Ferrier had induced in animals, by the same method of experimentation.

There are those who feel that further vivisecting should have then ceased, and that Mary Rafferty should have been allowed to die in peace. Such views, however, were not permitted by the experimenter to interfere with his zeal for scientific research. Other "observations: were made, and the needles were again passed into the brain evoking almost the same phenomena. The final experiments were thus described by the vivisector:

> Two days subsequent to observation No. 4, Mary was brought into the electrical room with the intention to subject the posterior lobes (of the brain) to galvanic excitation. The proposed experiment was abandoned. SHE WAS PALE AND DEPRESSED; HER LIPS WERE BLUE, AND SHE HAD EVIDENT DIFFICULTY IN LOCOMOTION. She complained greatly of numbness. . . . On further examination, there was found to be decided PARESIS and rigidity of the muscles of the right side. . . . She became very pale; her eyes closed; and she was about to pass into unconsciousness, when we placed her in the recumbent posture, and Dr. S. gave her, at my request, chloroform by inhalation.
>
> The day after observation No. 5, MARY WAS DECIDEDLY WORSE. She remained in bed, was stupid and incoherent. In the evening she had a convulsive seizure. . . . AFTER THIS, SHE LAPSED INTO PROFOUND UNCONSCIOUSNESS, AND WAS FOUND TO BE COMPLETELY PARALYZED ON THE RIGHT SIDE. . . . The pupils were dilated and motionless.

When did death come to her release? We do not know; the omission is significant; it may have been within a few moments. The next sentence in the report is headed by the ominous word, "AUTOPSY." The brain was taken out, and the track of the needles traced therein. One needle had penetrated an inch and a half. There was evidence of "INTENSE VASCULAR CONGESTION."

In cases like this, the investigation of a coroner apparently is not required. The experimenter himself was the physician to the hospital. He tells us of course that Mary's death was due to an extension of the disease, for the relief of which she had been led to the "Good Samaritan Hospital." Of the real cause of death, there was apparently but little doubt among scientific men. An English vivisector, Dr. David Ferrier, whose experiments upon monkeys had perhaps first suggested their repetition on a living human brain, questioned somewhat the propriety of the American experiments. In a letter to the London Medical Record, he referred to "the depth of penetration of the needles," the "occurrence of epileptiform convulsions FROM THE GENERAL DIFFUSION OF THE IRRITATION WHEN THE CURRENTS WERE INTENSIFIED," and declared that the "EPILEPTIC CONVULSIONS AND ULTIMATE PARALYSIS are clearly accounted for by the inflammatory changes" thus induced.

That the experiments had been to some extent injurious to his victim, the vivisector himself, in a letter to the British Medical Journal, very cautiously admitted. He regretted, he said, that the new facts which he had hoped would further the progress of Science were obtained of SOME injury to the patient. She was, however, "HOPELESSLY DISEASED,"—as if that fact tended to justify her martyrdom! "THE PATIENT CONSENTED TO HAVE THE EXPERIMENTS MADE." Is not this excuse the very height of hypocrisy? Twice, he had stated in his report of the case, that the young woman was "RATHER FEEBLEMINDED"; he suggests that this poor, ignorant, feeble-minded servant-girl was mentally capable of giving an intelligent consent to repeated experiments upon her brain, the possible result of which even HE could not foresee!

Who made these experiments? It was Dr. Roberts Bartholow, at that time the physician of the "Good Samaritan Hospital" in Cincinnati. His biographer says that he gained no credit "for his candour in reporting the whole affair,"—a hint, the significance of which for future experimenters, it is not very difficult to perceive. Yet his treatment of Mary Rafferty was no bar to his professional advancement. Not long after his victim was in her grave, one of the oldest medical schools in the country,—Jefferson Medical College of Philadelphia—offered him a professor's chair; and for several years he was Dean of the medical faculty of that institution.

It might seem impossible that any physician of the present day would care to come forward in defence of this experiment. Yet forty years after the deed was perpetrated, such justification was apparently attempted in an American journal, and republished in a pamphlet issued by the American Medical Association. It would seem at the outset that only by suppression of the worst facts relating to the case, could any defence be essayed. WAS THERE ANY SUCH SUPPRESSION OF MATERIAL FACTS? Let us see.

Did any injury to Mary Rafferty result from these experiments upon her brain? Bartholow himself admits some injury; he says that to repeat the experiments "would be in the highest degree criminal." The modern apologist, however, will have it otherwise. At the beginning of the experiment, she smiled as amused, and this, he tells us, "shows that she did not object, that the pain was not severe, AND THAT NO HARM WAS DONE HER." Is this a fair summary of the symptoms elicited during these experiments upon the brain? Why did the apologist mention only the "smile," and neglect altogether to mention the other symptoms reported by Dr. Bartholow? Why does he pass in silence her complain of "ACUTE PAIN IN THE NECK," the "GREAT DISTRESS" EXHIBITED, THE ARM AGITATED WITH CLONIC SPASM, THE FIXED EYES, THE WIDELY DILATED PUPILS, THE BLUE LIPS, THE FROTHING AT THE MOUTH, THE STERTOROUS BREATHING, THE VIOLENT CONVULSION lasting for five minutes and the succeeding unconsciousness lasting for twenty minutes? Why does the apologist leave unmentioned the symptoms following the subsequent experiments, the pallor and depression, the blue lips, the difficult in locomotion, the decided paresis and rigidity of muscles, the profound unconsciousness, THE FINAL PARALYSIS? Do omissions like these suggest an ardent desire to present the whole truth of the matter for the information of the public?

One the one side, stands a poor ignorant, feeble-minded Irish servant girl, full of faith and implicit trust in the benevolence of those about her; on the other a learned scientist, eager, as he says, "to ascertain how far the results of experiments on the brains of animals may be employed to elucidate the functions of the human brain," and her "consent" to procedures the purpose and dangers of which she knows nothing—to experiments involving her life, are suggested as a justification of whatever was done, and as a matter with which Society need have no concern!

Source: A. Leffingwell, *An Ethical Problem or, Sidelights upon Scientific Experimentation on Man and Animals*, 2nd edition (London: G. Bell and Sons LTD, 1916). Note: Some of the misspellings of the original document have been corrected to allow the excerpt to be read more easily.

THE TUSKEGEE EXPERIMENTS (1932)

Between 1932 and 1972, the United States Public Health Service organized the Tuskegee Study of Untreated Syphilis in black Americans, without their informed consent. In this letter, the researchers (using the name of the Macon County Health Department) ask the subjects to come into the Tuskegee Hospital for a lumbar puncture (spinal tap). They have the audacity to tell the subjects that they will be getting this "exam and treatment without cost." The researchers deceived the subjects by not telling them that they had syphilis, not telling them that they were subjects in a study, and not telling them that a lumbar puncture was for research only and had nothing to do with treatment. The researchers also actively prevented their subjects from getting treatment for their syphilis.

Macon County Health Department
Alabama State Board of Health and U.S. Public Health Service Cooperating with Tuskegee Institute

Dear Sir:

Some time ago you were given a thorough examination and since that time we hope you have gotten a great deal of treatment for bad blood. You will now be given your last chance to get a second examination. This examination is a very special one and after it is finished you will be given a special treatment if it is believed you are in a condition to stand it.

If you want this special examination and treatment you must meet the nurse at _____ on _____ _____ at _____M. She will bring you to the Tuskegee Institute Hospital for this free treatment. We will be very busy when these examinations and treatments are being given, and will have lots of people to wait on. You will remember that you had to wait for some time when you had your last good examination, and we wish to let you know that because we expect to be so busy it may be necessary for you to remain in the hospital over one night. If this is necessary you will be furnished your meal and a bed, as well as the examination and treatment without cost.

REMEMBER THIS IS YOUR LAST CHANCE FOR SPECIAL FREE TREATMENT. BE SURE TO MEET THE NURSE.

Macon County Health Department

Source: Macon County Health Department, "Letter to Subjects," n.d. Records of the USPHS Venereal Disease Division, Record Group 90, Box 239, National Archives, Washington National Record Center, Suitland, Maryland.

Further Reading

Altman, Lawrence K. 1987. *Who Goes First?: The Story of Self-Experimentation in Medicine.* New York: Random House.

Annas, George J., and Michael A. Grodin. 1992. *The Nazi Doctors and the Nuremberg Code: Human Rights in Human Experimentation.* New York: Oxford University Press.

Austin, Stephanie C., Paul D. Stolley, and Tamar Lasky. 1992. "The History of Malariotherapy for Neurosyphilis." *Journal of the American Medical Association* 268 (4) (July): 516–519.

Bliss, Michael. 1982. *The Discovery of Insulin.* Chicago: University of Chicago Press.

Bliss, Michael. 1992. *Banting: A Biography.* Toronto: University of Toronto Press.

Blue, Ethan. 2009. "The Strange Career of Leo Stanley: Remaking Manhood and Medicine at San Quentin State Penitentiary, 1913–1951." *Pacific Historical Review* 78 (2) (May): 210–241. doi:10.1525/phr.2009.78.2.210.

Braslow, Joel T. 1995. "Effect of Therapeutic Innovation on Perception of Disease and the Doctor-Patient Relationship: A History of General Paralysis of the Insane and Malaria Fever Therapy, 1910–1950." *American Journal of Psychiatry* 152 (5) (May): 660–665.

Carpenter, Kenneth J. 2008. "Harriette Chick and the Problem of Rickets." *Journal of Nutrition* 138 (5) (May): 827–832.

Cerletti, Ugo. 1950. "Old and New Information about Electroshock." *American Journal of Psychiatry* 107: 87–94.

Chernin, E. 1989. "Richard Pearson Strong and the Iatrogenic Plague Disaster in Bilibid Prison, Manila." *Reviews of Infectious Diseases* 11 (6): 996–1,004.

Chick, Harriette. 1976. "Study of Rickets in Vienna 1919–1922." *Medical History* 20: 41–51.

Clark, Ronald William. 1984. *J.B.S.: The Life and Work of J.B.S. Haldane.* Oxford: Oxford University Press.

Collins, W. 2013. "Origin of the St. Elizabeth Strain of *Plasmodium vivax*." *American Journal of Tropical Medicine and Hygiene* 88 (4) (April): 726. doi:10.4269/ajtmh.12-0351.

Dunn, Rob R. 2015. *The Man Who Touched His Own Heart: True Tales of Science, Surgery, and Mystery.* New York: Little, Brown and Company.

Emanuel, Ezekiel J. 2011. *The Oxford Textbook of Clinical Research Ethics*. Oxford: Oxford University Press.

Fletcher, William. 1907. "Rice and Beri-Beri: Preliminary Report on an Experiment Conducted at the Kuala Lumpur Lunatic Asylum." *Lancet* 1: 1,776–1,779.

Forssmann-Falck, Renata. 1997. "Werner Forssmann: A Pioneer of Cardiology." *American Journal of Cardiology* 79: 651–660.

Frankenburg, Frances R., and Ross J. Baldessarini. 2008. "Neurosyphilis, Malaria, and the Discovery of Antipsychotic Agents." *Harvard Review of Psychiatry* 16 (5): 299–307.

Frankenburg, Frances Rachel. 2009. *Vitamin Discoveries and Disasters: History, Science, and Controversies*. Santa Barbara, CA: Praeger/ABC-CLIO.

Hess, Alfred F., and M. Fish. 1914. "The Blood, the Blood-Vessels and the Diet." *American Journal of Diseases of Children* 8 (6): 385–405.

Hills, O. W., and E. Libert. 1951. "Clinical Aspects of Dietary Depletion of Riboflavin." *Archives of Internal Medicine* 87: 682–693.

Horwitt, M. K., and O. W. Hills. 1949. "Effects of Dietary Depletion of Riboflavin." *Journal of Nutrition* 39: 357–373.

Horwitt, M. K., and O. Kreisler. 1949. "The Determination of Early Thiamine-Deficient States by Estimation of Blood Lactic and Pyruvic Acids after Glucose Administration and Exercise." *Journal of Nutrition* 37 (4) (April): 411–417.

International Conference on the Insulin Treatment in Psychiatry, Max Rinkel. 1959. *Insulin Treatment in Psychiatry; Proceedings of the International Conference, Held at the New York Academy of Medicine, October 24 to 25, 1958*. New York: Philosophical Library.

Jones, James H. 1981. *Bad Blood: The Tuskegee Syphilis Experiment*. New York: Free Press.

Kreisler, Oscar, Erich Liebert, and M. K. Horwitt. 1948. "Psychiatric Observations on Induced Vitamin B Complex Deficiency in Psychotic Patients." *American Journal of Psychiatry* 105: 107–110.

Lebensohn, Zigmond M. 1999. "The History of Electroconvulsive Therapy in the United States and Its Place in American Psychiatry: A Personal Memoir." *Comprehensive Psychiatry* 40 (3): 173–181.

Lederer, Susan E. 1995. *Subjected to Science: Human Experimentation in America before the Second World War*. Baltimore: Johns Hopkins University Press.

Lederer, Susan E. 2002. "'Porto Ricochet': Joking about Germs, Cancer, and Race Extermination in the 1930s." *American Literary History* 14 (4) (Winter): 720–746.

Mashour, George A., Erin E. Walker, and Robert L. Martuza. 2005. "Psychosurgery: Past, Present, and Future." *Brain Research Reviews* 48: 409–419. doi:10.1016/j. brainresrev.2004.09.002.

Masterson, Karen M. 2014. *The Malaria Project: The U.S. Government's Secret Mission to Find a Miracle Cure*. New York: New American Library.

National Research Council (U.S.) Food and Nutrition Board. 1966. *The Food and Nutrition Board: Twenty-Five Years in Retrospect*. Washington, D.C.: National Academy of Sciences National Research Council.

Porter, Roy. 1997. *The Greatest Benefit to Mankind: A Medical History of Humanity*. New York: W. W. Norton.

Pressman, Jack D. 1998. *Last Resort: Psychosurgery and the Limits of Medicine*. Cambridge U.K.: Cambridge University Press.

Reverby, Susan, ed. 2000. *Tuskegee's Truths: Rethinking the Tuskegee Syphilis Study*. Chapel Hill: University of North Carolina Press.

Rosenfeld, Louis. 2002. "Insulin: Discovery and Controversy." *Clinical Chemistry* 48 (12): 2,270–2,288.

Shorter, Edward, and David Healy. 2007. *Shock Therapy: A History of Electroconvulsive Treatment in Mental Illness*. New Brunswick, N.J.: Rutgers University Press.

Slater, Leo B. 2006. "Chemists and National Emergency: NIH's Unit of Chemotherapy during World War II." *Bulletin for the History of Chemistry* 31 (2): 75–80.

Starr, Douglas. 2003. "Ethics: Revisiting a 1930s Scandal, AACR to Rename a Prize." *Science* 300 (5619) (April): 573–574. doi:10.1126/science.300.5619.573.

Stone, James L. 2001. "Dr. Gottlieb Burckhardt: The Pioneer of Psychosurgery." *Journal of the History of the Neurosciences* 10 (1) (March): 79–92. doi:10.1076/jhin.10.1.79.5634.

Valenstein, Elliot S. 1986. *Great and Desperate Cures: The Rise and Decline of Psychosurgery and Other Radical Treatments for Mental Illness*. New York: Basic Books.

Vollmann, Jochen, and Rolf Winau. 1996. "Informed Consent in Human Experimentation before the Nuremberg Code." *British Medical Journal* 313 (7070) (December): 1,445–1,449.

Wagner-Jauregg, Julius. 1922. "The Treatment of General Paresis by Inoculation of Malaria." *Journal of Nervous and Mental Disease* 33 (5) (May): 369–375.

Wortis, Joseph. 1959. "The History of Insulin Shock Treatment." In *Insulin Treatment in Psychiatry*, edited by Max Rinkel and Harold Edwin Himwich, 19–45. New York: Philosophical Library.

Era 4: World War II

INTRODUCTION

Human experimentation for many people now means the criminal acts carried out by Nazi physicians in World War II concentration camps. In 1933, the Nazi Party came to power in Germany, and in July of that year, the Nazis passed the Law for the Prevention of Genetically Defective Progeny, making it legal to sterilize people with supposedly hereditary illnesses such as "weak-mindedness," schizophrenia, alcoholism, deafness, and physical deformities. At the same time, the persecution of groups of people, such as Jews, Roma (Gypsies), homosexuals, and those with disabilities, increased. The Nazis thought that these groups should not be allowed to reproduce, or indeed to live, unless they could work as slaves. Within a few years, mass extermination began.

Heinrich Himmler (1900–1945), an architect of the Holocaust and chief of German police, was the leader of the Schutzstaffel (SS), a paramilitary unit. The SS was responsible for most of the Nazi war crimes and was an initiator of the medical experiments. Many of the people who served as administrators of the mass sterilizations and exterminations were physicians, including Ernst Grawitz (1899–1945) and Joachim Mrugowsky (1905–1948).

Experimentation in the German concentration camps was carried out on non-Aryan or "defective people." Because these people were not considered to be deserving of life, the Nazis did not think that medical experimentation on them needed to be conducted in an ethical manner. (In contrast, the Nazis believed that experimentation on animals did have to be carried out in a humane fashion.)

Some experiments were designed to protect the health and fitness of the German military. For example, concentration camp prisoners were put into low-pressure chambers to determine at what altitudes a pilot and his crew could survive if forced to eject from a plane in parachutes. Some prisoners were exposed to freezing temperatures to discover treatments for hypothermia, and others were given only seawater to drink to test ways of making it potable. Prisoners were exposed to phosgene and mustard gases to test antidotes. Some Nazi doctors also worked with German pharmaceutical companies, including Bayer and various medical institutes, to discover treatments for such infectious diseases as malaria, typhus, and tuberculosis.

One of the many horrifying aspects of the Nazi medical experiments was their personal nature. Some of the Nazi physicians personally supervised or directly caused the suffering of their subjects. German soldiers, in contrast, were disturbed by their massacre of populations. The military leadership was aware of this, and the soldiers' reluctance was, in part, a reason why the gas chambers were created—so that the German soldiers would not have to be so directly involved with the deaths of civilians.

It is difficult to understand how some German physicians, who presumably became doctors to diminish suffering, could have behaved with such cruelty. Nazi physicians came from one of the most civilized countries in the Western world—the home of Goethe and Beethoven. German technology and science were the envy of the world, and German medicine, in particular, was highly respected. Wilhelm Röntgen (1845–1923) had discovered X-rays. Robert Koch (1843–1910), along with the Frenchman Louis Pasteur (1822–1895), established the role of microbes in infections. Paul Ehrlich (1854–1913) developed salvarsan, the first treatment for syphilis. Medical students and physicians from the rest of the world came to Germany in the 1800s and early 1900s to study with these and other such renowned physicians.

The Nazi physicians could not claim that they did not know about medical ethics. Indeed, in 1900, the Prussian Ministry of Religion, Education, and Medical Affairs issued regulations stating that consent is needed in research procedures and that research could not be carried out on vulnerable patients. In 1931, Germany issued the most comprehensive research guidelines of the time, banning risky experiments on children or dying people.

The Nazis, interested in preventive medicine and health, conducted the first research in the world into the cancer-causing properties of cigarettes, asbestos, and X-rays. But their interest extended only to the health of the Aryan nation. The Nazi physicians may have believed what Hitler and Himmler preached—that Jewish, Roma, disabled, homosexual, and political prisoners were not truly human, but were more like cancers or infections that needed to be removed from the German Aryan nation. In addition, some of the Nazi physicians who participated in the experiments may have done so because of political ambition and anxiety to please their superiors. Some wanted to perform experiments that would lead to published papers that would further their careers.

After the war, revulsion at what the Nazis had done led to the Doctors' Trial, the first of 12 war crimes trials held at Nuremberg. An abundance of carefully preserved documentation as well as testimony by witnesses led to the conviction of most of the defendants, not one of whom admitted to any wrongdoing. Another result of the trial was the writing of the Nuremberg Code, the basis for our current research ethics.

Many German scientists and physicians, including those implicated in the medical experiments, were protected by the American military and brought to the United States by Operation Paperclip, which was designed in part to prevent such individuals from going to work for the Soviets during the early Cold War period. In some cases, the people were deported from the United States once their Nazi activities became known.

Another shocking combination of medical expertise and sadism was found in a large group of Japanese physicians working during the Sino-Japanese War and then during World War II. Microbiologist Shirō Ishii (1892–1951), of the Japanese army, experimented on prisoners of war, mostly Chinese, at Unit 731 in Pingfan, near Harbin, then in the puppet state of Manchuko, now in modern-day China. He and his colleagues performed operations on victims without anesthesia and killed several thousand people in the cruelest ways imaginable. Ishii used plane bombs and other techniques to spread smallpox, cholera, and plague in China, perhaps killing as many as 400,000 Chinese.

We know less about Unit 731 than we do about the German concentration camps for several reasons. Harbin, although a large multiethnic city, was isolated from the rest of the world. (The German concentration camps, in contrast, were very close to major population centers.) At the end of the war, Ishii instructed his subordinates to kill any remaining prisoners; there were, as far as we know, no survivors. Also, the hundreds of thousands of Chinese killed by plague and other infectious diseases may not have known that they were dying because of the actions of the Japanese.

Because of the Japanese skill at biological warfare, the United States, represented by General Douglas MacArthur, granted immunity to many of those responsible for Unit 731 so that the Americans, and not the Russians, could gain from Ishii's expertise in this area. The Americans working with the Japanese Unit 731 physicians were not, therefore, interested in discovering, examining, or publicizing the details of the Japanese war crimes. Indeed, the Americans discounted the subsequent Russian Khabarovsk trials of some of the Unit 731 participants as Communist propaganda.

The cruelty of the Japanese physicians of Unit 731 has been attributed to their reverence for the emperor, personal ambition, conviction of the superiority of the Japanese to other ethnicities, or fear of losing face. Some of the Japanese physicians went on to have successful careers after the war, apparently unhampered by their criminal activities of the past.

The Allied countries also carried out large medical experiments as part of the war effort, and in the United States, conscientious objectors volunteered to participate in some of them. These experiments, however, were different from those described above. In the Minnesota semistarvation experiment, which was carried out to work out how best to refeed starving soldiers and civilians in Europe, volunteers were enthusiastic about their involvement, grateful to be able to help the war effort, and fully informed.

Psychiatric patients, soldiers, prisoners, Quechua Indians, conscientious objectors, and medical students also participated in studies of antimalarial drugs carried out by the Allies. The best known of these studies took place at the Stateville Penitentiary in Illinois. Defenders of the Nazi physicians claimed that this latter group of experiments was similar to those carried out by the Nazis. But the Stateville prisoners were informed about the risks and benefits of the research and volunteered their involvement.

During World War II, the foundation for much Cold War experimentation was laid. Research into vaccines flourished. Franklin Delano Roosevelt appealed for donations to the National Foundation for Infantile Paralysis by comparing the fight against polio to the fight against the enemy abroad. One of the consequences of the Manhattan Project (1942–1946), which was established to develop nuclear bombs before the Germans could, was a large body of research that explored the health consequences of radiation and the use of radiation as a tool to explore human physiology and treat disease.

Medicine became more sophisticated. Some advances came from a tragedy unrelated to the war. A 1942 fire in Cocoanut Grove, a Boston nightclub, was one of the worst in U.S. history, killing 492 people and injuring about the same number. Oliver Cope (1902–1994) and Francis Moore (1913–2001) used new techniques in fluid resuscitation and burn care as well as a new antibiotic, penicillin, to treat some of the burn patients that were sent to the Massachusetts General Hospital. The patients treated with experimental techniques healed better than those treated with conventional techniques at other hospitals. Moore made other improvements in the care of patients with severe burns. He developed the practice of measuring body fluids and electrolytes so that they could be replaced accurately. He was also one of the first physicians to use radioactive dyes to locate abscesses and tumors in patients. The new technology as well as the experiments on both animals and humans—some in the laboratory and some in the "trenches"—revolutionized both burn care and surgery. Moore later became a leader in the field of liver transplants.

Work done during the World War II era also paved the way for heart surgery. For example, military surgeon Dwight Harken (1910–1993) removed shrapnel from the hearts of wounded soldiers. Until then, surgery on the heart was thought to be too dangerous. In 1944, at Johns Hopkins in Baltimore, Alfred Blalock (1899–1964), Helen B. Taussig (1898–1986), and Vivien Thomas (1910–1985) operated on a "blue baby" suffering from heart defects. By using the newly developed Blalock-Thomas-Taussig shunt, they redirected the blood flow so that unoxygenated blood traveled through the lungs and became oxygenated, thus allowing the formerly cyanotic, or "blue," baby to become healthy and pink.

Researchers during these years did not always heed the welfare or autonomy of the subjects. Nutrition experts in Canada began studies of the diets of the aboriginal people in Canada, but, in their experimental zeal, sometimes worsened the diet of those studied. In mid-20th-century American studies of vaccines, children and inmates in institutions were exposed to vaccines without their consent. These exposures seem questionable now but usually did not harm the subjects and were not done in an atmosphere of depravity and willingness to cause injury and death.

The activities that stand out as the worst, and those that still taint the concept of medical experimentation, are those carried out by the Nazis and Unit 731 physicians. Their experiments, often lethal, were performed by respected members of the medical establishment. They had a high mortality rate. The indifference of the physicians in the Nazi concentration camps and Unit 731 to the suffering of the subjects, and indeed their deliberate sadism, set these experiments apart from the others described in this book.

TIMELINE

1933	The Nazi Party comes to power in Germany.
1933	The first concentration camp is built in Dachau, Germany, the site of later medical experimentation, such as the exposure of inmates to freezing temperatures and conditions mimicking high altitudes.
1936–1945	In Japan, Unit 731 experiments in cruel ways on thousands of Chinese and prisoners of war.
1941	Medical experimentation begins in the Buchenwald concentration camp, including many trials of typhus vaccines.
1942	After a fire at a Boston nightclub, the Cocoanut Grove, Francis Moore (1913–2001) and Oliver Cope (1902–1994) experiment with new treatments for burns.
1942–1952	Canadian nutrition researchers maintain aboriginal communities on deficient diets.
1943	Albert Hofmann (1906–2008) of Sandoz Pharmaceuticals synthesizes and takes lysergic acid diethylamide (LSD) and describes vivid visual hallucinations.
1944	Malaria experiments begin at the Stateville Penitentiary in Illinois using convicts as the subjects.
1944–1945	Thirty-six conscientious objectors volunteer to live on a low-calorie diet in the Minnesota Starvation Experiment run by Ancel Keys.
1944	At Johns Hopkins in Baltimore, Alfred Blalock (1899–1964), Helen B. Taussig (1898–1986), and Vivien Thomas (1910–1985) operate on a "blue baby" suffering from heart defects and redirect blood flow to the lungs using the Blalock-Thomas-Taussig shunt.
1945	Schoolchildren in Nashville, Tennessee, are given lemonade containing radioactive iron in experiments designed to explore the absorption of iron.
1946–1947	At the Doctors' Trial in Nuremberg, 23 doctors and administrators are put on trial for medical atrocities.
1947	The Nuremberg Code is written in response to the atrocities described in the Doctors' Trial.

REFERENCE ENTRIES

AMERICAN EXPERIMENTS WITH MALARIA

The mosquito-borne illness malaria was a serious problem for the American military in World War II. In the quest for antimalarial drugs, American researchers and their international colleagues experimented on psychiatric patients, prisoners, conscientious objectors, soldiers, Arab villagers in Tunisia, medical students, and Quechua Indians in Peru.

Malaria is caused by one of several species of the parasite *Plasmodium*: *P. falciparum*, *P. vivax*, *P. ovale*, or *P. malariae*. These parasites have a complicated life cycle, involving stages in the anopheline mosquito (the vector) and the human (the host), and sexual and asexual forms. If a female anopheline mosquito carrying this parasite bites a person, *Plasmodium* sporozoites—which are the immature, infective, spore-like forms of the parasite—can be transmitted to that person. The sporozoites travel to the liver, where some stay dormant and some multiply to form merozoites, the next stage in the development of the parasite. The merozoites infect red blood cells, and some of them multiply in an asexual manner. The cells then burst, causing cycles of anemia, fevers, and chills in the human host. Other merozoites within the red cells develop into sexual forms known as gametocytes. A female anopheline, looking for a blood meal, bites an infected person and ingests the blood cells containing the gametocytes. In the mosquito gut, the gametocytes burst out of the human red blood cells and fuse with each other, forming zygotes that then develop into sporozoites. The sporozoites travel to the mosquito's salivary glands and infect the next person that the mosquito bites.

P. falciparum and *P. vivax* are the commonest causes of malaria in humans. Falciparum malaria is the more severe strain and can be fatal. Vivax malaria is less severe, but because it can be dormant in the liver for long periods of time, it can be difficult to eradicate.

Malaria has played a key role in military battles throughout history. The environmental damage that results from warfare—such as destruction of forests and degradation of the landscape—as well as the contact of troops without prior exposure to malaria to indigenous malarious populations, often led to a large number of malaria cases in armies. In Macedonia during World War I, for example, malaria immobilized French, British, and German armies for three years.

World War II was no exception. During this period, malaria continued to be problematic, as much of the fighting took place in malarious areas in Europe and the South Pacific. Quinine, a natural substance obtained from the cinchona tree, was the only antimalarial drug then available, but in 1942, supplies became limited after Japan conquered Java, home of cinchona plantations and the largest quinine factory in the world. Other antimalarial agents, such as atabrine, existed but were not very effective and had many side effects.

In the Pacific theater, malaria severely affected American and Filipino troops and contributed to General Douglas MacArthur's April 9, 1942, surrender of his army to the Japanese (who were also suffering from malaria). It continued to afflict the troops in the campaigns that followed in New Guinea and Guadalcanal, with some marines at Guadalcanal becoming ill with both falciparum and vivax malaria. Because the men had multiple attacks of malaria, the annual malaria rate was calculated at nearly 3,000 illnesses for every 1,000 soldiers. In May 1943, MacArthur famously said, "This will be a long war if for every division I have facing the enemy I must count on a second division in hospital with malaria and a third division convalescing from this debilitating disease!"[1]

During the Sicilian campaign in the summer and fall of 1943, malaria was also prevalent. When the German army retreated northward, they blew up drainage ditches and flooded the Pontine Marshes south of Rome, thus creating swamps—natural homes for mosquitoes—and making malaria far more common than would have been typical in this part of Italy.

Given the crippling threat on so many fronts, the American army formed malaria control units to eradicate mosquitoes. Because mosquito eggs hatch in stagnant water, one technique they used was to drain swamps and eliminate incidental containers of water, such as buckets or discarded tires. Once mosquito eggs have hatched into larvae, the larvae then become pupae that live in the water but need oxygen to live. So another step in malaria control was to spray water surfaces with kerosene. The kerosene deters mosquitoes from laying their eggs on the water, interferes with the access to oxygen of the larvae and pupae already there, and also may be directly toxic to the mosquitoes.

Several other chemical insecticides were also used. One was called copper acetate triarsenate, also known as Paris Green (so named because it was once used to kill rats in sewers in Paris and because of its emerald green color). "Bug bombs" using the chrysanthemum-derived insecticide pyrethrum and Freon as an aerosolizing agent were helpful. Then, once it became available in 1943, dichloro-diphenyl-trichloroethane (DDT) was very effective in lowering mosquito numbers.

In addition to the efforts to eliminate mosquitoes, there was also an educational campaign to help prevent or slow the spread of the disease. Soldiers were encouraged to wear long pants and long-sleeved shirts, not to go out at night when the mosquitoes were most active, to use bed nets, and to apply insect repellent to exposed skin.

At the same time, medical researchers were looking for new and more effective treatments for malaria. Currently available drugs had questionable efficacy and extremely unpleasant side effects. New drugs were tested on animals, particularly birds and dogs, but the effectiveness and toxicity of new drugs differed between malaria species and between hosts, so researchers were unsure how well the drugs would work in humans. Plus, *Plasmodium* could not be grown in culture. Testing therefore had to take place on humans.

One antimalarial drug, atabrine (also known as mepacrine or quinacrine), was synthesized by Bayer in Germany in 1931. It had a number of problems. Not only had the correct dosing not yet been determined, but the side effects were terrible: it made the skin yellow and led to stomach cramping, vomiting, and diarrhea. Soldiers often refused to take it. Because Winthrop, the American pharmaceutical company manufacturing atabrine, had links with Bayer, the German pharmaceutical company, there were also concerns about the quality of the Winthrop-made atabrine. The American military asked other companies to make "bootleg" versions of atabrine, but these pills too had a variety of puzzling side effects. In 1942, James Shannon (1904–1994), a nephrologist and future head of the National Institutes of Health (NIH), experimented with atabrine made by Winthrop, Abbott Laboratories, Imperial Chemical Industries in England, and Bayer's plant in Leverkusen, Germany.

Shannon gave the pills from these four manufacturers to healthy adults, including 250 Ohio State University medical students, 241 New Jersey State Reformatory prisoners, and 332 Sing Sing prisoners in New York. The research subjects reported side effects in confusing patterns. What was clear, though, was that no company made a "purer" or less toxic form of the drug.

In an attempt to account for the differing reactions to atabrine, Shannon, along with scientists at the Goldwater Memorial Hospital on Roosevelt Island in New York, approached the problem from a new angle. Using a new technique of measuring drug levels with a fluorometer, they found that absorption of atabrine differed between individuals and that effectiveness against the parasite was related to the blood level, not the dose. This work was some of the first showing the importance of blood levels of a drug. They performed these experiments (and others to do with dosing schedules) on more than 1,100 psychiatric patients in New York state hospitals, prison volunteers, and conscientious objectors.

Many other scientists were simultaneously working with atabrine and investigating possible new antimalarial drugs. G. Robert Coatney (1902–1990), a parasitologist, had been working at an NIH laboratory at the South Carolina State Hospital, where he learned about using malaria to treat neurosyphilis. Coatney moved to Washington, D.C., and developed the NIH's antimalarial clinical testing programs at a large psychiatric facility, St. Elizabeth Hospital (also known as St. Elizabeth's or St. Elizabeths). He also worked with a federal penitentiary in Atlanta, Georgia, that was close to the South Carolina State Hospital and another malaria research facility in Milledgeville, Georgia, so that he had a ready supply of malarial blood from patients with neurosyphilis who were being treated with malaria. He promised the convicts medical care, $50, a certificate signed by the surgeon general, and six months taken off their sentence if they volunteered for his studies, which involved being infected with malaria and then treated with new antimalarial drugs. He told them that he would begin with high doses of atabrine so that he could understand just how bad the side effects could be and that they would have to stay in the study for up to six months. Five hundred convicts signed consent.

During the war, Australian soldiers developed malaria at high rates while fighting in the Pacific. Brigadier Neil Fairley (1891–1966), director of medicine for the Australian army, established a research unit in Cairns, Queensland, to experiment with malaria treatments, in close conjunction with his American counterparts. Major Mabel Josephine Mackerras (1896–1971), an Australian zoologist, directed a number of research experiments in which anopheles pupae from Papua New

Guinea were collected and then grown in Cairns. Servicemen carrying *P. falciparum* or *P. vivax* gametocytes were exposed to these mosquitoes, which then infected malaria-free volunteers. Australian physicians tested the efficacy of atabrine under various conditions and showed that one tablet of atabrine a day would prevent acute attacks of malaria, cure those due to *P. falciparum*, and, while it was taken, postpone attacks of *P. vivax*. The Australians also tested atabrine, along with other drugs such as quinine and plasmaquine, on military volunteers exercising at high altitudes to test the effectiveness of drugs in possible combat situations.

The leading pharmaceutical chemists of the time worked in Germany. In the early 1930s, German scientists had found a promising drug, resochin, which they thought was too toxic to use. They altered the molecule, changing it to a substance that they named sontochin. A French doctor, Jean Schneider, working in Tunisia under the Vichy regime, organized a three-month experiment with sontochin and atabrine in seven northern Tunisian villages. In one village, he instructed the inhabitants to take a weekly dose of atabrine; in four villages, he distributed varying doses of sontochin; and in the remaining two villages, he didn't issue either drug.

In May 1943, after Tunis fell to the Allies, he turned over the results of his experiment—which showed the usefulness of sontochin—along with several thousand sontochin tablets to the Americans. American scientists altered the molecule and turned it back into resochin—the drug originally thought by the Germans to be too toxic to use. (The Americans had also earlier tested this molecule but had not realized its potential.) They renamed the drug chloroquine and began more tests.

In 1945, Rockefeller Foundation scientists tested the toxicity of chloroquine on Quechua Indians who lived and worked on an 18,000-acre sugar plantation in Peru in an almost feudal arrangement. The Quechua were told that they must take the drug; indeed, fieldworkers were not paid unless they took the weekly pill. It was also given to schoolchildren as young as six. The experiment was carried out from June to August, after the malaria season had already started, so that the effectiveness of chloroquine against malaria could not be tested. Eighty percent of the schoolchildren did become very ill from the drug, but they recovered when the dose, originally given at an adult strength, was lowered. The conclusion was that the toxicity of chloroquine was minimal and reversible.

Chloroquine was also tested on prisoners at Stateville, Illinois, and patients at the Boston Psychopathic Hospital (some with syphilis and some without) who had all been deliberately infected with malaria. Its toxicity was tested on conscientious objectors at the Massachusetts General Hospital and then on Australian soldier-volunteers by Fairley's group. In all of these groups, the toxicity of chloroquine was again found to be low.

As a result of these experiments, chloroquine became widely used as both a prophylactic and therapeutic agent for the treatment of malaria. It was cheap, effective, and—unlike what the German scientists originally thought—well tolerated. Unfortunately, *P. falciparum* and, to a lesser extent, *P. vivax* have developed resistance against this drug.

Malaria research during World War II was a large-scale scientific effort that involved thousands of experimental compounds and research subjects as well as collaboration between universities, hospitals, federal agencies, and pharmaceutical companies. This was the beginning of the industrialization of medical research. However, during those wartime years, it was not a pressing question as to whether prisoners, soldiers, or psychiatric patients could give informed consent to participate in such research.

Frances R. Frankenburg

Reference

1.   Russell, Paul F. "Malaria," 2.

AUSCHWITZ

Over a million people were killed during World War II at Auschwitz, a network of concentration camps located in modern-day Poland. Some of the prisoners were used as slave labor and others as subjects in medical experiments, such as sterilization by physicians Carl Clauberg and Horst Schumann. Bayer, the German pharmaceutical company, used prisoners as research subjects. Auschwitz was also the site of Josef Mengele's infamous experiments on twins and dwarfs.

Auschwitz was a group of concentration camps in southern Poland, situated some 37 miles west of Krakow. There were three separate concentration camps at the site: Auschwitz I (the main camp), Birkenau (Auschwitz II), and Monowitz (Auschwitz III). The largest of the three, Birkenau, was built to alleviate overcrowding at Auschwitz I; construction began in October 1941. Birkenau's "provisional" gas chamber, where prisoners were killed, was operational by early 1942. A second, larger gas chamber was constructed and became operational by June 1943. Prisoners were killed with a gas derived from prussic acid, but known by its brand name Zyklon-B. It was faster and more efficient than carbon monoxide, which had initially been used to murder prisoners in Nazi death camps. As many as 1 million people were exterminated at Birkenau between 1942 and late 1944, when the Germans suspended operations there.

The process of mass killing at Birkenau was virtually identical to that in other extermination facilities. Prisoners typically arrived by rail—in overcrowded boxcars—and were separated by gender upon arrival. They were then ordered to surrender all personal possessions, disrobe, and move toward "communal showers," a cruel euphemism for the gas chamber. Some people were "selected" by physician Josef Mengele (1911–1979) for experimentation, and some were selected to work. But most were killed. After the prisoners were killed by the poison gas, prison workers emptied the chamber of bodies and deposited them in large crematoria. By June 1943, Birkenau had four large crematoria that operated almost around the clock. The vast majority of prisoners were Jews from Central and Eastern Europe, although there were also a large number of Roma (Gypsies) as well.

Like most of the Nazi death camps, Birkenau was staffed with Schutzstaffel (SS) officials along with locally recruited police forces. Prisoners also helped run the facility. Orderlies (kapos) helped maintain order and discipline in the barracks, while crematoria personnel (sonderkommandos) helped process newly arrived prisoners and ready them for the gas chambers. They also gathered prisoners' personal possessions, removed any gold that gassed victims might have had in their teeth, and moved the corpses into the crematoria. Including prisoners, Birkenau may have had as many as 3,000 workers. Prisoners who served as workers were also killed on a regular basis, to be replaced by newly arriving prisoners.

Medical experimentation took place in Auschwitz I, the main camp. Horst Schumann (1906–1983), a German physician, worked at Auschwitz from 1941 to 1944. He irradiated both men and women to sterilize them. Subjects suffered radiation burns, and if they became too ill as a result of the radiation, they were gassed. If they survived, their testicles or ovaries were removed and examined. He also injected prisoners with blood taken from others ill with typhus.

Carl Clauberg (1898–1957) experimented with sterilization in part of Block No. 10 in the main camp by injecting chemical irritants into women's fallopian tubes. His experiments killed some of his subjects, and others were put to death so that autopsies could be performed.

Organized by the Bayer pharmaceutical company, SS camp physicians experimented with new drugs on the inmates. (Bayer also used many prisoners as slave labor.) Other experiments at Auschwitz included freezing (hypothermia) experiments and the experiments done by Mengele on twins.

The combination of mass murders and cruel experimentation makes Auschwitz a vivid symbol of humanity at its worst. The decision to send thousands of terrified people to the camp and then to "select" them for gassing, slave labor, or sadistic experimentation represents organized evil.

Paul G. Pierpaoli Jr.

BECKER-FREYSENG, HERMANN

Hermann Becker-Freyseng was a German physician who participated in medical experiments on concentration camp inmates before and during World War II.

Hermann Becker-Freyseng was born in Ludwigshafen, Germany, in 1910, and received his medical degree from the University of Berlin in 1935. The following year, he was given the rank of captain in the medical service and was posted to the department of aviation medicine, where he became an expert on the effects of high-altitude, low-pressure conditions on humans. In the meantime, he had become a member of the Nazi Party.

Becker-Freyseng conducted or supervised a number of experiments in the Nazi concentration camps. Through the use of various low-pressure chambers designed to mimic the effects of high altitudes on the human body, Becker-Freyseng and his colleagues killed a number of prisoners at the Dachau camp. In other experiments, he recorded the effects of extremely cold temperatures on the human body. He forced 40 prisoners to drink saltwater to measure their bodies' reactions. Some also had saltwater injected directly into their bloodstreams. The subjects were then subjected to liver biopsies—without the benefit of anesthesia—to measure that organ's reaction to the saltwater. All of the people involved ultimately died.

After World War II ended in 1945, Becker-Freyseng was taken into custody by U.S. occupation authorities who were interested in his knowledge of aviation. He was one of a number of German scientists involved in Operation Paperclip, which was designed in part to prevent such people from going to work for the Soviets during the early Cold War period. Nonetheless, he was put on trial for his medical experiments, and in 1946, during the Doctors' Trial, he was found guilty of war crimes and crimes against humanity and sentenced to 20 years in prison. While in prison, he contributed at least one chapter to a two-volume book, *German Aviation Medicine: World War II*, published under the auspices of the surgeon general of the U.S. Air Force in 1950. He was released in 1952 and died in 1961, in Heidelberg.

Paul G. Pierpaoli Jr.

BLOME, KURT

Kurt Blome was a German doctor and medical researcher who conducted or supervised unethical medical experiments on concentration camp inmates during World War II.

Kurt Blome was born in Bielefeld, Germany, on January 31, 1894. After his medical education and training, he was appointed deputy Reich health leader and head of cancer research in the Reich Research Council. The latter post was, however, a cover for Blome's other work. Beginning in 1943, Blome conducted experiments with bubonic plague on concentration camp inmates. He also experimented with various cancer-causing agents and biological and chemical substances. Among these were typhoid, cholera, anthrax, bubonic plague, malaria, and nerve agents such as sarin and tabun. Prisoners were routinely exposed to or infected with these various diseases and agents to test the efficacy of vaccines and antidotes. Many of Blome's experiments were conducted at the Dachau and Auschwitz concentration camps.

In May 1945, after the defeat of Germany, American military intelligence operatives arrested Blome in Munich. U.S. intelligence agents interrogated him because of their interest in his knowledge of chemical and biological warfare. In 1947, Blome was acquitted during the Nuremberg Doctors' Trial. It remains unclear whether American officials intervened in the judiciary process because they saw Blome as a potentially valuable scientist for U.S. weapons projects. Just two months after his acquittal, American chemical weapons experts interviewed him at great length. Blome was part of Operation Paperclip, the program in which German scientists worked for the United States so that Russia could not benefit from their expertise.

In 1951, Blome was asked to join the U.S. Army Chemical Corps, but he was denied a visa to work in the United States. He was later arrested by French officials, tried, and convicted of war crimes. Blome died on October 10, 1969.

Paul G. Pierpaoli Jr.

BRANDT, KARL

Karl Brandt was a German war criminal who served as Adolf Hitler's personal physician and participated in the Nazi T-4 "euthanasia" program, which systematically murdered handicapped and mentally challenged individuals and others deemed "unworthy of life." As the senior medical official in Germany during World War II, he had overall responsibility for the inhumane medical experimentation in the concentration camps and was the lead defendant in the Doctors' Trial. He was convicted and executed.

Karl Brandt was born in 1904 in Muhlhausen, Alsace-Lorraine, and received his degree in medicine from the University of Freiburg in 1929. Brandt became an adherent of "racial hygiene" policies, which were based on a pseudoscience that contended that medical professionals could treat a nation or racial group in the same way that they treated an individual by removing hereditary and other defects. In 1934, Hitler appointed him as his personal physician, and from that point on, Brandt became a member of Hitler's inner circle. He appears to have been both a believer in eugenics and a career-minded opportunist.

In 1939, a request from a German family for the mercy killing of their handicapped child served as the pretext for the initiation of the Nazi "euthanasia" program. Brandt, along with Philipp Bouhler, head of Hitler's Chancellery, was placed in charge of its planning and implementation. They received a rare explicit authorization from Hitler, allowing them to "grant mercy deaths" to "incurable" patients, as of September 1, 1939. Brandt and Bouhler then organized what became known as Aktion T-4, which referred to the mass murder of mentally ill and handicapped German adults and children. This program eventually expanded into the gassing of patients at six euthanasia centers throughout Germany. Patients were also murdered by starvation and lethal injection at other institutions. Public concern forced the program underground, but Brandt soon expanded it in 1941 to include other nationalities. As euthanasia slowed, its specialists brought their expertise in killing to the extermination of the Jews.

By 1942, the ambitious Brandt became chief of medicine and health for the Third Reich and the most powerful medical doctor in Germany. As such, he now presided over not just the "euthanasia" program, but also other Nazi criminal enterprises, including a wide variety of human experimentation projects carried out on concentration camp prisoners. Brandt sought increasingly more control over the medical establishment and health-related industries before falling out of favor with Hitler in 1944. He was then arrested by the Gestapo for allegedly planning to surrender to the Allies. Although Brandt escaped his Nazi death sentence, he was arrested by the Allies on May 23, 1945.

As the leading Nazi doctor and because of his involvement in a large number of medical criminal enterprises, Brandt was a main focus of prosecutors at the Nuremberg Doctors' Trial, which began in December 1946. Karl Brandt was found guilty of crimes against humanity and membership in a criminal organization and was executed on June 2, 1948, at Landsberg Prison in Landsberg am Lech, Germany.

Waitman W. Beorn

BUCHENWALD

Established in 1937, Buchenwald was a German concentration camp located near Weimar. Many of its prisoners worked as slave laborers. Physicians also used Buchenwald prisoners to test poisons, vaccines, and supposed "cures" for homosexuality.

Buchenwald was a Nazi concentration camp built in 1937 about five miles northwest of Weimar, Germany. Its first prisoners were male political prisoners; females were not imprisoned until late 1943 or early 1944. After the anti-Jewish pogrom of Kristallnacht in November 1938, 10,000 Jews were sent to Buchenwald, more than 200 of whom died almost immediately upon arrival. Other prisoners included criminals, Jehovah's Witnesses, Roma (Gypsies), military deserters, and, toward the end of the war, prisoners of war.

The camp was a source of slave labor for the German Reich. The prisoners worked in armaments and munitions factories and also in a stone quarry. Prisoners too weak to work were sent to "euthanasia" facilities in Bernburg, where they were killed.

In 1941, Nazi physicians began medical experimentation on prisoners at Buchenwald to test the efficacy of vaccines against diseases such as typhus, typhoid, cholera, and diphtheria. The typhus vaccines were of particular importance to the Nazis because German troops were dying of the illness in their fight with the Russians. Typhus, which is caused by a bacterium carried by lice, causes hallucinations, headaches, and high fevers. During the process of vaccine production, over 700 inmates were used as subjects and more than 150 died.

Later, in 1944, Danish physician Carl Vaernet (1893–1965) began experiments at Buchenwald in an attempt to "cure" homosexuality through gland implants and hormone injections. After the war, he continued his research while living in Argentina.

Between November 1943 and January 1944, physicians burned inmates with phosphorus taken from incendiary bombs to test various pharmaceutical preparations. Russian prisoners were poisoned with intravenous phenol or cyanide to see how long it would take for them to die. Those who did not die from the poisons were executed and then dissected.

As Russian forces spread across Poland, prisoners from the Polish concentration camps of Auschwitz and Gross-Rosen were marched west to join those already at

Buchenwald. On April 11, 1945, American soldiers liberated the camp. Between July 1937 and April 1945, 250,000 persons had been imprisoned in Buchenwald. About 56,000 prisoners died in the Buchenwald camp system.

Frances R. Frankenburg

DACHAU

Dachau, the first German concentration camp, was located about 10 miles from Munich, in southern Germany. Prisoners there were subjected to a variety of often deadly medical experiments, including extended exposure to low temperatures and infection with malaria. Some people were placed in low-pressure chambers to test the effects of high altitudes on German pilots; others were forced to drink seawater.

In Dachau, a pleasant suburb outside Munich, Germany, the first Nazi concentration camp was built in 1933, two months after Adolf Hitler took power. Dachau was used as a training camp for the Schutzstaffel (SS), who were instilled with the attitude that prisoners were *Untermenschen*, or subhumans.

During its 12 years of existence, Dachau was a camp for political prisoners, and its population was largely made up of dissidents, including socialists, Christian leaders, Jehovah's Witnesses, and people considered inferior, such as Roma (Gypsies), homosexuals, criminals, Jews, and Polish intellectuals. More than 3,000 clergy were imprisoned there, mostly Catholic, including bishops and one cardinal. The Vatican has beatified 6 imprisoned priests as martyrs, and the Serbian Orthodox Church recognized an imprisoned Serbian bishop as a saint.

Dachau was not an extermination camp, so German Jewish prisoners who arrived there were quickly shipped to death camps in Poland, such as Auschwitz-Birkenau. However, in 1944, Hungarian and other Jews were brought to Dachau to work as slave labor in munitions factories. At the time of liberation, about 30 percent of the camp population was Jewish. The "politicals" were made up of prominent leaders from every country invaded by the Nazis. In all camps, the prisoners formed an internal government, but at Dachau, the prisoners' previous political leadership experience made it possible to control the criminal element that preyed upon the weak in many other camps.

Among the 206,206 prisoners registered at Dachau during its existence, 31,591 deaths were recorded, though the number is certainly higher. This figure does not include the mass executions of Soviet and French prisoners of war who were dispatched by firing squads shortly after their arrival. It also does not include invalids or Jews shipped away and executed elsewhere. Most of the Dachau prisoners were used as slave labor, with almost 37,000 working in armament factories in 36 subsidiary camps. Both working and living conditions were harsh, with insufficient food, regular beatings, and unsanitary crowding. Each barracks housed some 1,500 people in unheated wooden buildings built for 200. By the end, in 1945, typhus was rampant in the camp, and the Red Cross tried to keep the prisoners from being freed before the American army arrived for fear of spreading the disease through the countryside.

Criminal and often lethal medical experiments were carried out on the prisoners. German SS physician Sigmund Rascher (1909–1945) conducted freezing experiments to determine the most effective means for treating German pilots who had ejected from their planes, crashed into the freezing waters of the North Sea, or were exposed in other ways to cold temperatures. For up to five hours at a time, inmates were put into tanks of icy water or kept outside in freezing temperatures. The doctors measured changes in the patients' heart rate, body temperature, muscle reflexes, and urination. Rewarming techniques, such as hot sleeping bags, scalding baths, or lying with naked women, were used. Some 80 to 100 patients died during these experiments. In other experiments, more than a thousand prisoners were infected with malaria, and some others with tuberculosis.

In 1942, Rascher and others, such as Hermann Becker-Freyseng (1910–1961), conducted high-altitude experiments in an attempt to find out how to protect German pilots forced to eject at high altitude. They placed prisoners in low-pressure chambers that simulated altitudes as high as 68,000 feet and monitored their responses. Of the 200 people subjected to these experiments, 80 died immediately, and the remainder were executed.

Later, from about July 1944 to about September 1944, scientists conducted experiments in the camp to study various methods of making seawater drinkable. About 40 Roma (Gypsies) were deprived of food and were allowed to only drink seawater.

On April 29, 1945, the camp, with more than 30,000 prisoners (almost 10,000 additional prisoners had been marched off three days earlier) was liberated by the American Seventh Army. Some American soldiers were so traumatized by what they saw that they shot a number of Nazi guards even after they had surrendered. The troops were never prosecuted. The shocked and infuriated American commanding officer ordered the citizens of Dachau to march through the camp to see its devastation so that they could never deny the evil that had existed among them. Forty camp staff were tried for war crimes, and 36 were sentenced to death. Rascher was executed on April 26, 1945, in unclear circumstances.

Becker-Freyseng was a defendant at the Nuremberg Doctors' Trial, where he was found guilty of war crimes and crimes against humanity even though he had earlier been recruited to work with the U.S. Army Air Forces.

Norbert C. Brockman

DOCTORS' TRIAL

Some of the perpetrators of the Nazi medical experiments were put on trial in 1946 in Nuremberg, Germany. The evidence of the Nazis' crimes against humanity led to the conviction of most of the 23 defendants and the establishment of a code of medical ethics.

During the years that the Nazis were in power in Germany, some German physicians participated in crimes against humanity in the form of pseudoscientific and often torturous and murderous medical experiments on prisoners in concentration camps. In total, as a result of the Holocaust and the Nazi regime, millions of people were killed who the Nazis thought were not worthy of life.

A trial of the Nazi physicians and administrators took place between December 9, 1946, and August 20, 1947. This was the first of 12 war crimes trials that the U.S. authorities held in their occupation zone in Nuremberg, Germany. Known officially as *United States of America v. Karl Brandt, et al.*, the Doctors' Trial was conducted by a U.S. military court. Twenty-three Nazi German defendants, 20 of whom were physicians, were charged with conspiracy to commit crimes; actual war crimes, including mass murder and torture of both prisoners of war and German citizens; and membership in a criminal organization. Some of the crimes involved Nazi medical experimentation that took place in concentration and death camps.

The judges were Walter Beals, Harold Sebrig, and John T Crawford. The prosecutors were Telford Taylor and James McHaney.

During the trial, which lasted almost 140 days, 84 witnesses gave testimony, and almost 1,500 documents were submitted describing mass murders of the mentally and physically unfit during the early years of the Nazi era and heinous medical experiments conducted at Nazi concentration and death camps.

The defense counsel (mostly German attorneys) presented several arguments to justify the doctors' actions: the doctors were forced to carry out orders; there was no international code of ethics, and therefore the entire trial was inappropriate; the subjects would have been executed anyway; the experiments would save other people from suffering; in some cases, the doctors were not even aware of the suffering; and in other cases, the doctor intended to sabotage the work of other Nazis. The defense also argued that the German doctors were not alone in their experimentation on prisoners and that other countries did it as well. An American medical expert, Andrew Ivy, testified that in experiments involving American prisoners, such as the malaria experiments at Stateville Penitentiary, the prisoners were voluntary subjects who gave full consent. Ivy actually misled the court by suggesting that an American code of ethics had already been debated and issued, when such was not the case at the time.

None of the defendants admitted guilt or expressed any remorse. Seven were acquitted, seven were hanged, and the rest were sent to prison for varying lengths of time. The defendants and their eventual sentence are as follows: Hermann Becker-Freyseng (20 years in prison, lowered to 10, released in 1952); Wilhelm Beiglböck (15 years in prison, lowered to 10); Kurt Blome (acquitted); Victor Brack (hanged); Karl Brandt (hanged); Rudolf Brandt (hanged); Fritz Fischer (life in prison, lowered to 15 years, released in 1954); Karl Gebhardt (hanged); Karl Genzken (life in prison, lowered to 20 years, released in 1954); Siegfried Handloser (life in prison, lowered to 20 years, released in 1954); Waldemar Hoven (hanged); Joachim Mrugowsky (hanged); Herta Oberheuser (20 years in prison, lowered to 10 years, released in 1952); Adolf Pokorny (acquitted); Helmut Poppendick (10 years in prison, released in 1951); Hans Wolfgang Romberg (acquitted); Gerhard Rose (life in prison, lowered to 20 years, released in 1955); Paul Rostock (acquitted); Siegfried Ruff (acquitted); Konrad Schäfer (acquitted); Oskar Schröder (life in prison, lowered to 15 years, released in 1954); Wolfram Sievers (hanged); and Georg August Weltz (acquitted). The three who were not physicians were Victor Brack (SS colonel); Rudolf Brandt (personal administrative officer to Heinrich Himmler, head of the SS); and Wolfram Sievers (SS colonel and director of the Institute for Military Scientific Research). There was only one woman, Herta Oberheuser.

One of the outcomes of this trial was the Nuremberg Code, a list of 10 principles applying to human experimentation.

Frances R. Frankenburg

HOFMANN, ALBERT

During World War II, chemist Albert Hofmann accidentally discovered the hallucinogenic effects of lysergic acid diethylamide (LSD)—the 1960s counterculture drug—while working in a sober Swiss pharmaceutical company research laboratory. A series of self-experiments with LSD confirmed the surprising mind-altering properties of this fungus-derived molecule.

Albert Hofmann (1906–2008) was born in Baden, Switzerland. After finishing his chemistry studies at the University of Zurich in 1929, he joined the Sandoz Company pharmaceutical research laboratory in Basel. At that time, the head of the laboratory, Arthur Stoll (1887–1971), was working on the identification and isolation of biological substances that had medical effects, such as the foxglove plant (that produces digitalis); Mediterranean squill (that produces cardiac glycosides); and *Claviceps purpurae*, a fungal parasite that afflicts rye plants, particularly in cold, damp weather. *Claviceps* can produce an "ergot," a dark purplish sclerotium or hard mass of mycelium that replaces the grain of the rye plant. Midwives and doctors had been using ergot extracts to stop postchildbirth bleeding and diminish the pain of migraine headaches. But in the wrong dosage, ergot can be poisonous, leading to hallucinations, gangrene, and convulsions. Ergot poisoning, for example, may have been involved in the set of painful symptoms known as St. Anthony's Fire, a disease that occurred in the Middle Ages, and it has been implicated in the events surrounding the suspected witchcraft in Salem, Massachusetts, between 1692 and 1693.

In 1918, Stoll isolated ergotamine, the first ergot alkaloid. Later, in the early 1930s, scientists at the Rockefeller Institute of New York isolated and characterized the nucleus common to all ergot alkaloids, lysergic acid. Other researchers showed that the compound in ergot that stopped bleeding, ergobasine, when broken down, yielded lysergic acid and propanolamine.

Hofmann produced a new series of lysergic acid compounds he hoped would have useful or interesting pharmacological properties. In 1938, he produced the 25th substance in this series of derivatives—lysergic acid diethylamide, abbreviated to LSD-25, or, as the years went by, simply LSD. He paid little attention to it at the time.

Five years later, he returned to LSD-25. On April 16, 1943, after some hours of working in his laboratory, he became restless and dizzy and went home. There he experienced two hours of "an uninterrupted stream of fantastic pictures, extraordinary shapes with intense kaleidoscopic play of colors."[1] He guessed, correctly, that this experience might have been due to an accidental exposure to LSD.

Three days later, on April 19, he deliberately took 250 micrograms of LSD. This self-experiment has become one of the most famous in history. Once again, he experienced distortions in his perception. He wrote that "kaleidoscopic, fantastic images surged in on me, alternating, variegated, opening and then closing themselves in circles and spirals, exploding in colored fountains, rearranging and hybridizing themselves in constant flux."[2] His superiors at Sandoz were amazed that such small quantities of the drug could have powerful effects and tried it themselves, with similar results. As is now well-known, LSD is a powerful mind-altering molecule.

Hofmann continued his work. He became interested in "magic mushrooms" and in the late 1950s was the first to synthesize psilocybin, the active agent of these mushrooms. He later studied the morning glory seeds that were used by the Mazatec people (indigenous inhabitants of southern Mexico) to induce visions. He discovered that the substance responsible for the morning glory–induced hallucinations was actually an ergot alkaloid, hitherto only known to be produced by fungi.

It is remarkable that, during the chaos of World War II, Swiss scientists investigating and experimenting with a cereal fungus would have produced the prototypical drug of the 1960s counterculture movement.

Frances R. Frankenburg

References
1. Hofmann, "LSD—My Problem Child."
2. Ibid.

MENGELE, JOSEF

Josef Mengele was a German physician who experimented on concentration camp inmates. His activities epitomized the cruelty of the Nazi physicians.

Josef Mengele (1911–1979) was born in 1911, in Gunzburg, Bavaria. He began studying medicine in 1930, with a special interest in anthropology and genetics, and obtained his medical degree in 1938. He also joined Germany's National Socialist Party led by Adolf Hitler. Mengele became a research assistant at an institute for heredity and racial purity at Frankfurt University and joined the elite Schutzstaffel (SS) within the National Socialist Party. In 1940, he volunteered for the German army and took part in the invasion of the Soviet Union before an injury rendered him unfit for military service.

In May 1943, Mengele voluntarily became the senior physician in the women's section of the Auschwitz concentration camp. One of his duties was to examine arriving prisoners and decide whether they were to be sent to the gas chambers or to forced labor. This was known as "making selections." A number of the prisoners also became the subjects of Mengele's medical experiments. Auschwitz provided him with many research subjects, especially Roma (Gypsies), deformed people, and twins. Mengele's particular interest was twin research, reflecting his interest in genetics. He experimented on almost 1,500 pairs of twins, many as young as 9 or 10. Mengele's crude surgery included blood transfusions, attempts to change eye color, amputations, and deliberate infections.

Mengele exemplified many of the paradoxes found among the Nazi physicians. He was reported to always be immaculate in his personal appearance, to be devoted to his research, and to often be whistling airs from classical music. At times, he could be charming and was well regarded by his superiors. But survivors of Auschwitz described him as a person who coldly tortured people and sent others to their deaths in a casual, almost amused manner. He became known as the "Angel of Death."

Mengele continued his experiments until the advance of the Red Army forced him to leave Auschwitz on January 17, 1945. U.S. forces captured him, but he managed to escape, despite being listed as a war criminal. He returned to Gunzburg and, in 1948, with financial assistance provided by his family, was able to travel to and settle in Argentina under an assumed name. In 1956, Mengele returned to Germany and married for a second time. In 1961, he fled to Paraguay. Fearing capture in Paraguay, he fled again in 1978, this time to Brazil. He died in 1979.

Martin Moll

MINNESOTA STARVATION EXPERIMENT

Ancel Keys is known for his invention of nonperishable rations (known as K-rations), which were widely used in World War II, as well as his observational Seven Countries Study, in which he showed the benefits of what we now know as the Mediterranean diet. Toward the end of World War II, he directed a study of semistarvation using conscientious objectors as research subjects, with the goals of increasing the understanding of the effects of semistarvation and understanding how best to refeed civilians who had experienced starvation during the war.

Ancel Keys (1904–2004) was a physiologist who earned a PhD in oceanography and biology from the Scripps Institute in California and then another PhD in physiology from King's College at the University of Cambridge. While studying at the Harvard Fatigue Laboratory in 1935, he led a group of 10 men as part of the International High Altitude Expedition to study the effect of extreme climates on human physiology. The small group traveled to a small miners' village named 'Quilcha in the Chilean Andes. For six months, they assessed their own adaptation to hypoxia, low barometric pressure, and cold. In 1939, he moved to Minnesota and established the Laboratory of Physiological Hygiene at the University of Minnesota School of Public Health and was its director for 33 years.

During World War II, he developed nonperishable rations for paratroopers that were small enough to fit into an army jacket pocket. General George S. Patton learned about them, and as a result, they were eventually used throughout the military, becoming known as K-rations.

As World War II ended, millions of civilians and soldiers were facing starvation, so Keys organized a project in which he could systematically study the effects of starvation in isolation from the other problems that were affecting civilians in Europe. He also assessed the best ways of feeding people who had experienced starvation. This time, he did not use himself or his colleagues. Instead, he recruited 36 conscientious objectors, all screened for physical and mental health, from the Civilian Public Service (CPS) and the Selective Service System. The subjects were single men between the ages of 20 and 33. Fifteen were members of the three historic peace churches: Brethren, Friends (Quakers), or Mennonite. Many had been doing menial and unpaid work in CPS camps and were eager to participate in a project that would help others.

From November 1944 to October 1945, they participated in Keys's study of human starvation at the University of Minnesota. The study took place underneath the university's football stadium, where there was a dormitory, laboratory, and office space and a kitchen. The volunteers were fully informed of all the procedures at the beginning of and throughout the trial. Careful physical examinations were done both before and during the study: their weight was followed carefully, as was their ability to lift weights or run on a treadmill. Bloodwork was performed, and the quality of their semen was examined. Their hearing, vision, fitness, and mental acuity were also regularly evaluated.

During the first 12 weeks, they ate 3,200 calories a day. In the next 24 weeks, or the semistarvation phase, they were fed about 1,600 calories a day, enough to lead to a loss of a quarter of their body weight. Keys fed them what was available in Europe at the end of the war: potatoes, rutabagas, turnips, cabbage, bread, and macaroni. In the 12 weeks that followed the semistarvation phase, he experimented with a number of restricted rehabilitation diets in which men received different amounts of food. In the final 8 weeks they were allowed to eat whatever they wanted. At all phases, the men were encouraged to work and to be physically active. Some took classes at the university; one volunteer taught French to others. They were asked to walk about 22 miles a week.

While their caloric intake was being restricted, Keys noted a range of physical changes. The subjects' temperatures, respiratory rates, and heart rates all fell. Their ankles, knees, and faces became edematous, or swollen. They complained of feeling cold, dizzy, and tired. Their hair fell out. Their muscular strength and endurance decreased, but their hearing improved.

The men experienced psychological changes as well. They became depressed and lost interest in outside events or sexual activity. They reported a sense of loss of concentration and intellectual ability, although there was no change in their performance on intelligence tests. They stopped attending or teaching classes. Four men withdrew from the experiment. Unable to cope with the incessant hunger, three cheated and ate additional food. After the first incident, Keys established a "buddy system" in which none of the participants were allowed to leave the study area alone. One subject developed hematuria (blood in his urine) and had to leave the study. Another cut off three of his fingers while chopping wood; whether this was accidental is difficult to determine, but he was allowed to continue participating in the study.

Keys and his colleagues discovered that to recover from starvation the men needed about 4,000 calories a day, about 800 more calories than they were consuming during the first 12 weeks. What's more, he found that vitamin and protein supplements were not helpful in recovery, and for many months after the experiment ended, the men reported feeling persistent hunger. There were no obvious long-term deleterious health effects from the study.

To help in the refeeding of European civilians, Keys and his colleagues released the results from the study in the form of two pamphlets as quickly as they could. In *Experimental Starvation in Man*, a 48-page pamphlet published in October 1945, before the study was even finished, he described his work, but he could not yet give practical advice. A few months later, in January 1946, two of his colleagues, both conscientious objectors and psychologists, Harold Guetzkow (1915–2008) and Paul Bowman (1914–2008), published a 72-page pamphlet titled *Men and Hunger: A Psychological Manual for Relief Workers*. In it, they emphasized how psychologically difficult it was for starving people to stand in line or to have to witness strength and vitality in others. Eventually, Keys and his colleagues published a two-volume book called *The Biology of Human Starvation* in 1950. It emphasized the importance of providing abundant calories to those who had been starved. Keys also noted that it would be impossible to inculcate ideas of democracy among people who were still suffering from the effects of starvation because of their overwhelming preoccupation with food.

In this book, Keys remarked that many of the psychological changes that he observed could also be useful in understanding some of the symptoms of anorexia nervosa, the disorder in which people deliberately restrict their caloric intake. People with anorexia are commonly preoccupied with food. Indeed, Keys reported that the subjects of his experiment also became increasingly interested in recipes, cooking, and food as the experiment progressed. After the study ended, three former subjects even became chefs.

After the war, his interest in nutrition continued, but in a different direction. He noticed that in many European countries, where food supplies were limited, heart attacks seemed rare. At the same time, by reviewing obituaries, he saw that many Minnesotan businessmen, presumably eating well, seemed to die prematurely of heart attacks. Keys became interested in the connection between cholesterol and heart disease and studied this in the Hastings Insane Asylum. (Little more is known about this.) There he put some subjects on low-fat diets and compared them to subjects eating an equal number of calories but more fat. Compared to other subjects, the serum cholesterol of those eating the low-fat diet fell.

In 1947, Keys began a 40-year-long study of 286 Minneapolis businessmen in which he found links between smoking, high blood pressure, serum cholesterol, and heart attacks. Then, in 1958, he began the well-known Seven Countries Study (SCS), which established the value of what has come to be known as the Mediterranean diet. In this prospective epidemiological study of diet in 16 cohorts, comprising nearly 13,000 men in the United States, Italy, Greece, Yugoslavia, Finland, the Netherlands, and Japan, he found that people living in countries where there was a diet low in animal or saturated fats and high in fresh vegetables, fruit, and nonfat milk products had fewer cardiac problems. He showed that the amount of saturated fat in the diet is associated with the blood levels of cholesterol. In Finland, for example, he noticed that farmers and woodcutters were often of normal weight and seemingly fit. But they had high levels of animal fat in their diet and correspondingly high levels of serum cholesterol and heart disease. (He colorfully described them as buttering their cheese.)

Keys followed the findings of his experiments and observations by eating a Mediterranean diet himself. In their later years, he and his wife lived part-time in Pioppi, an Italian seaside village 100 miles south of Naples. He died at the age of 100. The SCS has been criticized for its methodological shortcomings, but the Mediterranean diet continues to be promoted by many nutritionists and physicians.

Keys's book about starvation remains a classic because of its thoroughness and also because it is unlikely that the experiment will ever be repeated. Although the subjects all volunteered and gave informed consent, the conditions under which they volunteered were highly unusual. Many of the conscientious objectors were unhappy with the menial duties that they had been assigned in CPS camps. Some felt guilty or embarrassed that they were not contributing to the war effort, but they were aware of the scientific and humanitarian value of the study and were proud to be able to participate.

Frances R. Frankenburg

NUREMBERG CODE

The Nuremberg Code is a code of medical ethics developed as a result of the Doctors' Trial.

Between December 1946 and August 1947, the American authorities at Nuremberg tried 23 participants in the Nazi human experiments in what has become known as the Doctors' Trial. It was the first of 12 war crimes trials.

In May 1947, Dr. Leo Alexander, an American physician who was acting as a medical adviser to prosecutors at the Doctors' Trial, submitted to the court six principles he believed should govern all future medical research. On the day the Doctors' Trial ended, the judges, in their verdict, added four more principles to Alexander's six. The resulting Nuremberg Code was one of the first documents that prescribed the norms of medical research involving human subjects.

The first principle of the Nuremberg Code, and the longest, begins by saying that "the voluntary consent of the human subject is absolutely essential." The rest of the code, in brief, holds that those conducting the research must take all precautions to minimize or mitigate pain or injury to participants; researchers must be willing to stop or interrupt experiments when participants appear to be in danger or pain; participants themselves must be able to opt out of an experiment if they believe it necessary; experiments must be structured to yield tangible results with wide applications; experiments must not be random or unnecessary; experiments must be conducted only by qualified scientists and physicians; and all experiments must be structured so that no permanent harm is inflicted on participants.

Many nations subsequently adopted the Nuremberg Code to guide their own medical experiments, and the June 1964 Helsinki Declaration, which was based on the code, codified the principles for the international medical community. The Helsinki Declaration was written by the World Medical Association (WMA) and has been continually revised over the years.

Paul G. Pierpaoli Jr.

NUTRITION RESEARCH IN CANADA'S ABORIGINAL COMMUNITIES

Between 1942 and 1952, Canadian researchers performed nutrition experiments on malnourished aboriginal populations in Manitoba and at six residential schools. The researchers used at least 1,300 aboriginal people—most of them children—as subjects to investigate the effectiveness of vitamin supplements. In some cases, the people were intentionally fed poor diets.

In the 1940s, aboriginal populations in Canada were malnourished and ill. This was due to a number of factors, including residual effects of the Great Depression, the weakening of the fur trade, and the decrease in relief provided by the Canadian federal government.

In 1942 a group of medical experts traveled to the aboriginal communities in Northern Manitoba to document the high rates of malnutrition. This work was sponsored by the Canadian Indian Affairs department, the New York–based Milbank Memorial Fund, the Royal Canadian Air Force (RCAF), and the Hudson's Bay Company. One of the RCAF physicians was Frederick Tisdall (1893–1949), Canada's leading nutrition expert and coinventor of Pablum, a processed cereal for infants that was nutritious and easily prepared and digested. The researchers linked the malnutrition to a tuberculosis epidemic and cases of blindness in Norway House, a large Cree community in northern Manitoba. At the time, researchers calculated the local people were living on fewer than 1,500 calories a day. Normal, healthy adults generally require at least 2,000 calories.

As part of their work, the researchers studied 300 malnourished aboriginal people. They gave nutritional supplements—including riboflavin, thiamine, or ascorbic acid—to 125 of the subjects and considered the other 175 as controls.

None of the Cree subjects were informed that they were participating in the two-year study. No results of that study are available.

In 1947, plans were developed for research on about 1,000 aboriginal children in six residential schools in British Columbia, Ontario, Nova Scotia, and Alberta. This research was led by federal nutrition expert Lionel Pett (1909–2003), who had already carried out surveys on nutrition in low-income communities in Edmonton.

In a school in Port Alberni, British Columbia, the children received 8 ounces of milk a day for two years, although the recommended amount was more than twice that amount. The goal was to get a baseline reading for when the allowance was increased to 24 ounces. At another school, children were divided into one group that received vitamin, iron, and iodine supplements and one that received no supplements.

One school reduced amounts of vitamin B_1 to create another baseline before levels were boosted. A special enriched flour that could not be legally sold elsewhere in Canada under food adulteration laws (the flour contained bone meal) was provided to children at another school. At St. Paul's Residential School in southern Alberta, the children's poor diet was maintained so that they could serve as controls. During that time, dental services were withdrawn from schools participating in the study because dental caries and gingivitis are indicators of dietary problems, and the researchers did not want dental treatment distorting their results.

The researchers studied nutritional deficiencies without consulting or getting consent from any of the people involved or, in the case of the children, their parents. They made no attempt to improve the nutrition of people already suffering ill effects from their inadequate diets, and in some cases, they deliberately maintained or worsened the poor diets and dental care of those involved. As far as is known, these studies did not lead to a better understanding of the effects of malnutrition or vitamin deficiency, nor did they lead to improved nutrition for Canada's aboriginal people.

Frances R. Frankenburg

OBERHEUSER, HERTA

Herta Oberheuser was a German medical doctor who conducted cruel and sadistic medical experimentation on concentration camp inmates.

Herta Oberheuser (1911–1978) was born in 1911 in Cologne and received her medical degree in Bonn in 1937, with a specialty in dermatology. Following the completion of her medical training, the 26-year-old Oberheuser joined the Nazi Party as an intern and later as a physician for the League of German Maidens. By 1940, Oberheuser had been assigned as assistant physician to Karl Gebhardt, chief surgeon of the Schutzstaffel (SS) and personal physician to Reichsführer SS Heinrich Himmler.

The May 27, 1942, assassination of German security police chief Reinhard Heydrich, who died because of infections sustained in the attack on him, led to the establishment of a branch of the Hohenlychen Sanatorium close to the Ravensbrueck concentration camp where infections could be studied. Gebhardt and Oberheuser used the camp's inmates as subjects for their medical experiments.

On July 27, 1942, 75 women at Ravensbrueck were ordered to the commandant's headquarters. Oberheuser examined the women and evaluated their suitability for the experiments. Those chosen had their legs cut and bacteria placed in the wounds. The subsequent infections were then treated with new sulfonamide drugs. All of the experiments were conducted without the subjects' consent.

The results of the initial experiments were disappointing because they failed to replicate actual combat injuries. Later experiments sought to correct this. Inmates were subjected to gunshot wounds infected with dirt and foreign material; they also endured severed muscles and broken bones. Wounds were then injected with bacteria, causing gas gangrene and tetanus. Prisoners who survived these experiments were often crippled for life.

Oberheuser also conducted experiments involving bone and muscle transplantation. She also oversaw the transfer of inmates to the Hohenlychen Sanatorium, where unnecessary amputations and transplants were conducted. The goal of these experiments was to provide "spare parts" for wounded German soldiers. Once a subject's usefulness had passed, Oberheuser killed the person with injections of gasoline. She is also reported to have removed limbs and organs from children while they were still alive.

Following the end of the war, Oberheuser was the only woman to stand trial at the Nuremberg Doctors' Trial. On August 20, 1947, she was found guilty for her part in conducting human experimentation at Ravensbrueck and at Hohenlychen. Originally sentenced to 20 years, her sentence was later reduced to 10 years. However, she ended up only serving 5 years and was released in 1952. She returned to practice as a doctor, establishing a family medical practice in Stocksee, Germany. In 1958, her medical license was revoked after she was recognized by a former Ravensbrueck inmate. Oberheuser died in 1978, in Linz am Rhein, West Germany.

Robert W. Malick

RAVENSBRUECK

Located outside of Berlin, Ravensbrueck was a Nazi concentration camp for women where medical experimentation took place.

The Ravensbrueck concentration camp was located 56 miles north of Berlin, Germany, on swampy land near the Havel River. On May 15, 1939, the first prisoners arrived, 867 women transferred from the Lichtenburg camp. Ravensbrueck was staffed by 150 female Schutzstaffel (SS) supervisors (Aufseherinnen), male guards, and male administrators. In 1942 and 1943, the camp served as a training base for women supervisors, and 3,500 women were trained there for work in Ravensbrueck and other camps.

In late 1939, the camp held 2,000 prisoners. By late 1942, there were 10,800, and by 1944, the main camp contained 26,700 female prisoners and several thousand female minors grouped in a detention camp for children. Most of the camp was evacuated in March 1945 as the Russians approached, and 24,500 prisoners were marched into Mechlenburg. When Ravensbrueck was liberated by Soviet troops on April 29 and 30, they found 3,500 ill and famished females.

Over the course of its existence, at least 107,000 women were interned in Ravensbrueck and its satellite detention centers, most of which were industrial slave-labor sites. Approximately 50,000 inmates died while imprisoned there due to overwork, exposure, malnutrition, disease, and abuse.

Medical experimentation began at Ravensbrueck in 1942. It included deliberate mutilation and infections to test sulfonamide antibiotics. Bone and muscle were removed from women, usually with no anesthetic agents, to allow the study of regeneration of bone, muscle, and nerves. Limbs were removed. One of the goals of the experiments was to be able to replace limbs or other body parts for wounded German soldiers.

Two of the Nazi physicians who worked at Ravensbrueck were Carl Clauberg (1898–1957) and Herta Oberheuser (1911–1978). Clauberg was a Nazi physician who experimented in Block 10 at Auschwitz, Ravensbrueck, and Dachau to try to find cheap and efficient ways of sterilizing women. At Ravensbrueck, he sterilized over a hundred Roma (Gypsy) women. He was captured by the Soviet Union, put on trial, sentenced to 25 years, and then released and returned to West Germany. He was rearrested in 1955 but died in 1957 before his second trial.

Oberheuser, the only female physician to be tried at the Nuremberg Doctors' Trial, worked at the Ravensbrueck concentration camp from 1940 to 1943, where she inflicted wounds on adults and then contaminated them. She operated on children without anesthesia and killed them. She was convicted, received a 20-year sentence, and was released early in 1952 after only 5 years in prison. She practiced medicine in Germany for the next 6 years until a former prisoner at Ravensbrueck recognized her. Her license to practice medicine was then revoked.

Ravensbrueck is infamous now for the brutality of the slave labor and experimentation and the involvement of so many women as both the victims and the perpetrators of the atrocities.

Bernard A. Cook

STATEVILLE PENITENTIARY MALARIA EXPERIMENTS

In the 1940s, researchers from the University of Chicago used prisoners at Stateville Penitentiary and patients at a nearby psychiatric hospital as subjects in malaria experiments. At the Nuremberg Doctors' Trial, in an attempt to justify the Nazi physicians' actions, it was argued that what had been done in the concentration camps was similar to these American experiments.

Experimental research in malaria requires the participation of human subjects because there are no good animal models. Beginning in 1944, the University of Chicago and the U.S. Army organized a series of experiments to investigate the illness in a clinical research unit at the Stateville Penitentiary, located about 30 miles from Chicago. Alf S. Alving, a nephrologist who was newly interested in malaria, directed the project. The researchers liked the idea of using prisoners at Stateville because the inmates were young and healthy. They also were captive, and so could be easily controlled and followed, which was ideal for this kind of study. Some of the prisoners said that they were pleased to help in the war effort.

Alving and his colleagues wanted to test the efficacy and toxicity of antimalarial medications. Over 400 prisoners provided blood for the anopheles mosquitoes that are vectors for *Plasmodia*, the parasites that cause malaria. Other prisoners worked as technicians for the experiment. In the first studies, all of the subjects were white males who were expected to be in Stateville for at least 18 months. (Black Americans were not included because of genetic differences in their response to the two most common types of malaria, falciparum and vivax. In particular, black Americans who carry the sickle cell trait are less susceptible to falciparum malaria, and those with a particular blood group known as Duffy negative are more resistant to vivax malaria.) Researchers explained the purpose of the studies to the prisoners, and they signed consent forms, which read in part, "I assume all the risks of this experiment and declare that I absolve the University of Chicago and all the technicians and researchers who take part in the experiment, as well as the government of Illinois, the directory of the State penitentiary and every other official, even as concerns my heirs and representatives, of any responsibility."[1] Many of the men hoped that by volunteering their sentences would be shortened, although this was not promised to them.

In most instances, the prisoners were exposed to malaria via bites from infected mosquitoes. But in a few cases, mosquitoes were killed, and their salivary glands, containing *Plasmodia* parasites, were dissected, cut up, and suspended in a solution that was then injected into the prisoners' veins, under their skin, or into their lymph nodes. After they became ill, they received experimental treatments in the form of chloroquine, which Alving was studying at the time. (Chloroquine was an antimalarial drug that German chemists in the 1930s had researched and rejected as being too toxic. The Americans, who had earlier tested the molecule without realizing its potential, began new tests on it toward the end of World War II.) Alving found that the Stateville convicts tolerated and responded to it when it was administered once a week at low doses.

In a separate incident, a strain of *Plasmodium vivax*, one of the parasites that causes malaria, was isolated from a patient who was thought to have become ill with malaria in New Guinea. This strain of malaria, known as the Chesson strain, was difficult to treat and was maintained by infecting psychotic patients at the Manteno State Hospital in Manteno, Illinois, with the parasite.

In contrast to many other wartime studies, the experiments at Stateville were well publicized. In the June 1945 issue of *Life* magazine, the prisoners were described as voluntary subjects who were proud to be contributing to the war effort. Nathan Leopold (1904–1971)—an infamous prisoner who, along with Richard Loeb (1905–1936), murdered 14-year-old Bobby Franks in 1924—was pleased with his participation and even wrote about the experience in detail in his autobiography, *Life Plus 99 Years*.

The publicity, however, had an unexpected outcome in Germany. At the 1946 Doctors' Trial at Nuremberg, in an attempt to show that there was no internationally recognized code of ethics related to medical research, the defenders of the Nazi physicians compared the American use of prisoners at Stateville to the German doctors' experimentation on prisoners in the concentration camps.

In Germany, Claus Schilling (1871–1946), a physician who at one point had worked at the Rockefeller Foundation in Berlin and who had a lifelong interest in tropical diseases, had been testing antimalaria vaccines in psychiatric patients in Italy beginning in the 1920s. At first, he gave malaria to patients already ill with neurosyphilis as a form of therapy, but then he infected patients no matter what their diagnosis so that he could see the effects of malaria. He then continued his work at the Dachau concentration camp, where he carried out malaria experiments on about 1,200 inmates between 1941 and 1945. This work consisted of infecting people with malaria and testing synthetic antimalarial drugs in high and sometimes lethal doses.

Other similar experiments were carried out in the Buchenwald camp. German physician and expert in tropical medicine Gerhard Rose (1896–1992) also tested antimalarial drugs on mentally ill Russian prisoners of war in a psychiatric clinic in Thuringia, which is located in central Germany. After the Americans liberated Dachau, Schilling was put on trial there for his role in these experiments. He was found guilty of committing war crimes and hanged.

Subsequently, the lawyers who defended the 23 Nazis at the better-known Doctors' Trial at Nuremberg compared the medical research done on malaria in the German concentration camps to that done by Americans in prisons, in an attempt to show that there was no internationally recognized code of ethics related to medical research. (Rose was tried at the Doctors' Trial and sentenced to life in prison but released in 1955).

Andrew Ivy (1893–1978), one of the physicians testifying for the prosecution at the Doctors' Trial, testified that the comparison was baseless because the Stateville prisoners volunteered and gave written informed consent. Ivy also told the court that he had chaired the committee appointed by Illinois governor Dwight Green to consider the conditions under which prisoners could be used ethically as subjects in the medical experiments. However, the committee had not actually been formed until after the war, and it had never met. The lawyers defending the Nazis asked Ivy if the committee had been formed because of the Nuremberg trials, and he replied that it had not. Commentators described Ivy's response as "flirting with perjury."[2] Eventually, the committee did actually meet and generate a report supporting the ethical nature of the wartime research on Illinois prisoners.

Alving continued working after World War II to find better treatments for soldiers suffering from malaria in Korea and Vietnam. He tested a new antimalarial drug, primaquine, unusual in its broad spectrum of activity. It eliminates the *Plasmodia* parasites from the liver and can also be used prophylactically. However, about 10 percent of black Americans treated with primaquine developed a dangerous hemolytic anemia. Alving discovered that the hemolytic anemia was caused by glucose-6-phosphate dehydrogenase deficiency, the most common enzyme pathology, which is more common in black Americans than other groups. This discovery led to a new field in pharmacology—pharmacogenetics.

Frances R. Frankenburg

References
1.   Harcourt, "Making Willing Bodies."
2.   Harkness, "Nuremberg and the Issue of Wartime Experiments," 1,674.

UNIT 731

Unit 731 was the name for the Japanese army's secret biological warfare units. Between 1936 and 1945, medical experimentation of the cruelest nature took place in these units.

Lieutenant Colonel Shirō Ishii (sometimes referred to as Ishii Shiro) (1892–1951) established Unit 731, officially known as the Epidemic Prevention and Water Purification Bureau in Harbin, Manchuria, in 1936. Most of Unit 731's work took place in a 150-building complex called Ping Fan, about 14 miles from Harbin. Smaller units were located in Nanking, Beijing, Guangzhou, and Singapore. As part of Unit 731, up to 20,000 medical and scientific personnel experimented on prisoners and produced and spread bacteria that caused anthrax, bubonic plague, cholera, dysentery, tetanus, typhoid, typhus, and other infectious diseases.

To develop methods to disperse biological agents and enhance their effectiveness, Unit 731 infected prisoners of war. Unit personnel referred to the prisoners—mostly Chinese, Koreans, and Soviets—as *maruta* (logs) because the Japanese had told the local Chinese that the Unit 731 facility was a lumber mill. American, British, and Australian prisoners were also used as human guinea pigs. After infecting a prisoner, researchers might then cut open his body, sometimes while he was still alive, to determine the effects of the disease. No anesthetics were employed, as these might have affected the results. Medical researchers also confined infected prisoners with healthy ones to determine how rapidly diseases spread.

In addition, Unit 731's doctors conducted experiments on compression and decompression and the effects of extreme cold on the body, subjecting prisoners' limbs to ice water and then amputating them. Up to 10,000 prisoners died in these experiments.

The Japanese army also repeatedly conducted field tests using biological warfare against Chinese villages. Japanese aircraft spread plague-infected fleas over Ningbo (Ningpo) in Zhejiang (Chekiang) Province in eastern China in October

1940. Japanese troops also dropped cholera and typhoid cultures into wells and ponds. In 1942, germ-warfare units deployed dysentery, cholera, and typhoid in Zhejiang Province. Smallpox was spread as well. Although the exact numbers are impossible to determine, some researchers estimate that over 400,000 Chinese civilians were killed by Japanese germ warfare.

At the end of the Pacific War, Ishii and other researchers escaped to Japan. They left behind their laboratory equipment as well as plague-infected mice that produced outbreaks of the disease in the Harbin area between 1946 and 1948. No prisoners survived.

After the Japanese surrender, the United States did not bring Ishii and his colleagues before the International Military Tribunal for the Far East (the Tokyo War Crimes Trials) for their crimes. Instead, they were granted immunity in exchange for providing information on the experiments to U.S. authorities, which Washington considered invaluable in its own biological warfare program. The Soviet government did prosecute 12 members of the unit at Khabarovsk in December 1949, all of whom admitted their crimes. They were convicted and received sentences ranging from 2 to 25 years in a labor camp.

Many of the Japanese physicians who worked in Unit 731 went on to have prestigious roles in universities and the newly established Japanese National Institute of Health.

Kotani Ken

DOCUMENTS

THE ACTIVITIES OF UNIT 731 (1942)

Frank James, an American prisoner of war (POW), describes three horrifying encounters with Unit 731. The caliper-measurements of the POWs and the interrogation about their ethnic background is of course reminiscent of the Nazis' fascination with ethnicity, as displayed by many "researchers" associated with the Kaiser Wilhelm Institute of Anthropology, Human Heredity, and Eugenics. The Nazis believed in the racial superiority of the Aryans, and in a similar way the Japanese considered themselves superior to non-Asians and non-Japanese Asians. The United States government did cover up Japan's human experiments as is claimed here. General Douglas MacArthur, Supreme Allied Commander in Japan, with the support of the Joint Chiefs of Staff protected Japanese scientists from war-crimes prosecution in exchange for information about biological weapons. Although not clear from this passage, most of the victims of Unit 731 were Chinese soldiers and civilians.

Testimony of Frank James
Committee on Veterans' Affairs
Subcommittee on Compensation, Pension, and Insurance
September 17, 1986

Mr. Chairman and distinguished members of this subcommittee, I thank you for this opportunity to speak on the subject of the use of American prisoners of war as guinea pigs for the purpose of biological warfare research by the Japanese Army Unit 731. I was one of the POWs captured by the Japanese armed forces after the fall of Bataan and Corregidor in the Philippines during the early part of 1942. Of the Americans captured, more than 1,000 were moved by ship in 1942 from the Philippines to Manchuria. This group was joined en route in Korea by some British and Australian soldiers captured in Singapore. These men were used as slave laborers, working from daybreak to darkness, 7 days a week, in the Japanese factories located in Mukden and Harbin, Manchuria.

Upon arrival at Mukden on November 11, 1942, we were met by a team of medical personnel wearing masks. They sprayed liquid into our faces and we were given injections. This group (Unit 731) left the camp and returned only two more times, to my knowledge.

The following three-month period after our arrival in Mukden, no medication was issued to the sick POWs. They were placed in four so-called hospital wards, with the worst cases placed in Ward 4, under the care of an Australian doctor, Major Brennan. Ward 4 had the highest death rate.

During this three- or four-month period in the winter of 1942, some 300 American POWs (or, captives, as they were regarded) had died, out of the original group that left Pusan.

Over 200 of the dead at Mukden were stored above ground in an old wooden building during the winter months. As spring approached, the bodies began to thaw, so burial details were organized to thaw out the permafrost on the ground and dig graves for the dead. A team of Japanese medical personnel (Unit 731) arrived with an autopsy table for taking specimens. The table was installed in the wooden building where the dead were stored and two POWS were selected to work with the team.

I was one of those two men.

Our duties were to lift the bodies off the tables the bodies that had been selected. These had been identified by a tag tied to the big toe, which listed the POW's number. The Japanese then opened the bodies (head, chest and stomach) and took out the desired specimens, which were placed into containers and marked with the POW's number. The specimens were taken away by the Japanese medical group.

Later, the group returned to Mukden again to perform what seemed to be psycho-physical and anatomical examinations on selected POWs. I was one of them.

The exams included the following: Upon entering the room, we were required to walk in footprints that had been painted on the floor, which led to a desk, at which a Japanese medical person sat. He observed us as we walked. We were also asked questions about our national origin and "American" was not accepted as an answer. It had to be "Scot," or "French" or "English" or whatever the ethnic background was. I remember being asked whether I was getting enough steak, and I answered, "What's that?"

The medical person also measured my head, shoulders, arms and legs with calipers, and asked many questions about the medical history of my family.

The impact of being used as a guinea pig for biological weapons testing may never be known unless the documents that Unit 731 turned over to the American Occupation Forces under General MacArthur—in exchange for immunity from prosecution at the War Crimes Tribunal—are released. Medical information pertaining to the health of each POW should be released to him, his doctor and the Veterans Administration.

In summation, Mr. Chairman, I appreciate the opportunity to be heard before this august body. I can assure you that I am as patriotic an American as can be found in our wonderful United States of America. I have always taught my daughters to be thankful that our founding fathers had the foresight to create a lasting nation, founded upon the common man and ensuring his personal rights, including the pursuit of happiness.

Yet the evidence I have given today might sound vindictive. That is not my purpose, although I admit to feeling anger about what I have learned since the war about the dealings of MacArthur and his staff on this matter.

I request that whatever documents pertaining to myself and other POWs, and the research into the immune system, be released. I am specifically desirous of obtaining the photograph taken of me by Unit 731, in early 1943. At that time, I had lost all body hair, weighed about 80 pounds and wore only a sweater. Above my head was a sign with my POW number—1294.

I have repeatedly attempted to get included in my VA health records the diseases from which I suffered during my time as a POW, but I always get the same answer from the Army or the VA: No medical evidence exists! So, by God, if there is documentation about the health of an American POW with the Mukden number of 1294, I want help to dig this information out. One thousand two hundred and forty-three days of my life are a void in the official medical records.

To this day, I can still see those half-frozen, half-thawed intestines of the bodies that the Japanese medical personnel opened on that autopsy table.

Thank you very much for this opportunity to speak.

Source: Treatment of American Prisoners of War in Manchuria: Hearing before the Subcommittee on Compensation, Pension, and Insurance of the Committee on Veterans' Affairs, House of Representatives, 99th Congress, 2nd sess., September 17, 1986 (Washington, D.C.: Government Printing Office, 1986).

THE NUREMBERG CODE (1948)

On December 9, 1946, an American military tribunal began criminal proceedings against 23 German physicians and administrators for their willing participation in war crimes and crimes against humanity. Among the charges were that German physicians experimented on thousands of concentration camp prisoners. The experiments were sadistic and often lethal, and the prisoners did not give their consent. The American judges and physicians who were present at the trial wrote the Nuremberg Code in 1948. This code was the first international document outlining the absolute importance of voluntary participation and informed consent. The influence of this code on global human-rights law and medical ethics has been immense.

Nuremberg Code
Directives for Human Experimentation

1. The voluntary consent of the human subject is absolutely essential.

   This means that the person involved should have legal capacity to give consent; should be so situated as to be able to exercise free power of choice, without the intervention of any element of force, fraud, deceit, duress, over-reaching, or other ulterior form of constraint or coercion; and should have sufficient knowledge and comprehension of the elements of the subject matter involved, as to enable him to make an understanding and enlightened decision. This latter element requires that, before the acceptance of an affirmative decision by the experimental subject, there should be made known to him the nature, duration, and purpose of the experiment; the method and means by which it is to be conducted; all inconveniences and hazards reasonably to be expected; and the effects upon his health or person, which may possibly come from his participation in the experiment.

   The duty and responsibility for ascertaining the quality of the consent rests upon each individual who initiates, directs or engages in the experiment. It is a personal duty and responsibility which may not be delegated to another with impunity.

2. The experiment should be such as to yield fruitful results for the good of society, unprocurable by other methods or means of study, and not random and unnecessary in nature.

3. The experiment should be so designed and based on the results of animal experimentation and a knowledge of the natural history of the disease or other problem under study, that the anticipated results will justify the performance of the experiment.

4. The experiment should be so conducted as to avoid all unnecessary physical and mental suffering and injury.

5. No experiment should be conducted, where there is an *a priori* reason to believe that death or disabling injury will occur; except, perhaps, in those experiments where the experimental physicians also serve as subjects.

6. The degree of risk to be taken should never exceed that determined by the humanitarian importance of the problem to be solved by the experiment.

7. Proper preparations should be made and adequate facilities provided to protect the experimental subject against even remote possibilities of injury, disability, or death.

8. The experiment should be conducted only by scientifically qualified persons. The highest degree of skill and care should be required through all stages of the experiment of those who conduct or engage in the experiment.

9. During the course of the experiment, the human subject should be at liberty to bring the experiment to an end, if he has reached the physical or mental state, where continuation of the experiment seemed to him to be impossible.

10. During the course of the experiment, the scientist in charge must be prepared to terminate the experiment at any stage, if he has probable cause to believe, in the exercise of the good faith, superior skill and careful judgement required of him, that a continuation of the experiment is likely to result in injury, disability, or death to the experimental subject.

Source: "Trials of War Criminals before the Nuremberg Military Tribunals under Control Council Law No. 10," vol. 2 (Washington, D.C.: U.S. Government Printing Office, 1949), 181–182.

Further Reading

Alving, A. S., B. Craige Jr, T. N. Pullman, C. M. Whorton, R. Jones Jr, and L. Eichelberger. 1948. "Procedures Used at Stateville Penitentiary for the Testing of Potential Antimalarial Agents." *Journal of Clinical Investigation* 27: 2–5.

Annas, George J., and Michael A. Grodin. 1992. *The Nazi Doctors and the Nuremberg Code: Human Rights in Human Experimentation*. New York: Oxford University Press.

Barenblatt, Daniel. 2004. *A Plague upon Humanity: The Secret Genocide of Axis Japan's Germ Warfare Operation*. New York: HarperCollins Publishers.

Berghoff, Robert S., Morris Fishbein, George Fox, Ralph Gallagher, Andrew C. Ivy, Kaywin Kennedy, and Oscar Mayer. 1948. "Ethics Governing the Service of Prisoners as Subjects in Medical Experiments. Report of a Committee Appointed by Governor Dwight H. Green of Illinois." *Journal of the American Medical Association* 136 (7) (February): 457–458.

Comfort, Nathaniel. 2009. "The Prisoner as Model Organism: Malaria Research at Stateville Penitentiary." *Studies in History and Philosophy of Biological and Biomedical Sciences* 40: 190–203. doi:10.1016/j.shpsc.2009.06.007.

Cope, Oliver. 1943. "Care of the Victims of the Cocoanut Grove Fire at the Massachusetts General Hospital." *New England Journal of Medicine* 229 (4): 138–147.

Emanuel, Ezekiel J. 2011. *The Oxford Textbook of Clinical Research Ethics*. Oxford: Oxford University Press.

Gold, Hal. 1996. *Unit 731: Testimony*. Tokyo: Yenbooks.

Harcourt, Bernard E. 2011. "Making Willing Bodies: Manufacturing Consent among Prisoners and Soldiers, Creating Human Subjects, Patriots, and Everyday Citizens—The University of Chicago Malaria Experiments on Prisoners at Stateville Penitentiary." Working Papers at Chicago Unbound. Last modified May 2011.

Harkness, John M. 1996. "Nuremberg and the Issue of Wartime Experiments on US Prisoners. The Green Committee." *Journal of the American Medical Association* 276 (20) (November): 1,672–1,675. doi:10.1001/jama.276.20.1672.

Hofmann, Albert, and Jonathan Ott. 1990. *LSD, My Problem Child: Reflections on Sacred Drugs, Mysticism, and Science*. Mt. View, CA: Wiretap. http://search.ebscohost.com/login.aspx?direct=true&scope=site&db=nlebk&db=nlabk&AN=2009172.

Hornblum, Allen M. 1997. "They Were Cheap and Available: Prisoners as Research Subjects in Twentieth Century America." *British Medical Journal* 3215: 1,437–1,441.

Kalm, Leah M., and Richard D. Semba. 2005. "They Starved So That Others Be Better Fed: Remembering Ancel Keys and the Minnesota Experiment." *History of Nutrition* 135: 1,347–1,352.

Katz, Jay, Alexander Morgan Capron, and Eleanor Swift Glass. 1972. *Experimentation with Human Beings; The Authority of the Investigator, Subject, Professions, and State in the Human Experimentation Process*. New York: Russell Sage Foundation.

Lerner, Barron H. 2007. "Subjects or Objects? Prisoners and Human Experimentation." *New England Journal of Medicine* 356 (18): 1,806–1,807.

Lifton, Robert Jay. 1986. *The Nazi Doctors: Medical Killing and the Psychology of Genocide*. New York: Basic Books.

Masterson, Karen M. 2014. *The Malaria Project: The U.S. Government's Secret Mission to Find a Miracle Cure*. New York: New American Library.

Mosby, Ian. 2013. "Administering Colonial Science: Nutrition Research and Human Biomedical Experimentation in Aboriginal Communities and Residential Schools, 1942–1952." *Histoire sociale/Social History* 46 (91): 145–172.

Proctor, Robert N. 1988. *Racial Hygiene: Medicine under the Nazis*. Cambridge, MA: Harvard University Press.

Proctor, Robert. 1999. *The Nazi War on Cancer*. Princeton, N.J.: Princeton University Press.

Russell, Paul F. 2015. "Volume VI. Communicable Diseases. Malaria. Chapter 1. Introduction." U.S. Army Medical Department Office of Medical History. Accessed January 18, 2015.

Shuster, E. 1997. "Fifty Years Later: The Significance of the Nuremberg Code." *New England Journal of Medicine* 337: 1,436–1,440.

Slater, Leo B. 2006. "Chemists and National Emergency: NIH's Unit of Chemotherapy during World War II." *Bulletin for the History of Chemistry* 31 (2): 75–80.

Spitz, Vivien. 2005. *Doctors from Hell: The Horrific Account of Nazi Experiments on Humans*. Boulder, CO: Sentient Publications.

Tucker, Todd. 2006. *The Great Starvation Experiment: The Heroic Men Who Starved So That Millions Could Live*. New York: Free Press.

Era 5: Cold War

INTRODUCTION

After World War II ended, the hostility between the Western powers and the Soviet bloc grew. The Soviet blockade of Berlin, the 1949 Soviet explosion of its own nuclear bomb, and then the Korean War all increased the tensions between the former Allies. During the struggles of the next four decades, known as the Cold War, each side feared that the enemy would use radioactive, chemical, or biological weapons against large populations. These fears led to experimentation with new weaponry—both in how to use it and how to defend against it.

The world had been appalled at the human medical experimentation that took place in Germany and Japan before and during World War II, and the Nuremberg Code had been written as a reaction to the Nazi experimentation in particular. The first principle of that code emphasized the importance of informed consent. Nonetheless, much of the medical experimentation of the Cold War was performed in secrecy and without consent from the subjects.

Of all of the experimentation that took place in those years, that which involved radiation was perhaps the most shocking when the extent of it was revealed to the public. Radiation is complex, difficult to understand, and usually imperceptible. Visible light, microwaves, and radio waves are types of radiation that are familiar, fairly well understood, and medically harmless; they occupy a small part of the spectrum of radiation.

The radiation relevant to medical experimentation is ionizing radiation that forces electrons out of atoms to create ions. Ionizing radiation includes alpha radiation (helium nuclei or clusters of two neutrons and two protons); beta radiation (high-speed electrons); gamma rays and X-rays (photons, or energy without charge or mass); and neutron radiation. The dangers of ionizing radiation became apparent early in the history of its use. Wilhelm Röntgen (1845–1923) discovered X-rays in 1895, and it was not long before it became clear that X-rays led to burns, ulcers, and skin cancers. Radiologists and radium dial painters ("the radium girls") alike developed cancers. (Young women working in a factory in New Jersey painted numbers on the dials of wristwatches using radioactive paint and licked the tips of the brushes to get sharp points.) Clarence Dally (1865–1904), who worked with X-rays with Thomas Edison, died from probable radiation-induced cancer in 1904. Marie Curie (1867–1934), the great physicist who developed the theory of radioactivity and discovered two elements, polonium and radium, developed disfigured hands and died of probable radiation-induced leukemia.

The acute effects of radiation are burns, caused by beta radiation, or radiation sickness, following exposure to large amounts of radiation. Other consequences of ionizing radiation occur only after a latency period of some years and consist mostly of an increase in the number of cancers, particularly leukemias and thyroid cancers, due to damage to the cell's genetic material.

Many of the scientific experiments in this era involved nuclear devices because the American military wanted to learn how to make "better" atomic and nuclear bombs. In one series of experiments in the 1940s and 1950s, bombs were detonated over the Marshall Islands to study their effects on ships. Scientists also wanted to measure how much radiation would be released as a result of thermonuclear detonation and to study the effects of the radiation on animals. The Marshallese on the island where the bombs were dropped were evacuated, but they were not fully informed of the risks both to their homes and to their health and have since claimed that they were used as guinea pigs. The American soldiers exposed to the bombs over Hiroshima and Nagasaki, those who cleaned up ships involved in the Marshall Islands blasts, and those who were exposed to later experimental blasts in Nevada have been called "atomic veterans."

Some research during the Cold War period used radiation as a medical tool. For example, physician John Lawrence (1904–1991) worked closely with his brother, Ernest Lawrence (1901–1958), a physicist, to devise medical treatments using radiation or radioisotopes to treat cancers. The use of total body irradiation (TBI) to treat cancer was seen as helpful at first, and is still used today at times, but also became controversial when some physicians in Cincinnati were accused of using it experimentally, perhaps with the goal of testing radiation's effect on the body rather than treating cancer.

The Manhattan Project (1942–1946), the effort to build an atom bomb before the Germans did, exposed thousands of scientists and workers to the possible dangers of radiation. Scientists conducted animal experiments to try to understand how radioactive substances acted in the body, but different animal species responded differently. It became clear that human experiments were needed. Plutonium, a new radioactive element, was involved in the manufacture of the atom bomb. Physician Joseph Hamilton (1907–1957), working at the University of California at San Francisco and at Berkeley, and others injected plutonium into people without informing them so that researchers could better understand the medical effects of exposure to this little-understood element.

Thousands of people were exposed to radiation in other studies. The exact number and the harm suffered are difficult to determine, however, because of the poor record keeping and the deliberate secrecy of many of the experiments. Perhaps unsurprisingly, people were usually not informed that they were subjects in radiation experiments. The experiments were kept secret so as not to alarm the subjects or the public—but also to avoid lawsuits.

One set of experiments on nutrition, in contrast, was not hidden. In 1946, the Manhattan Project, shortly to be subsumed by the Atomic Energy Commission (AEC), announced an isotope distribution program as a top priority. Radioisotopes were used as tracers in medical experiments. The program was designed in part to polish the image of the AEC. Radioisotopes were made available at low cost to researchers and free of charge altogether for cancer research. Nutrition scientists were quick to see the value of radioactively tagged food, which could help them study the absorption of various nutrients. The amount of radiation needed for such studies seemed so small that the researchers did not think that they needed to tell the subjects that they were participating in experiments. Experiments done on schoolchildren, pregnant women at Vanderbilt University, and boys at the Fernald School in Massachusetts had not been secret, but the subjects (or their parents) had not been informed. When these studies were publicized by Eileen Welsome (b. 1951) and other journalists, they did not seem as innocent to the general public as they had seemed to researchers a few years earlier.

Other experiments carried out during the Cold War years concerned biological and chemical warfare. Researchers were looking for drugs that could be used as truth drugs or incapacitants. In an unlikely series of events, the Central Intelligence Agency became interested in the possible military use of such psychedelic drugs as lysergic acid diethylamide (LSD), which were more commonly associated with long-haired youths rejecting mainstream culture than with national security.

Most subjects in these experiments did not give informed consent and were deceived in multiple and repeated ways. Yet, there were documents outlining principles of ethical research and the importance of informed consent. The Judicial Council of the American Medical Association (AMA) wrote in 1946 that experimentation on humans must be preceded by experimentation on animals, that the human subject should give consent, and that the experiments should be carried out with proper medical protection and management.

In April 1947, Carroll Wilson, general manager of the AEC, wrote two letters articulating the ethics of research on human subjects, explaining that (1) there must be a possibility that a patient could be helped by the research; (2) two doctors had to document that the patient understood and agreed to the experiment; (3) research on patients could only proceed if there was a chance that it could help the subject; (4) informed consent from the patient and next of kin had to be complete and written; and (5) consent could be rescinded. While the impact of these two letters is not clear, they do provide evidence that the ideas of informed consent are not that new. Notably, Wilson used the term "informed consent" perhaps for the first time in the history of written regulations of experimentation.

In 1953, Secretary of Defense Charles Wilson issued a memorandum known as the Wilson Memorandum, again insisting that subjects had to sign consent and that the signature had to be witnessed. He added that the research had to be approved of by the secretary of defense and that prisoners of war could not be used.

The secrecy of the experiments of this time and the disappearance of records suggest that at least some of the researchers knew that the experiments were ethically questionable.

Some have argued, despite the letters and memorandum mentioned above, that the research ethics of the past were different from those of today and that earlier researchers should not be held to modern standards. In the past, most physicians worked in a paternalistic way, seldom telling patients what they, the doctors, felt would not be helpful and what might upset them. Physicians carrying out experiments or treatments alike rarely explained them in detail to the subjects or their patients. The report from the AMA, moreover, was hidden in a long committee report in the *Journal of the American Medical Association*; it is doubtful that many people read it. The guidelines issued by Carroll Wilson of the AEC were not promulgated.

Finally, the Wilson Memorandum was actually a secret document. Many military personnel involved in medical experiments did not even know of its existence. Apologists for the researchers have also argued that these experiments rarely caused harm and that the secrecy was warranted because they were carried out in the midst of great and justifiable concern about the safety of scientists, soldiers, and the citizenry.

In addition to the large amounts of research on radiation, dramatic advances were made in vaccine development during these years. The National Foundation for Infantile Paralysis (NFIP), one of the first patient advocacy groups, organized a large experiment—perhaps the largest of its kind—with the killed polio vaccine prepared by Jonas Salk (1914–1995). Other experts, namely polio expert Albert Sabin (1906–1993), used a weakened (attenuated) live vaccine and worried that the NFIP and Salk were acting too quickly and putting people at risk. Salk's vaccine worked well, but when the vaccinations were scaled up, this in itself—not fully appreciated at the time—became a different type of experiment. Killing the virus in small lots is easier to do than killing it in large lots, and the mistakes that the pharmaceutical companies made led to some cases of paralysis and even death. Vaccine experiments, as with the earlier radiation experiments, were often carried out on institutionalized children. Such children were also used in investigations of ringworm, acne, and thyroid hormones.

It was some decades before the basic principles of the Nuremberg Code were accepted by researchers. The World Medical Association met in Helsinki in 1964 and issued guidelines based on the Nuremberg Code. A distinction was made between therapeutic experimentation and research with no immediate clinical benefit, and guardians were allowed to give consent on behalf of individuals who could not understand the issues involved.

The medical community was slow to take these ethical concerns seriously. In the late 1960s, physicians Henry Beecher (1904–1976) and Maurice Pappworth (1910–1994) described how some English and American physicians were continuing to experiment on subjects without gaining their consent. In 1972, the public at large was shocked to learn about the Tuskegee Study of Untreated Syphilis—in which black Americans with syphilis were either not treated or undertreated for their illness—which was supported by the United States Public Health Service. There was a wide gap between the medical and nonmedical communities in how they understood the importance of consent.

The National Research Act in 1974 mandated the formation of institutional review boards (committees that reviewed research) and established the National

Commission for the Protection of Human Subjects of Biomedical and Behavioral Research (known as the National Commission) that issued the influential Belmont Report (1979), suggesting that all human experimentation had to be founded on respect for persons, beneficence, and justice.

In the 1960s and 1970s, prisoners were widely used in research, with about 90 percent of all pharmaceutical research being done on prisoners. This fact came to the attention of a civil rights activist of the time, Jessica Mitford (1917–1996), who wrote a scathing expose of the American penal system in a book titled *Kind and Usual Punishment: The Prison Business*. One chapter was devoted to experiments on prisoners. She pointed out that the prisons were so poorly and inhumanely run that sometimes being a medical guinea pig meant an improvement in living conditions. Some prisons and prison doctors made a lot of money from experimentation. Mitford described the work of one physician who used prisoners in Oklahoma, Arkansas, and Alabama for drug and blood plasma studies in mostly unregulated conditions. In one prison in Alabama, almost a third of the subjects studied developed viral hepatitis compared with 1 percent of other prisoners. Mitford's revelations (and those of others) led the National Commission to write a report in 1976 highly critical of research in prisoners. Federally funded research using prisoners was effectively banned in the United States in 1978.

Experiments continued to be carried out on vulnerable populations. One of the most important changes in the way that people treated sex and family life was the introduction of the oral contraceptive pill. The clinical trials—experiments of a sort—that established the "pill's" safety and effectiveness were carried out on poor women, many illiterate, in Puerto Rico, because the trials could never have been carried out on the mainland. These women were willing to take a pill that prevented pregnancy but had no idea that that the pill was still experimental.

In sum, the horrors of the German concentration camps did not substantially affect the researchers of the Cold War, who saw the Nazi physicians as sadistic and themselves as scientists intent on making medical discoveries or protecting their countries. Yet, the combination of rapid technological advances in radiation physics, vaccine, and antibiotic development and the availability of large numbers of potential subjects in prisons and other institutions meant that human experimentation was taking place on an altogether unprecedented scale—and not always with the greatest of care for the research subjects.

TIMELINE

1945–1947	American scientists investigating medical effects of nuclear bombs inject plutonium into 18 people without their consent.
1945–1963	Harris Isbell (1910–1994) conducts experiments on mind-altering drugs at the Lexington Narcotic Farm. He is partially funded by MKULTRA, a secret project run by the Central Intelligence Agency (CIA).

1946	The Manhattan Project, a program with the goal of producing nuclear weapons for the Allies, begins to distribute medical isotopes to researchers with the aim of showing that radioactivity can be used for medical as well as military purposes.
1946	The Judicial Council of the American Medical Association (AMA) declares that human subjects of experimentation must give consent, that experimentation on humans must be preceded by experimentation on animals, and that the experiments should be carried out with medical protection and management.
1946–1948	Physicians working for the United States Public Health Service expose uninformed Guatemalan citizens to sexually transmitted diseases.
1946–1949	Researchers at Vanderbilt University give 700 pregnant women radioactive iron to test iron absorption in pregnancy.
1946–1953	The Massachusetts Institute of Technology and Quaker Oats collaborate in giving members of the "science club" at the Fernald State School in Massachusetts cereal containing radioactive iron and calcium in order to study the absorption of these minerals.
1946–1958	The United States Army detonates bombs in the Marshall Islands, beginning with Operations Crossroads in 1946, in which bombs are detonated over the Bikini Atoll in the Marshall Islands and in a lagoon, the first of 66 peacetime nuclear explosions in which the amount and effect of released radioactivity is examined.
1947	Carroll Wilson, general manager of the Atomic Energy Commission (AEC), writes that there must be a possibility that a patient can be helped by the research, two doctors must document that the patient understood and agreed to the experiment, research on patients can only proceed if there was a chance that it could help the subject, informed consent from the patient and next of kin has to be complete and written, and the consent can be taken back.
1947	English physicians organize the first major double-blind trial by assigning patients with tuberculosis to active treatment with streptomycin, or bedrest, using random numbers.

1950	The United States Navy sprays *Serratia* and *Bacillus* germs over San Francisco as a way of testing the country's susceptibility to biological warfare.
1952	Jean Delay (1907–1987) and Pierre Deniker (1917–1998) use chlorpromazine as a single drug to treat a man with mania, the first time that a drug has been shown to have antipsychotic properties.
1953–1973	Project MKULTRA, a secret program of the Central Intelligence Agency (CIA), experiments with mind control, sometimes on unsuspecting American and Canadian citizens.
1953–1957	Physicians at the Massachusetts General Hospital (MGH) collaborate with the AEC in administering uranium to comatose patients.
1953	Secretary of Defense Charles Wilson issues a secret memorandum known as the Wilson Memorandum, again insisting that the subjects have to sign consent and the signature had to be witnessed. Research has to be approved of by the secretary of defense, and prisoners of war cannot be used.
1954–1973	Conscientious objectors who are Seventh-day Adventists join Operation Whitecoat and participate in medical experiments rather than become combatants.
1954	Jonas Salk (1914–1995) and the National Foundation for Infantile Paralysis organize a large clinical trial in the United States to test the Salk polio vaccine, a killed-polio vaccine.
1954–1956	Chester Southam (1919–2002) injects elderly and terminally ill patients at the Jewish Chronic Diseases Hospital with live cancer cells to test their immunity without obtaining informed consent.
1956–1971	Saul Krugman (1911–1995) and colleagues infect children at the Willowbrook State School in New York with hepatitis viruses; there are concerns about the adequacy of the consent and the ethics of the experiments. Their work leads to important advances in the understanding and treatment of hepatitis.
1957–1961	MKULTRA funds some of the brainwashing experiments of Donald Ewen Cameron (1901–1967), a psychiatrist who is the director of the Allan Memorial Institute in Montréal.

1960–1972	Eugene Saenger (1917–2007) at the University of Cincinnati conducts total- or partial-body irradiation of patients with cancer in conjunction with the Department of Defense.
1961–1963	Timothy Leary (1920–1996) organizes the Harvard Psilocybin Project and conducts experiments with the psychoactive substance with 32 prison inmates in Concord, Massachusetts, and 20 theology students and professors attending a Good Friday service at the Marsh Chapel of Boston University.
1963–1971	Carl Heller and Alvin Paulsen irradiate the testicles of prisoners in Oregon and Washington with the support of the AEC.
1964	The World Medical Association, meeting in Finland, passes the Helsinki Declaration addressing research ethics.
1966	Henry Beecher (1904–1976), an American anesthesiologist and medical ethicist, describes 22 medical experiments carried out by American physicians, without consent, in an influential *New England Journal of Medicine* article.
1967	In Cape Town, South Africa, Christiaan Barnard (1922–2001) transplants a heart from a young woman killed in a car accident into a middle-aged man suffering from heart disease, and he lives for 18 days. This is the first heart transplant.
1967	Maurice Pappworth (1910–1994), an English physician and medical ethicist, writes *Human Guinea Pigs: Experimentation on Man*, describing experiments carried out in England and the United States that had no therapeutic reason or informed consent.
1968	The Ad Hoc Committee of the Harvard Medical School to Examine the Definition of Brain Death, headed by Henry Beecher, defines death as the cessation of brain function.
1972	Jean Heller of the *New York Times* describes the Tuskegee Study of Untreated Syphilis and shocks the public.
1973	Jessica Mitford (1917–1996) writes a book, *Kind and Usual Punishment: The Prison Business*, about abuses taking place in American prisons, including unethical medical experimentation.

1974   The National Research Act creates the National Commission for the Protection of Human Subjects of Biomedical and Behavioral Research, also known as the National Commission, and requires that research projects funded by the Department of Health, Education, and Welfare be reviewed by institutional review boards (IRBs) and, in 1979, that all federally funded research be reviewed by IRBs.

1975–1976   The Rockefeller Commission and Church Committee investigate the activities of the CIA, including the secret program MKULTRA.

1979   The National Commission prepares the Belmont report, or Ethical Principles and Guidelines for the Protection of Human Subjects of Research, outlining three basic principles for ethical research: respect for persons, beneficence, and justice.

1984   Barry Marshall (b. 1951) drinks *Helicobacter pylori* to prove that this bacterium can live in the stomach and cause ulcers, and in 2005, along with J. Robin Warren (b. 1937), receives the Nobel Prize in Physiology or Medicine.

REFERENCE ENTRIES

AMERICAN BACTERIAL ATTACKS ON U.S. CITIES

While investigating the possibility of being attacked by biological agents, the United States Army released bacteria and fluorescent compounds over parts of the United States. The best known of these releases was a mock biological attack on San Francisco in which the military secretly sprayed the city with *Serratia* bacteria and other agents thought to be harmless. Some people, unwitting subjects, may have become ill because of this experiment.

During the 1940s and 1950s, the U.S. Army wanted to determine whether an enemy could attack American cities using biological weapons such as bacteria. To find out if such an assault could be successfully carried out, the army launched its own simulated bacterial assaults by releasing bacteria in various parts of the country to measure how widely the bacteria might spread. Not many details about these staged assaults are known.

Many of these releases occurred at the Dugway Proving Grounds in Utah, where the human population was small. Other releases or staged assaults occurred in more densely populated locations, including the Pentagon, where, in August 1949, bacteria were intentionally introduced into the air-conditioning ducts.

Later, over the course of a week in September 1950, as part of an operation called "Sea Spray," a Navy ship sprayed *Serratia* and *Bacillus* microbes—bacteria not believed to pose any danger to humans—over San Francisco from giant hoses on the deck of the ship. To better track the spread of the spray, researchers added zinc cadmium sulfide particles, which are easily traced because they fluoresce under ultraviolet light. The mist of bacteria was hidden by the San Francisco fog.

Two weeks later, 11 men and women were hospitalized in San Francisco with fever and other symptoms, which was subsequently diagnosed as pneumonia caused by exposure to bacteria believed to be *Serratia marcescens* (a common variety of *Serratia* that rarely can cause human illnesses). One person died. Doctors reported this unusual outbreak in a medical journal.

Although the San Francisco attacks were the most dramatic, in other parts of the country army researchers conducted similar mock attacks without the cover of Bay Area fogs. Bacteria were released in cities in the Northeast and along the Pennsylvania Turnpike. Zinc cadmium sulfide particles released over the Midwest were transported, presumably by winds, as far east as New York State. As far as we know, no civilians were aware of or harmed in these exercises.

In May 1965, the army released *Bacillus globigii* (a bacterium not known to cause human illness) at Washington's National Airport and its Greyhound bus terminal. More than 130 passengers carried the bacteria to almost 40 cities throughout the United States in the next two weeks.

In 1966, military researchers spread *Bacillus subtilis* (also known as hay bacteria and thought to be harmless) in the New York City subway system by dropping bacteria-filled lightbulbs onto the tracks in stations in midtown Manhattan. The bacteria spread throughout the subway system. As a result, army officials concluded in a January 1968 report that a subway attack could possibly expose Americans to infectious microorganisms. In 1969, President Richard Nixon ended offensive germ-warfare activity and the stockpiling of biological agents.

The press found out about these biological warfare tests in the 1970s. In 1977, the army testified in Senate hearings that between 1949 and 1969, air tests of biological agents were conducted 239 times. In 80 experiments, the army researchers used live bacteria thought then not to be harmful to human health. Other experiments involved the use of inactive substances. Army officials denied that the 11 cases of pneumonia and 1 death in San Francisco were caused by their experiments, blaming the infections on hospital-acquired infections. There is some similarity to the experiments carried out at Porton Down, in England, in which the British military exposed its own population to various substances to explore England's susceptibility to biological warfare.

The army had conducted these experiments to devise ways of protecting the American population from attacks by the enemy, but the public recoiled at the idea of serving as uninformed research subjects.

Frances R. Frankenburg

ATOMIC VETERANS

American military servicemen were exposed to radiation during and after the bombing of Hiroshima and Nagasaki and during peacetime nuclear detonations between 1945 and 1962. Some of the exposures suffered by the "atomic veterans," as they became known, were experimental.

The term *atomic veterans* refers to the almost half a million American veterans who were exposed to military radiation between 1945 and 1962. Two hundred thousand American World War II veterans took part in the occupation of Hiroshima or Nagasaki after the August 1945 bombing or were prisoners of war in this area before 1946. Another 200,000 military personnel participated in aboveground nuclear tests between 1945 and 1962 designed to investigate the effects of nuclear bombs. About 2,000 to 3,000 of this latter group were subjects of research, some of it medical.

One of the first such postwar exposures took place during Operations Crossroads, a series of peacetime nuclear detonations at Bikini Atoll in the Marshall Islands in 1946. The first detonation of a nuclear bomb there took place on July 1, 1946. One of the purposes of the detonation was to see what happened to ships in the Bikini lagoon. Just six days after the explosion, 4,900 military men were assigned to clean or decontaminate the ships. They were warned about the dangers of radioactivity, although it is not clear how effectively the warnings were delivered. A few wore radiation monitors, most of which did not work, and a few wore protective clothing.

On August 10, Colonel Stafford Warren—the chief of the Radiological Safety Section of the Joint Task Force for Operation Crossroads—insisted, against the wishes of the navy, that the decontamination work be stopped because of the unexpected extent of the contamination of the ships and the danger it posed to the servicemen. (Warren had been chief of the medical section of the Manhattan Project and was in charge of both radiation safety at the first American nuclear test, Trinity, in July 1945, and on-ground inspections at Hiroshima.) While not technically subjects of medical research, these military personnel later came to feel that they had unknowingly participated in experiments in which their health could have been harmed.

More nuclear tests were carried out at the Nevada National Security Site (NNSS), an unpopulated area in Nevada set aside for the testing of nuclear devices. At the NNSS, the military conducted a series of exercises—named the Desert Rock exercises—between 1951 and 1957. Desert Rock exercises were designed to test the knowledge and attitudes of soldiers to nuclear explosions, while other exercises examined the medical effects of the blasts on the soldiers.

Some of the NNSS medical studies investigated flash blindness, which is the temporary or permanent loss of vision that occurs when a person is exposed to an extremely high-intensity light flash—such as that which occurs during a nuclear blast. This loss of vision is sudden and can be hazardous, particularly for pilots who may be blinded in midflight. In these studies, the military personnel were informed about the reasons for the tests and may have volunteered to participate.

In 1951, during Operation Buster-Jangle at the NNSS, which included the exercise known as Desert Rock I, subjects flew 15,000 feet above and 9 miles away from three detonations so that the effects of the explosions on their vision could be tested. A year later, during Operation Tumbler-Snapper, 12 subjects witnessed detonations from a trailer 10 miles away. Half of the subjects wore protective goggles. Two subjects in the group who did not wear goggles developed retinal burns. In 1953, these tests were repeated. No records of consent exist, but some of the participants do remember providing written consent. As a result of these experiments, protective eyewear was improved.

Another group of NNSS experiments involved about a dozen pilots flying through a mushroom cloud, the large cloud that forms as a result of a nuclear explosion. This kind of experiment was known as "cloud penetration" and was done because the unmanned drones that had previously been used to obtain air samples after a blast were found to be ineffective. General Ernest A. Pinson, who directed these experiments, insisted on flying through the clouds himself. In 1955, during Operation Teapot, the first deliberately planned "early cloud penetration," the pilots swallowed capsules that measured internal radiation and then flew into clouds immediately after the detonation of a nuclear device. In the subsequent Operation Redwing in 1956, the pilots did not use the usual filters in the planes so that they could measure the effects of inhaling particles from the unfiltered ambient air.

The results of these experiments were interpreted as evidence that it was not particularly dangerous to fly through a mushroom cloud, nor were filters or other special equipment needed to protect the pilot and crew. The experiments also showed that measurements of external exposure were sufficient, as the internal and surface measurements of radiation were identical.

When it comes to military medical research, the usual ethical concerns related to medical experimentation are difficult to define because soldiers are typically expected to follow orders, no matter what the danger. Indeed, almost by definition of their work, soldiers are routinely exposed to hazards. In this case, the pilots did not sign written consent, as the tasks seemed more occupational than experimental.

After much deliberation, the Department of Defense (DoD) decided that the guidelines for medical experimentation should be the same whether or not the subject is a member of the military. The DoD decided to use the Nuremberg Code as a basis for its own rules with respect to medical research. Secretary of Defense Charles Wilson issued a memorandum to this effect in 1953, but the document was classified as top secret until 1975, which explains why not all military people involved in medical experiments—including the organizers of the cloud penetration experiments—knew of its existence.

The harm done to the atomic veterans has been difficult to estimate. Complete details of the actual exposure to radiation are not available. Not all of the personnel involved in the peacetime tests wore film badges or dosimeters (devices that measure or monitor cumulative radiation dose), and in any case, these devices were not always accurate. Many records have been lost, and some were classified as secret, either because of security concerns or possibly because of fears of veterans making legal claims as a result of the radiation exposure.

There was one study of the effects of radiation on 46,000 personnel; however, it was flawed because it had misidentified and excluded large numbers of subjects.

A further complication is that some of the veterans had taken an "oath of secrecy" forbidding them to reveal any details of their service. The results of the research, therefore, are not conclusive. But the overall impression that most researchers have is that there has not been a clear increase in cancer risk among these personnel, expect possibly for a small increase in leukemia.

In 1996, the Repeal of Nuclear Radiation and Secrecy Agreement Laws was passed, allowing veterans to reveal details about their military involvement in nuclear testing so that, if appropriate, they would be able to obtain a service-connected disability. To get that disability, however, a veteran has to go through a "dose reconstruction," estimating how much radiation he or she received. This is a painstaking process that can take over a year.

Despite the lack of clear evidence, surviving atomic veterans who have completed the dose reconstruction and who have certain illnesses are eligible for compensation. The illnesses presumed to be related to exposure to ionizing radiation are the following: cancers of the bile ducts, bone, brain, breast, colon, esophagus, gallbladder, liver (if primary), lung, pancreas, pharynx, ovary, salivary gland, small intestine, stomach, thyroid, and urinary tract as well as leukemia (but not chronic lymphocytic leukemia), lymphoma (but not Hodgkin disease), and multiple myeloma.

While the exposure of members of the military to the peacetime detonations has not clearly been shown to be harmful, the atomic veterans were often inadequately educated about the risks they might have been taking. In the medical experiments, there was usually little informed consent. The exposure to radiation could have led to long-term effects or it could have been relatively safe, but the consequences will never be known for certain because of the inadequate record keeping and lack of follow-up.

Frances R. Frankenburg

AVERSION THERAPY IN SOUTH AFRICA

During the apartheid era in South Africa, some soldiers may have been the subjects of experiments, including the attempted conversion of homosexuals to heterosexuality.

During the apartheid era, the government of South Africa maintained a large military force, and beginning in 1967, conscription became universal for young white men. Universal conscription meant that not all of the conscripts were ideal soldiers, and so the military authorities became concerned about a number of issues among these conscripts, including homosexuality, drug abuse, and the refusal to fight. Publicity surrounds the actions of one military psychiatrist in particular who dealt with some of the soldiers from these groups.

Aubrey Levin (b. 1938) joined the South African Defence Force (SADF) in 1969 as a psychiatrist and colonel. Two years later, he became director of the the SADF's Drug Rehabilitation Program at One Military Hospital, also known as the

Voortrekkerhoogte military hospital, in Pretoria. He directed Ward 22 in that hospital from 1969 to 1974 and treated or experimented on recruits whom he considered to be "deviant." These were soldiers who were identified as homosexual, those who smoked marijuana, and those who did not want to serve in the army. The "therapy" for the gay soldiers (mostly male) was known as aversion therapy and included receiving painful electric shocks on the arms while being shown pictures of naked men. Such therapies were designed to eliminate any homosexual impulses.

Conscripts who smoked marijuana or used other drugs were sent to Greefswald, a military detention camp, where they were assigned to forced labor. Some of the recruits reluctant to fight were subjected to "narcoanalysis," that is, questioning while under the influence of barbiturates.

Between 1971 and 1989, Levin is reported to have arranged for as many as 900 homosexual soldiers, mostly 16- to 24-year-old males, to be subjected to "gender reassignment" surgeries, usually against their will. Some are reported to have died, and often the surgery was reported to have been incomplete. The soldiers were discharged with no follow-up and with little ability to complete or reverse the process. Little is known about what happened to the people reported to have undergone these procedures.

Levin was a well-established and respected psychiatrist in South Africa. For some years, he was also the director of mental health in the Department of Health Services and Welfare and professor of psychiatry at the University of the Orange Free State.

In 1994, the apartheid era ended in South Africa with the election of Nelson Mandela as president. A year later, the South African government created a Truth and Reconciliation Commission (TRC) to investigate violence and human rights abuses under apartheid. At that time, Levin left the country and moved to Canada, where he worked as a psychiatrist. In June 1997, the Health and Human Rights Project submitted a report to the TRC naming Aubrey Levin as a key figure in the "torture" of gay men in the military as part of a military scheme to "reprogram" gay recruits with electric shock treatment.

The nature of the work done on Ward 22 is not clear. Some of the recruits are said to have deliberately claimed that they were gay so they did not have to serve in the army, and some may actually have wanted gender-reassignment surgery. Aversion therapy was not supported by all of the South African military or the psychiatrists there; indeed, some military officers and psychiatrists in South Africa were openly gay at that time. Some have suggested that the work was carried out to ensure that white men continued to procreate. Little can be said about the work's contribution to advancing medical science because no publications are known to have arisen from it. In general, it has been perceived as punitive to those who may have been subjected to it.

When questioned about his South African work, Levin admitted to using what he called mild electric shocks in some cases. He said that on rare occasions he used barbiturate-aided psychotherapy to help recruits who were struggling with various issues. But he denied ever harming or experimenting on the soldiers. Levin's character and reliability were damaged by his 2013 conviction of sexual assaults on some of his male patients in Canada.

Whatever the exact nature of the work, it seems possible that at least some of the soldiers underwent cruel and medically unjustifiable procedures. The soldiers were vulnerable, in that they had an unusual status of being considered at once prisoner, patient, and "deviant." In fact, the procedures might be considered a clearer example of poor treatment rather than experimentation. There is also no evidence of informed consent for the experiments, if they can be considered as such, or for the treatments.

Frances R. Frankenburg

BEECHER, HENRY

Henry Beecher was an American physician best known for his description of the placebo response and his scathing review of unethical American medical experiments. These influential articles are, in part, responsible for the common use of a placebo control in clinical experiments and trials and with the formation of institutional review boards. Beecher, however, had a more complicated approach to experimentation than is suggested by these two well-known articles. He had little faith in institutional reviews or rules, and in his earlier years, he collaborated with doctors who had worked in concentration camps and also experimented with mescaline and lysergic acid diethylamide on unwitting subjects for the Central Intelligence Agency.

Harry Unangst (1904–1976) was born in Kansas and changed his name to Henry Knowles Beecher in his twenties. He studied at the University of Kansas and did his medical training at Harvard Medical School. He also studied for four years in the physiology laboratory of Nobel Prize–winner Augustus Krogh (1874–1949) in Denmark, returning to Boston in 1936 to become an anesthesiologist at the Massachusetts General Hospital. During World War II, he served as a physician in North Africa and Italy, where he treated over 200 soldiers with serious wounds. He noted that few of the wounded asked for pain relief, so he became interested in how a person's psychological state might affect his or her perception of pain.

In 1947, two years after the end of the war, the chief of the United States Medical Intelligence Branch sent information to Beecher about experiments carried out at the Dachau concentration camp using the cactus-derived hallucinogen mescaline and experiments at the Mauthausen concentration camp with the hallucinogen lysergic acid diethylamide (LSD). Mescaline had been the drug of choice for the German secret police, the Gestapo. Kurt Plötner, a Nazi physician who had worked at Dachau, gave mescaline to Jewish and Russian prisoners in an exploration of drugs that could be employed as an aid in interrogations. Beecher became interested in this area of research.

Beecher worked for the European Command Interrogation Center at Camp King in Germany. Also at Camp King were soldiers who had worked with the

Gestapo and former Nazi physicians, including Kurt Blome. Blome, who had been tried but acquitted of war crimes, was part of Operation Paperclip, the program in which German scientists worked for the United States after World War II, so that the Soviet Union could not benefit from their expertise. He, along with other former Nazi doctors and Americans, interrogated Soviet defectors and double agents.

In 1951, Beecher began to pursue secret research for the American military, and possibly the Central Intelligence Agency (CIA), testing both mescaline and LSD on subjects without their knowledge. He described their resulting paranoia and panic. He carried on this work in secret for over a decade. Although there is no evidence that Beecher worked directly with Blome, he did work with General Walter Schreiber, the former medical chief for the Wehrmacht who had experimented on concentration camp inmates. Beecher described him as helpful. Beecher published very little about his work with LSD. It was only after much of the CIA and other military documentation was declassified that scholars became aware of the extent of this work.

Beecher also pursued research on his observation that wounded soldiers were able to withstand injuries without asking for pain relief. How much pain a person suffers from a wound is affected not just by the severity of the wound but also by the person's state of mind. The stress of battle can cause a person to ignore what in other situations might be experienced as agonizing pain.

Another state of mind, quite different from that associated with the traumas of war, is the belief that one is receiving assistance. Beecher investigated the surprising effects of a placebo—a drug with no physiological activities. In an influential 1955 article, he reviewed 15 studies and found that a third of patients improved with the placebo. He made the important point that placebo-reactors, as he called the subjects who responded to placebo, are not those with "imaginary" pain. Placebo can relieve pain arising from clear physical causes. He also noted that placebo can even cause adverse side effects and lead to measurable physiological reactions, such as a decrease in the production of gastric acid. Experiments are now often done in a double-blind manner with a placebo control, due in part to the argument of this influential article.

Beecher's work also played a role in the creation of the institutional review boards, which are committees established by institutions to review research. In 1959, he published an article in the *Journal of the American Medical Association* about the questionable research ethics of physicians. Then, in 1966, he published his most influential article in the *New England Journal of Medicine*, "Ethics and Clinical Research." In this article, he described 22 examples of American medical experimentation that had been done without consent that put the patients' lives at risk. He did not name the investigators, but the editors of the journal knew the full details of the experiments and were able to verify and confirm what Beecher had written. The research had been carried out at prestigious and respectable institutions. Beecher blamed the unethical work on the amount of money involved and the professional ambition of the physicians. He wrote that patients, "if suitably approached," will agree to do what their physicians ask them to do. In the studies that he described, however, it seemed unlikely that the subject or the guardian would have agreed to the experiment if the physician had informed him or her clearly of the risks involved. A "suitable approach" to the patients also means, from the point of view of the ambitious physician-researchers, argued Beecher, withholding information about possible dangerousness.

In one study he mentioned, children described as "mental defectives or juvenile delinquents" were given a new antibiotic to treat their acne so that possible liver dysfunction caused by the antibiotic could be assessed. In another, patients were exposed to lengthy periods of anesthesia, and their hearts were catheterized or their livers biopsied for research—not for their benefit. In the Willowbrook experiment in Staten Island, children were deliberately infected with hepatitis, and at the Jewish Chronic Diseases Hospital in Brooklyn, live cancer cells were injected into 22 subjects.

This article and other publications, such as Maurice Pappworth's book *Human Guinea Pigs: Experimentation on Man*, played a part in the formation of federal regulations concerning human experimentation that mandated signed informed consent and the formation of institutional review boards. But the result was not what Beecher wanted. He did not think, for example, that the Nuremberg Code was either necessary or helpful. He thought that the code's first principle—that the patient be able to understand the experiment—was too idealistic, as it was unlikely that patients could understand medical or research procedures. He wrote that to obtain truly informed consent is difficult (although a worthy goal) because the patients usually are not physicians or scientists and making decisions when ill is difficult. Also, the hazards of any experiment may not be known with any certainty. Nor did Beecher believe in regulation. He thought that physicians should be ethical and that regulation itself could not guarantee such behavior. Beecher wrote that the answer was to rely on the "safeguard provided by the presence of an intelligent, informed, conscientious, compassionate, responsible investigator."[1]

It is difficult to reconcile Beecher's concerns about ethical experimentation with his history of collaboration with physicians who had worked in the concentration camps and his secret work with mescaline and LSD on subjects without their knowledge—work that we only know about because the formerly secret government documents have been declassified.

Beecher made one more contribution of note to medicine: the determination of when a patient could be considered dead. This decision became more difficult when people who could not breathe on their own started to be kept alive by ventilators. It was particularly fraught if the person was a potential organ donor and, in some senses, seemed to be dead—that is, the individual's heart was still beating, but he or she had no brain function. In terms of organ donation, the sooner such a person can be declared dead, the better shape their organs will be in and the more successful transplantation will be.

In 1968, Beecher headed a committee at Harvard that decided a person could be considered dead if that individual had severe brain damage and no brain activity as measured by an electroencephalograph or neurological exam, even if the person's heart were still beating. This decision made organ transplantation easier but has also proven to be controversial. Not all people are comfortable with the idea that a person who still has a pulse is dead, even if that person cannot breathe on their own and does not seem to have a functioning brain.

Frances R. Frankenburg

Reference

1.   Beecher, "Ethics and Clinical Research," 1,360.

BELMONT REPORT

The goal of researchers who perform experiments on humans is to make discoveries. The welfare of the researchers' subjects is not always the first priority and is sometimes put in jeopardy. One of the most significant pieces of American legislation regulating scientific research was the 1974 National Research Act, which led to the creation of the National Commission for the Protection of Human Subjects of Biomedical and Behavioral Research. This commission produced a number of reports, the most important of which was the Belmont Report of 1979.

Following the revelations concerning the Tuskegee Study of Untreated Syphilis (1932–1972), in which black Americans with syphilis were either not treated or inadequately treated, and after concerns about fetal research were raised in the Kennedy hearings of 1973 and in articles and books written by physicians detailing unethical human experimentation, the Nixon Administration passed the National Research Act of 1974.

The National Research Act required that research projects funded by the Department of Health, Education, and Welfare (DHEW) have "institutional review boards" (IRBs) to ensure that the research complied with federal requirements and, in particular, that human participants faced minimal risks and gave adequate informed consent before the research could receive DHEW funding.

This act also created the National Commission for the Protection of Human Subjects of Biomedical and Behavioral Research, composed of two bioethicists, three physicians, two biomedical researchers, three lawyers, and one public member. The commission's job was to review the protection of the rights and welfare of people who were the subjects of federally funded research. DHEW was required to respond to the commission's recommendations.

Over the course of its existence, from 1974 to 1978, the commission prepared 17 reports. The first one, in 1975, was about fetal research. In 1976, it considered the question of research in prisoners and commented on the poor conditions in prisons and the potential for abuse of authority. This report, issued in 1978 as Subpart C, was controversial because it placed so many restrictions on the use of prisoners in medical research that this practice was effectively banned. In 1978, the commission issued a report on IRBs, expanding the 1974 regulations that required IRBs for DHEW-funded projects to regulations that required IRBs for all federally funded research projects.

The commission was also asked to prepare a report about the ethics of research. For three days in February 1976, it met at the Belmont House, a conference center of the Smithsonian Center located in Elkridge, Maryland. The commission continued to work on this report over the next two years, finishing in June 1978. It was published in 1979 and is now known as the *Belmont Report* or *Ethical Principles and Guidelines for the Protection of Human Subjects of Research*—probably the commission's most important product. *The Belmont Report* addressed the boundaries between practice and research and the necessity of obtaining informed consent. And, most importantly, it outlined three basic ethical principles that must guide all research:

1. Respect for persons: People should make their own decisions. If a person is not capable of doing that, or has, in the words of the report, "diminished autonomy," he or she should be "protected." Even those who are incapable of making their own decisions should give their assent to the study, while their health care proxy should give the informed consent with the person's best interest in mind.
2. Beneficence: Human subjects should not be harmed, and the research should maximize benefit and minimize risk.
3. Justice: Benefits and risks of research should be distributed fairly. The commission noted that in the 19th and early 20th centuries, the burden of serving as research subjects fell unfairly on the poor. The commission warned against selecting people to be subjects based on convenience or the vulnerability of the subject. Studies should, when possible, include people of all ages and from a range of ethnicities and circumstances.

Frances R. Frankenburg

BOSTON PROJECT

From 1953 to 1957, in what was known as the Boston Project, physicians at the Massachusetts General Hospital injected dying patients with uranium as part of a "dual experiment" serving both the interests of the atomic energy community, which was concerned about occupational hazards, and the medical community, which was looking for new treatments for brain tumors.

In the 1950s, the Atomic Energy Commission (AEC) wanted to discover how the human body handles uranium so that they could create safety standards for their workers who were exposed to it. To do so, the Health Physics Division at the AEC Oak Ridge National Laboratory (ORNL) in Tennessee paired with neurosurgeon William Sweet (1910–2001) at the Massachusetts General Hospital (MGH). Sweet, who had trained at Harvard Medical School and spent more than 60 years at MGH, advanced the field of neurosurgery, both in clinical care and basic research. He was one of the coinventors of the first human positron imaging device, a forerunner to positron emission tomography, or PET scanning. He was interested in using radioisotopes both to localize and to treat brain tumors, and he used phosphorus-32, obtained from ORNL, to locate brain tumors. The isotope localized in brain tumors but could only be detected when the skull was opened, so it was not very useful. Sweet had also explored isotopes of boron and arsenic, hoping that they would localize in tumors and emit positrons or alpha radiation that would destroy the tumors. These therapies did not work, so he then turned to uranium as a possible treatment of brain tumors, particularly the untreatable and highly malignant glioblastoma.

The goals of ORNL and Sweet were different, but they could both be accomplished by injecting uranium into MGH patients with glioblastomas. The use of patients near death meant that the ORNL scientists did not have to be concerned about any long-term effects of the uranium and that they would be able to examine tissue obtained at autopsy to find out how the body handled uranium and measure its distribution throughout the body.

The goal of Sweet and MGH, in contrast, was to discover whether uranium localized in the brain tumors. If it did, physicians could inject a uranium isotope, uranium-235, into a person with a glioblastoma. Uranium-235 is fissile, meaning that it can be broken apart by thermal neutrons. (This isotope was used in the "Little Boy" bomb detonated over Hiroshima during World War II.) If uranium-235 in the brain tumor was exposed to a neutron beam to "activate" the uranium, the energy released could theoretically destroy the tumor.

Between 1953 and 1957, 11 patients at MGH were injected with various isotopes of uranium. The researchers discovered that the uranium localized in the human kidney at higher concentrations than it did in small animals and caused chemical, rather than radioactive, toxicity. This meant that the existing standards for acceptable uranium levels might have been too high. The uranium did not concentrate in tumor tissue, indicating that there would not be a role for uranium in tumor therapy.

There were many problems with this "dual experiment." First, it had been hastily organized, and was not preceded by the usual type of animal experiment. Next, there is no evidence that a protocol was ever written. The AEC supervised most radioisotope experiments (that involved low levels of radioactivity), but because this experiment was different—having to do with the highly radioactive uranium—it was, ironically, not supervised in the same way. Indeed, it seems not to have been supervised very closely at all.

The two groups involved also had different attitudes toward the uranium. ORNL scientists handled it carefully. The uranium was accounted for down to a milligram level and was accompanied by armed guards. Once the uranium reached MGH, however, this caution disappeared, and the MGH scientists handled it more casually. The groups also differed in the doses they wanted to use. Sweet wanted to use high doses, while ORNL wanted to use cumulative low doses, approximating occupational exposure. The ORNL ended the project when they discovered that Sweet was using doses many times higher than the permissible body burden.

Another problem is that there is no documentary evidence of informed consent. Sweet told the Advisory Committee on Human Radiation Experiments that he did obtain consent from the patients or their families and that he had given them all the information that he had about the experiment. But no evidence exists to support his claim.

Additionally, the experiments were not well conducted. In the first few experiments, the stopcocks in the injection tube did not work correctly. With the last three patients, the patient seemed to excrete more uranium than was reported to have been injected.

Finally, the selection of the patients was flawed. Although all of the patients were supposed to have been terminally ill and to have a malignant brain tumor, at least 1 of the 11 patients in the experiment did not have a brain tumor. This man had been brought into the hospital unconscious and had a subdural hematoma, not a brain tumor. He was given uranium and might have suffered from some kidney damage as a result. One other patient recovered and went home. The families of three patients refused to allow autopsies so we cannot be certain of the diagnosis in these cases.

The idea of a single experiment answering the questions of two quite different sets of investigators was appealing, but it turned out to be unworkable. Not much was learned from the administration of radioisotopes into ill patients. Whether the patients or their families actually did give consent or whether the patients were harmed remains unknown.

Frances R. Frankenburg

CAMERON, DONALD EWEN

Donald Ewen Cameron was the director of the Allan Memorial Institute in Montréal, a psychiatric research center. He used intensive electroconvulsive therapy and drug-induced comas in a form of "brainwashing." Some of his work was funded by the Central Intelligence Agency.

Donald Ewen Cameron (1901–1967) was born in Scotland and graduated from Glasgow University with his medical degree in 1924. He studied at the Phipps Institute in Baltimore with renowned psychiatrist Adolf Meyer (1866–1950) and then spent a year studying in Zurich. In 1929, he moved to Canada and became director of admissions at the Brandon Mental Hospital in Brandon, Manitoba. While there, he treated the patients with the methods of the time, including malariatherapy, insulin shock, and lobotomies. After seven years, he accepted a position as director of research at the Worcester State Hospital in Massachusetts. After another two years, he moved to Albany, New York, where he became professor of neurology and psychiatry at Albany Medical College.

In 1943, the Rockefeller Foundation helped to establish a psychiatric institute affiliated with the medical school at McGill University in Montréal. Although there were some areas of neurological and psychological academic strength in Montréal—neurologist Wilder Penfield (1891–1976) was making advances in the control of seizures and in mapping the brain, while psychologist Donald

O. Hebb (1904–1985) was exploring the surprisingly potent effects of sensory deprivation—there was little expertise in psychiatric research or training. The only English-speaking psychiatric facility was a large asylum at Verdun. Cameron was selected to be the first director of the newly established Allan Memorial Institute at McGill, known as "the Allan."

For 20 years, he was head of the Allan—which quickly became a center for psychiatric teaching, research, and clinical care—as well as chairman of the department of psychiatry at McGill. In many ways, he was an excellent choice. He instituted liberal policies such as never locking the doors in the facility. He developed the concept of a day hospital, in which patients could get intensive psychiatric treatment but not have to be hospitalized. He built up the psychiatry residency program at McGill. He was known to his admiring colleagues as the "Chief." He was skilled at grantsmanship, meaning that he had the ability to write grants that would be approved and funded. He wrote extensively and was well regarded by his peers, and in 1961, he was a founding member and president of the World Psychiatric Association. He was also the president of the American and Canadian psychiatric associations and brought conferences to Montréal, including the first North American psychopharmacology conference. Because of his international reputation, he was invited in 1945, along with other psychiatrists, including Jean Delay (1907–1987)—one of the first psychiatrists to use the antipsychotic medication chlorpromazine—to examine Adolf Hitler's deputy Rudolf Hess at the Nuremberg Trials. They concluded that Hess was fit to stand trial.

Cameron was interested in advancing psychiatry and to that end carried out an ambitious—and increasingly controversial—program of experimentation at the Allan. In the early 1950s, he began to use some relatively new technology of the time—audiotapes—to speed up what he saw as the tedious process of psychotherapy. He taped psychotherapy sessions and then repeatedly played a patient's statements back to him or her. When this technique didn't produce results, he began to use more aggressive techniques, including electroconvulsive therapy (ECT).

At that time, most patients with depression were treated with ECT two or three times over a period of a few weeks. However, some psychiatrists had started experimenting with ECT at a higher frequency. For example, in England, Robert Russell and Lewis Page treated patients with ECT once or twice a day—or even more often. Cameron adopted this "Page-Russell technique," which is also known as "regressive ECT" because the person undergoing the ECT treatments becomes confused to the point of being incontinent and needing to be fed. Cameron called the results "annihilation."

He also drugged his patients into prolonged and heavy periods of sleep. While they were in these states, he played tapes to them for hours at a time. The tapes often consisted of derogatory comments. The hope was that this process would erase existing harmful or unpleasant memories or patterns of bad behavior or break down their resistance to psychotherapy. He called this technique "depatterning," and once it was accomplished, he thought that the patient would become a "blank slate" on which to rebuild the "psyche" by "psychic driving" using "psychic implants."

His work attracted the interest of John Gittinger (1917–2003), a psychologist who worked for MKULTRA, a secret program run by the Central Intelligence Agency (CIA) that investigated mind control. The goal of MKULTRA was to investigate mind control, or brainwashing, both to be able to defend Americans against enemy agents and also to obliterate memories among CIA agents who no longer needed to know military secrets or who might be defectors. Gittinger asked a colleague to suggest to Cameron that he apply for funding from the Society for the Investigation of Human Ecology (SIHE), a "front" for the Central Intelligence Agency. Cameron, always looking for financial support for his research, asked the SIHE to support his work in investigating the effects of "repetition of verbal signals" and devising ways to "inactivate" the person while he or she was exposed to "psychic driving." The CIA approved his application for funds in February 1957 and paid Cameron about $19,000 a year for four years, beginning in 1957. His work was known as Subproject 68 of MKULTRA.

Cameron performed many experiments on patients at the Allan in the guise of treatment. He took Hebb's work on sensory deprivation much further than Hebb had done. In Hebb's experiments, graduate students volunteered to spend time in sensory-deprivation rooms. The subjects wore goggles and earphones. The students could not bear the isolation for more than a few days before becoming so distressed that the isolation, originally intended to last for weeks, was ended. On one occasion, Cameron put a 52-year-old woman who suffered from anxiety in a "box" for 35 days, where she was subjected to "prolonged sensory isolation." He experimented with lysergic acid diethylamide (LSD), paralytic drugs, and electroshock. He attempted to "depattern" over 50 patients by combining electroshock therapy and drug-induced coma-like states with "psychic driving." Some people were put to sleep for one to two months, with taped messages being played for hours at a time, being woken only to eat or to relieve themselves.

Cameron's work was not kept secret, either from his colleagues or the public. He openly described his treatments to the physicians who referred patients to him. He told the popular press that he was using brainwashing techniques on his patients, not to extract secrets from them or to indoctrinate them into carrying out sinister tasks but to help them. Hebb and others at McGill, including Penfield, disapproved of what Cameron was doing, but there is no record of anyone attempting to stop him. Hebb, who also had connections with the CIA, later said that Cameron's work made no sense at all and that his work was "criminally stupid."[1]

The CIA stopped funding Cameron in 1961, but the Canadian government continued to support his work. In 1963, Cameron announced at a conference that his experiments had not been successful, and he stopped his work in this area. A year later, he left the Allan and moved back to Albany, where he worked for the Veterans Administration, dying in 1967. His successor at the Allan, Robert Cleghorn, ended the practice of multiple ECT treatments and, presumably, Cameron's other practices.

Cameron's experiments would never have come to such wide attention and outrage had it not been for the discovery years later of his connection with the

CIA and his controversial treatment of Velma Orlikow, the wife of a member of the Canadian Parliament. Velma (known as Val) Orlikow was a Winnipeg, Manitoba, woman who developed a serious postpartum depression in the mid-1950s. She had gone to the Mayo Clinic in nearby Minnesota for treatment but did not improve. Desperate for help, she went to the Allan. On 14 occasions, Cameron gave her LSD combined with either a stimulant or a "depressant" medication and then left her alone while a tape recorder played back excerpts from previous therapy sessions. She disliked these "treatments," such as they were, but felt unable to stop them. Cameron would cajole her to continue by saying to her—as he said to many of his female patients—"Lassie, don't you want to get well, so you can go home and see your husband?"[2]

He also treated her insomnia with the highly addictive barbiturates and withheld them unless she cooperated with his suggestions. At one point, she was discharged from the hospital but stayed in Montréal by herself so that she could continue her treatment with him. After returning home to Winnipeg, she made a suicide attempt and returned once again to the Allan. Her husband, David, at that time a practicing pharmacist, and his brother continued to give her barbiturates.

Meanwhile, her husband became active in politics. Representing Winnipeg, he was a member of the Canadian Parliament between 1962 and 1988. Val Orlikow remained depressed. While they were living in Ottawa, they periodically drove across the border to Lake Placid, New York, where Cameron lived so that she could continue seeing him. She did this until he ended his treatment with her in 1967. Afterward, she remained depressed and unable to lead an active life.

In the late 1970s, David Orlikow read an article in the *New York Times* about the recently discovered mind-control activities of the CIA. He discovered that one of the physicians who had received funding from the CIA was Cameron. Val Orlikow was horrified to realize that Cameron might have been experimenting on her without her knowledge or consent and with the involvement of the United States government.

As a result, the Orlikows found a Washington-based attorney, Joseph Rauh, a political activist and civil rights lawyer. Rauh was willing to sue the CIA, claiming that it had been negligent in funding these harmful experiments. The case was complicated, however, because the years in which Orlikow had been treated by Cameron did not correspond with the years he received SIHE funding. However, eight other patients had stories somewhat similar to Orlikow's, and their years of treatment corresponded with Cameron's SIHE funding.

They joined her as plaintiffs. One man who had gone to the Allan for treatment of alcoholism was treated with barbiturates and put to sleep for 36 days. Another who had a complaint of leg pain was diagnosed as having a psychosomatic disorder. He was "depatterned" with intensive electroshocks and LSD and put into a drug-induced sleep for 23 days. A young doctor was admitted and "depatterned" with electroshock treatments and barbiturates. Following these experiments, many of the patients suffered from severe amnesia, and at least one person was diagnosed with a severe organic brain syndrome. The Canadian government did not wholeheartedly support the Orlikows' suit, fearing perhaps the political repercussions of backing a challenge to the CIA. The CIA, for its part, did not want to admit to anything.

During the hearings that ensued, psychiatrists testified as to the nontherapeutic nature of Cameron's work. A bioethicist pointed out that the patients had seen Cameron for treatment and had never agreed to be experimental subjects or given informed consent. The CIA and another bioethicist argued that it was common for researchers at the time to not obtain informed consent. The suit was settled out of court. In the 1980s, other patients who had been treated by Cameron during the years after the CIA had stopped their support sued the Canadian government; each of the victims was awarded $100,000 in compensation.

In retrospect, the combination of Cameron's administrative power and his willingness to harm people in the service of making discoveries to bring him fame was dangerous. Cameron's experiments were performed on a population that was vulnerable because of their psychiatric illnesses and without their consent—or even awareness that they were subjects of an experiment.

The patients, their families, and other Canadians did not protest against Cameron's work until the connection with the CIA was made. Yet, Cameron might well have proceeded with his work without the CIA funding because of his determination to advance psychiatry. The Canadian outrage at the cruelty of his work, though well deserved, was fueled by a resentment of American interference with the treatment of Canadian patients and revulsion at the nature and secrecy of the MKULTRA projects.

Frances R. Frankenburg

References

1. Streatfeild, *Brainwash*, 228.
2. Marks, *The Search for the "Manchurian Candidate,"* 149.

CARDIOPULMONARY RESUSCITATION

If a person suddenly stops breathing and his or her heart stops beating, occasionally he or she can be revived by cardiopulmonary resuscitation (CPR), a combination of chest compressions, establishment of an airway, and rescue breathing. Many experiments establishing the best way to perform CPR were carried out on anesthetized and paralyzed patients who were not breathing on their own.

Reviving a person who has suddenly stopped breathing or who has had a cardiac arrest is now a well-accepted medical activity and is known as cardiopulmonary resuscitation (CPR). *Cardiopulmonary* refers to the heart (cardio) and lungs (pulmonary); *resuscitation* means the revival of someone who is unconscious or who is not breathing or does not have a beating heart. The cardiac part of CPR involves chest compressions. The pulmonary part of CPR involves moving air through the airway, or the passage between the nose, mouth, and lungs, so that oxygen can reach the lungs. The development of CPR had several false starts, and the development of the pulmonary and cardiac parts of CPR proceeded along slightly different tracks before being joined in the 1960s.

Airway and Rescue Breathing

The first organized attempts to help people who had stopped breathing to breathe again began in Europe in the 1700s because of interest in preventing drowning deaths. These attempts included various ways of moving air into the lungs of a drowning victim, including mouth-to-mouth breathing. But in the 1770s, the use of exhaled air as a way of resuscitating people fell into disfavor. Around that time, Swedish chemist Carl Wilhelm Scheele (1742–1786) had discovered oxygen, and French chemist Antoine Lavoisier (1743–1794) had named it and shown its importance in breathing. Expired, or exhaled, air was not thought to contain enough oxygen to keep a person alive. As an alternative, some people advocated the use of a bellows as a way of forcing air into the lungs. People also found mouth-to-mouth breathing unacceptably intimate and worried that germs could be transmitted from the victim to the rescuer.

There were sporadic accounts of mouth-to-mouth breathing rescues. Midwives (and later obstetricians) long used this technique on newborn babies who failed to breathe. With the invention of anesthesia in the mid-1800s, anesthetists sometimes supported an overly sedated and nonbreathing patient with expired air through an endotracheal tube. But mouth-to-mouth, mouth-to-tube, and other kinds of rescue breathing remained uncommon until the mid-20th century.

In 1861, a young English physician named Henry Robert Silvester (1829–1908) developed a mechanical way of moving air in and out of the lungs of a person who had stopped breathing. He put the person on his or her back and then lifted both arms upward to cause inspiration and, applying pressure, folded the person's arms on his or her chest to cause the person to exhale. Colonel Holger Louis Nielsen (1866–1955), in Denmark, invented a different version of artificial respiration in which the person lay face down. These resuscitation techniques and other variations were used for the next hundred years to revive people.

During a poliomyelitis epidemic in Minnesota in 1946, patients with spinal-bulbar paralysis caused by poliomyelitis were ventilated with tank respirators, or "iron lungs." If the equipment failed, the paralyzed person was unable to breathe. Anesthesiologist James Elam (1918–1995) often performed mouth-to-nose or mouth-to-mouth respiration to keep the patients alive for up to three hours at a time.

In 1954, Elam expanded on this work and performed a number of experiments with postoperative patients. The patients were deliberately kept paralyzed for a longer period than they would have been otherwise so that the experiment could be carried out. Defying the belief that had held since the 18th century, Elam showed that a doctor breathing into a nonbreathing postoperative patient through a mask or tracheal tube could indeed provide that patient with sufficient oxygen. Whether these patients knew about the prolonged paralysis or gave consent is not known. Later, he began to work with Peter Safar (1924–2003), another anesthesiologist.

In 1956, Safar, Elam, and other colleagues, including Martin McMahon, chief of the Baltimore firefighters, began a series of experiments on volunteers. On weekends, they used operating rooms at the Baltimore City Hospital to determine the effectiveness of mouth-to-mouth ventilation compared to the Silvester and Holger Nielson techniques. They worked with "rescuers" and "volunteers." Most of the rescuers were nonmedical people, including a 10-year-old boy, a 70-year-old person, Boy Scouts, Safar's wife (not a physician), and firefighters. The volunteers were physicians, medical students, and one nurse; some of them volunteered several times. The volunteers agreed to undergo the actual resuscitation. Although no mention is made of written consent, the volunteers, all medical personnel, understood what they were undergoing.

The researchers anesthetized and paralyzed the volunteers for several hours. The paralytic medication stopped them from breathing but did not affect their hearts. Then the rescuers practiced resuscitating them. The experiments were filmed.

Safar and colleagues showed that artificial breathing worked best when the rescuer extended the person's neck and pulled the jaw up, using the techniques today known as "head tilt" and "jaw thrust." These maneuvers prevent the tongue from falling into the airway and obstructing it. Professionals performing the Silvester or Holger Nielsen method achieved poorer results than the rescuers, untrained in medicine, performing mouth-to-mouth or mouth-to-airway ventilation. Safar and Elam measured carbon dioxide and oxygen levels in both the volunteers and rescuers and once again showed that the rescuer's expired air contained enough oxygen to oxygenate another person sufficiently to keep that person alive. (Safar and McMahon also developed a pocket-size S-shaped breathing tube, or airway, that allows the rescuer to ventilate the unbreathing person without mouth-to-mouth contact. This device further helped to maintain the airway, or to keep it open.)

Meanwhile, Archer Gordon (1921–1994), a cardiologist, had been evaluating methods of artificial respiration for some years. He experimented on corpses from the wards of Cook County Hospital in Chicago and concluded that a modified Nielsen procedure was the best and that mouth-to-nose or mouth-to-mouth was too difficult to teach. Later, Elam convinced Gordon to test his conclusions by more experiments. Gordon experimented with mouth-to-mouth techniques on infants and small children who had been put under general anesthesia for circumcision and indeed became convinced of the superiority of mouth-to-mouth ventilation. He joined Elam and Safar in working to convince others of the rediscovered benefits of mouth-to-mouth rescue breathing. (In his 1958 description of these experiments, no mention is made of consent on behalf of the children.)

Chest Compressions

The development of chloroform anesthesia in the mid-1800s increased the number of sudden cardiac arrests during surgery, probably due to chloroform-induced cardiac arrhythmias. In the late 1800s and early 1900s, Friedrich Maass, a German surgeon, and George Washington Crile (1863–1943), an American surgeon, revived people whose hearts had stopped during anesthesia, by performing closed chest compression in humans. This technique, however, did not become widely used at this time. Instead, when such arrhythmias occurred, other physicians would sometimes open the chest and manually squeeze the heart rhythmically to restart the heart. This major medical intervention, known as "open chest cardiac massage," was impossible outside of an operating room.

Closed chest compressions finally became an accepted part of medical practice because of the work of people interested in the electrical system of the heart. This system organizes a regular rhythmic pumping. William Bennett Kouwenhoven (1886–1975) was an electrical engineer who, together with another electric engineer, Guy Knickerbocker, and physician James Jude at Johns Hopkins University, was studying fibrillation, or an irregular heart rhythm. Kouwenhoven, Knickerbocker, and Jude explored ways of defibrillating, or shocking, the heart back into a regular rhythm. (The work on defibrillation was funded by electrical companies because of an increasing number of electrocutions due to exposure to capacitators, transmission wires, or other electrical machinery.) In 1958, when working with dogs, they forcefully applied heavy defibrillation paddles to the chest of a dog, and even before applying a current, a pulse in the femoral artery appeared. This accidental or serendipitous observation led to the rediscovery of chest compressions. Further experimentation in dogs answered such questions as how fast, where, and how deep to press. (The team went on to make advances in defibrillation of the heart.)

Chest compressions help to circulate blood throughout the body, even when the heart is not pumping. Pushing down on the chest forces blood through the heart and to the rest of the body. When the person performing the compressions releases his or her pressure on the victim's chest, the chest expands and creates a negative pressure that pulls blood back into the heart, ready for the next compression. The alternating positive and negative pressure are needed to keep the blood circulating throughout the body.

Cardiopulmonary Resuscitation

In the 1960s, cardiopulmonary resuscitation (CPR) was established by the integration of chest compressions with mouth-to-mouth ventilation. This widely accepted and fairly simple procedure does not require sophisticated medical training or equipment. At first the sequence for CPR was ABC: airway, breathing, compressions. However, in 2010, the sequence was changed to CAB—putting the emphasis on chest compressions. As of 2016, the emphasis in CPR is on doing high-quality chest compressions and getting a defibrillator as quickly as possible. Closed chest compressions are of value mainly as a way of keeping the person alive until the heart can be defibrillated or restored to a regular rhythm.

In summary, although some details of cardiopulmonary resuscitation were worked out through experimentation on animals, the definitive experiments with maintaining the airway and rescue breathing were carried out on surgical patients who had been anesthetized and paralyzed. Often little mention is made of consent. Other experiments involved laypeople, including Boy Scouts, practicing on paralyzed volunteers who were medical professionals and did understand what they were undergoing.

Frances R. Frankenburg

CIA AND MIND CONTROL

During the Cold War, the Central Intelligence Agency (CIA) became apprehensive about the possibility of the enemy using brainwashing drugs to control human behavior. The CIA conducted a series of secret experiments, as part of a project called MKULTRA, to gain its own expertise with mind control, or brainwashing.

During the Cold War, the U.S. government was concerned about the possible use of "brainwashing drugs" by countries such as China and the Soviet Union. Government officials wondered whether Hungary's Cardinal József Mindszenty (1892–1975) had been brainwashed by the Russian Communists and whether American prisoners of war in North Korea had been brainwashed by their Chinese captors. Both Mindszenty and the American POWs had confessed to crimes that they had almost certainly not committed.

With the goal of understanding how various drugs might control human behavior, the Central Intelligence Agency (CIA), directed by Allen Dulles, established Project Bluebird in April 1951. Bluebird became known as Artichoke on August 20, 1951, and then MKULTRA (sometimes spelled MK-ULTRA) in April 1953. MKULTRA was led by Sidney Gottlieb (1918–1999), an American biochemist who was interested in anything that could change a person's thinking. In particular, he was intrigued by the psychedelic agent lysergic acid diethylamide (LSD) because of its powerful effects on the mind. At one point, Gottlieb recruited a well-known New York magician, John Mulholland, to prepare a manual to teach CIA agents how to slip LSD or other drugs into drinks of enemy agents to "incapacitate" them. LSD is ideal for these purposes because it can be used in small quantities and is colorless, odorless, and tasteless.

The CIA organized secret experiments to determine the possible effectiveness of psychedelics and other drugs in the use of brainwashing. The CIA tested LSD and other drugs on many people, such as narcotics addicts, federal prisoners, terminally ill cancer patients, and college students, without their consent. In 1953, Gottlieb surreptitiously gave LSD to CIA agent Frank Olson while investigating reactions to the drug, and a short while later, Olson fell from a hotel window and died. Whether his death was related to the LSD and whether it was murder or suicide continues to be debated.

Over the course of its existence, MKULTRA worked with about 80 institutions, including universities and prisons. Two prominent psychiatrists at the New York State Psychiatric Institute, supported by CIA funds and interested in the effects of mescaline, treated a depressed patient with increasing doses of derivatives of this psychedelic agent; he died as a result of the experiment.

Another institution involved in these experiments was the Lexington Narcotic Farm in Kentucky, established in 1935 as an addiction treatment center. Research was carried out at a part of the farm known as the Addiction Research Center (ARC). From 1945 to 1963, ARC's director was Harris Isbell (1910–1994), a respected medical scientist who worked for MKULTRA. As part of the MKULTRA experiments, about 300 patients were given LSD, often in high doses and for lengthy periods of time to test its effects.

Perhaps the most infamous mind-control experiments conducted with the help of the CIA were those done by psychiatrist Donald Ewen Cameron (1901–1967) in Canada. For 20 years, he carried out experiments at the Allan Memorial Institute, the main psychiatric hospital at McGill University in Montréal. Cameron held many prestigious positions in psychiatry, including the presidency of the World Psychiatric Association and the American and Canadian psychiatric associations.

He developed the concept of "psychic driving," which fascinated the CIA. He thought that he could erase existing memories and rebuild the psyche completely. MKULTRA paid over $60,000 to support his work at the Allan Memorial Institute, which included experiments with LSD, paralytic drugs, and electroshock. He put subjects into drug-induced comas and played tape loops of noise or repetitive statements. His patients were unaware that they were experimental subjects and instead thought they were receiving psychiatric treatments to help their conditions. After MKULTRA stopped funding Cameron, the Canadian government supported his work. In the 1980s, patients who had been treated by Cameron sued the Canadian government. Each of the victims was awarded $100,000 in compensation.

One unexpected consequence of the CIA's interest in LSD was that the experiments it sponsored introduced some people to the drug, who then promoted its use. In 1960, Stanford University student Ken Kesey (1935–2001) was paid $75 to take part in some CIA-funded and Stanford-organized LSD experiments at the Veterans Administration (VA) hospital in Menlo Park. He liked his experiences with LSD, dropped out of his Stanford writing program, became an attendant at the VA hospital, and wrote successful novels, including *One Flew Over the Cuckoo's Nest* (later adapted into an Academy Award–winning film) and *Sometimes a Great Notion*. He also formed the Merry Pranksters, a group of people who drove across America under the influence of various drugs, and organized a series of parties known as "acid tests." Tom Wolfe (b. 1931) described these parties in his 1968 book *The Electric Kool-Aid Acid Test*.

Many details of these experiments will probably never be known. Gottlieb retired from the CIA in 1972, noting that his work had not been useful. In 1973, Richard Helms, then the CIA director, destroyed many MKULTRA records.

But despite the destruction of files and the secrecy of the work, details began to emerge in the 1970s. In the mid-1970s, two governmental agencies investigated the activities of the Central Intelligence Agency (CIA), including MKULTRA. These investigations came about because, in December 1974, the *New York Times* reported that the Central Intelligence Agency (CIA) had carried out illegal activities during the 1960s. In 1975, in response to these reports, President Gerald Ford established the President's Commission on CIA Activities Within the United States. (Because this commission was headed by then Vice President Nelson Rockefeller, it is now known as the Rockefeller Commission of 1975.) The commission issued a report later that year in which it described abuses by the CIA, including mail opening and surveillance of domestic dissident groups and some issues relating to the assassination of President John F. Kennedy. The commission briefly discussed the activities of MKULTRA.

The second body was an 11-member Senate committee, chaired by Frank Church of Idaho, officially known as the United States Senate Select Committee to Study Governmental Operations with Respect to Intelligence Activities, and unofficially known as the Church Committee. The committee reviewed the files of the Rockefeller Commission and then went on to review files from the Federal Bureau of Investigations, CIA, Internal Revenue Service, and other federal agencies. Members of the committee interviewed 800 people and conducted over 250 hearings. The committee issued 14 reports in 1975 and 1976.

Both investigative bodies were aware of the existence of MKULTRA, but because most of the records had been destroyed, little of value emerged from these investigations. There was enough evidence, however, for the Church Committee to condemn the project because of its covert use of uninformed citizens as research subjects.

More details were revealed when John D. Marks, a former State Department officer, using the Freedom of Information Act, obtained boxes of MKULTRA records that had mistakenly not been destroyed because officials thought that they contained only financial records. Marks also conducted many interviews of his own and wrote a 1978 book detailing MKULTRA activities, *Search for the "Manchurian Candidate": The CIA and Mind Control: The Secret History of the Behavioral Sciences*, a comprehensive account of the CIA's experiments.

There is no evidence that the MKULTRA experiments were of any practical use or ever used against American enemies.

Frances R. Frankenburg

DECLARATION OF HELSINKI

The World Medical Association (WMA) was established in 1947. At its 1964 assembly in Helsinki, it issued the Declaration of Helsinki, a modified form of the 1947 Nuremberg Code addressing research ethics, and the first attempt of the international research community to regulate itself. Many revisions have followed.

The Nuremberg Code, written in 1947 in reaction to the crimes committed by the Nazi physicians before and during World War II, outlined the ethical aspects of human research. The code was admired, but it had little impact in the few years after it had been written. Many physicians felt that the Nuremberg Code was addressed to barbaric physicians and had little relevance for them. Yet, during the next two decades, some physicians continued to perform research studies of an ethically questionable nature.

The World Medical Association (WMA), established in 1947, is an international association that represents national medical associations. The WMA is primarily interested in medical ethics, public health, and the professional freedom of physicians. In 1948, it issued the Declaration of Geneva, outlining the ethical duties of physicians. In 1964, during its assembly in Helsinki, Finland, the WMA addressed one of the areas of confusion in the Nuremberg Code: whether or not the rules applied in the same way to both healthy volunteers and ill subjects. Many doctors had claimed that they were surely allowed to differentiate between patients and research subjects and to have more freedom with respect to the former.

To resolve this confusion, the Declaration of Helsinki created two categories of research: Clinical Research Combined with Professional Care and Non-therapeutic Clinical Research. In the first case, physicians only had to get consent "when consistent with patient psychology."[1] In the words of Helsinki, "In the treatment of the sick person the doctor must be free to use a new therapeutic measure if in his judgment it offers hope of saving life, re-establishing health, or alleviating suffering."[2] For research without clinical care, fully informed consent was needed.

In both categories, Helsinki allowed a legal guardian to give consent for a subject who was unable to give informed consent. To some, this was considered a move away from the insistence of the Nuremberg Code that the subject himself or herself give consent. To others, it meant that groups of people formerly denied the possibility of participating in research now had that opportunity.

Since 1964, the Declaration of Helsinki has been amended seven times, most recently in October 2013. The first revision, in 1975, doubled the length of the 1964 version and clearly stated that control groups should receive the "best proven diagnostic and therapeutic method."[3] This statement has been used to criticize the use of placebos or less-effective treatments in studies in third-world countries. Others have suggested that this requirement is too rigorous and does not acknowledge the real-world situation—that many people simply have no access to the best therapies.

The 1975 Declaration of Helsinki also addressed some elements of ethical research missing in the Nuremberg Code in that it mandated attention to preservation of confidentiality. The 1975 version also stated that "concern for the interests of the subject must always prevail over the interests of science and society."[4] The 1975 revision is also notable for its introduction of the requirement for an overseeing "independent committee" to review research proposals, similar to what is known in the United States as an institutional review board.

The Helsinki document had more impact than the Nuremberg Code, perhaps because it was written by the global medical community and not solely in response to Nazi acts of evil.

Frances R. Frankenburg

References

1.   Declaration of Helsinki I, 18th World Medical Assembly, Helsinki, Finland, June 1964. In Annas and Grodin, *The Nazi Doctors*, 331–333.

2. Ibid.
3. Declaration of Helsinki II, 29th World Medical Assembly, Tokyo, Japan, October 1975. In Annas and Grodin, *The Nazi Doctors*, 333–336.
4. Ibid.

DEVELOPMENT OF CHLORPROMAZINE

Before the development of chlorpromazine, there was no effective treatment of psychotic illnesses. A fortunate experiment by a French surgeon-anesthetist led to the discovery of the first antipsychotic agents.

The development of chlorpromazine, the first effective antipsychotic medication, has been described as serendipitous because the investigators involved had not been looking for a psychiatric medication, but rather a safe antihistamine to be used in anesthesia. Patients under general anesthesia sometimes experienced severe loss of blood pressure, or shock. Because histamine lowered blood pressure, it was hypothesized that the release of histamine was the cause of anesthesia-related shock. It was then a natural next step to postulate that antihistamines could prevent surgical shock.

By 1945, the Rhône-Poulenc laboratories in France had synthesized clinically useful antihistaminic molecules. Paul Charpentier, a Rhône-Poulenc chemist, used a phenothiazine molecule to synthesize promethazine, later known in the United States as Phenergan (an antihistaminic drug used to treat allergies and motion sickness). He gave this molecule to naval surgeon-anesthesiologist Henri Laborit (1914–1995) to test as a preoperative sedative and "autonomic stabilizing agent." Laborit administered promethazine to his patients before surgery in an attempt to prevent surgical shock. He found it (like the other antihistamines) to be sedating and came to value its sedating property over its specific antihistaminic property.

In October 1950, Rhône-Poulenc began to study phenothiazines specifically with respect to their central nervous system activity. Charpentier synthesized chlorpromazine in 1950 by adding chlorine to another phenothiazine called promazine. Rhône-Poulenc sent samples of chlorpromazine to Laborit. After administering the new agent, Laborit found that he was able to use smaller doses of anesthetic while at the same time achieving deeper and more prolonged anesthesia. Laborit and his anesthesiologist-collaborator Pierre Huguenard used what is called a "lytic cocktail"—a mixture of drugs designed to produce sedation and analgesia—to produce "artificial hibernation," or reduced metabolism, in presurgical patients. By combining several agents (in varying combinations), including barbiturates, opiates, curare, chlorpromazine, or promethazine, smaller amounts of each drug could be used. In 10 to 15 minutes after the administration of the "cocktail," hypothermia was induced with the use of icepacks, and the surgery then proceeded. At that time, hypothermia and "artificial hibernation" were thought to make surgery a safer and more tolerable procedure by lowering the metabolic needs of the body. Hypothermia is still sometimes used today in the treatment of cardiac arrest and brain injury.

Laborit also experimented with preoperative intravenous doses of 50 to 100 milligrams of chlorpromazine (with no other agents) and found that his patients were calm, tranquil, and alert. Despite his original interest in these drugs as antishock agents and potentiators of anesthesia, Laborit appreciated the significance of the patient's "désintéressement" in his or her surroundings and concluded that chlorpromazine might have uses in psychiatry. This surgeon-anesthetist's experiment would turn out to be a key event in the history of psychopharmacology.

Psychiatrists at the military hospital where Laborit worked took advantage of the sedative and apparent antianxiety effects of the new drug to potentiate the effects of a barbiturate to successfully treat a young man diagnosed with acute mania. In February 1952, Jean Delay (1907–1987) and Pierre Deniker (1917–1998), at Hôpital Sainte Anne, near Paris, were the first psychiatrists to use chlorpromazine as a monotherapy for mania and other "excited" states. Delay and Deniker convened meetings, wrote articles, and fostered much of the excitement that led to the development of the new field of effective medications to treat psychotic illnesses.

The introduction of chlorpromazine to North America began in Montréal. In the spring of 1953, psychiatrist Heinz Lehmann (1911–1999), working at the Verdun Protestant Hospital (now called the Douglas Hospital), first administered chlorpromazine to student nurses. Even though some nurses collapsed because of low blood pressure, Lehmann was not deterred and went on to treat manic patients with chlorpromazine with good results. He used doses as high as 800 milligrams a day, while Delay and Deniker were using about 150 milligrams a day. (In general, European psychiatrists continue to use psychiatric medications at lower doses than American psychiatrists.) Lehmann noted that some patients with chronic schizophrenia had accidentally been left on large doses of chlorpromazine. To his surprise, about one quarter of the patients seemed to improve. This accidental experiment was the first long-term use of the medication.

The effectiveness of chlorpromazine allowed thousands of formerly confined psychotic patients to leave asylums and led to the involvement of large pharmaceutical companies in the development of more psychiatric medications and antipsychotic agents.

Frances R. Frankenburg

FERNALD STATE SCHOOL

Between 1946 and 1953, the Massachusetts Institute of Technology (MIT)—with support from Quaker Oats and as part of research authorized by the Atomic Energy Commission—carried out some controversial nutrition experiments at a Massachusetts residential school called the Fernald State School. Young boys who were members of a so-called science club were fed oatmeal containing radioactive isotopes so that the researchers could study the absorption of calcium and iron.

In 1848, Samuel Gridley Howe (1801–1876), an abolitionist, educator, physician, and philanthropist, established the Massachusetts School for the Feeble-Minded to help disadvantaged children lead better lives—the first such institution in the United States. In 1925, its name was changed to the Walter E. Fernald School, in honor of its third superintendent, Walter E. Fernald (1859–1924). The school was located in Waltham, about 12 miles northwest of Boston. By mid-20th century, the school had developed a mixed population: some of the children suffered from developmental disabilities, and others were there because their families, for various reasons, could not manage to raise them. The higher-functioning boys worked in the fields around the school, in the kitchen, or on weaving machines.

In the 1940s, radioisotopes were used in many experiments to study various aspects of nutrition. Institutionalized people were ideal subjects because their diet could be closely monitored. The Massachusetts Institute of Technology carried out several of these experiments at the Fernald School with the authorization of the Atomic Energy Commission (AEC). Congress had established the AEC in 1946 to develop a variety of uses of nuclear science and technology that had hitherto been used to make bombs. Around this time, a "science club" was established at Fernald. Those boys selected to join the club were offered larger portions of food, parties, and trips to Boston Red Sox baseball games. However, the boys did not study science or perform experiments; they were the subjects of experiments. Once chosen, their membership and participation in the experiments were mandatory.

One study was sponsored by the food company Quaker Oats. In the late 1940s, there was concern about the nutritional value of the cereals, as some research showed that plant-based grains contained high levels of phytate, a substance that when consumed inhibited the absorption of iron and calcium. When Quaker discovered that MIT was interested in investigating how minerals and vitamins are absorbed, they offered to help to fund the research to gain some commercial advantage over their rivals and to prove the nutritional value of their oatmeal.

Between 1946 and 1953, researchers gave over 70 members of the Fernald "science club" iron-enriched cereals and calcium-enriched milk for breakfast. To track absorption of the minerals, radioactive iron and calcium tracers were given orally or intravenously. Blood was taken from the boys on a regular basis, and their urine and feces were collected.

The parents or guardians of the children were informed about these studies in misleading language. In November 1949, the school superintendent sent parents a letter describing a special diet for the boys that was rich in iron and vitamins and required some blood tests. Parents and guardians were asked to sign an enclosed form to grant permission for the boys to participate. In May 1953, the school sent the parents another letter, again making it seem that they were interested in improving the nutrition of the students. This letter required the parents to do nothing—unless they objected to the study. They were not informed of the use of radioisotopes.

The children were probably not harmed by the radiation in these studies, as the amount of radioactivity they were exposed to was very low. Nonetheless, the study personnel did not inform the boys or their parents and guardians of the nature of these experiments. The researchers did not choose to use themselves, their own children, or other children in institutions, such as those at expensive boarding schools. Instead, they chose disadvantaged and developmentally disabled children and then provided parents and guardians with an incomplete explanation of the studies. Critics have suggested that most people, if informed of the true nature of these studies, would not have participated or allowed their own children to be involved. Many have also noted that the use of institutionalized children, while convenient for the researchers, did not seem fair or ethical. Indeed, a 1995 class-action lawsuit resulted in a 1998 district court decision awarding the subjects a $1.85 million settlement from MIT and Quaker Oats.

The oatmeal studies are the best documented of these kinds of radioisotope studies, but other such experiments were done at Fernald and similar schools in Massachusetts, including studies of thyroid function at the Wrentham State School that involved the administration of radioactive iodine. In the history of medical experimentation, the use of institutionalized children as unwitting subjects was not unusual.

Frances R. Frankenburg

HEART SURGERY AND TRANSPLANTATION

Heart surgery, including heart transplants, an example of the success of modern medicine, required much innovation and experimentation.

For a long time, the heart seemed an impossible candidate for surgery. The heart is full of blood, making it difficult for surgeons to see or feel what they were doing once inside that organ. The rapid heartbeat hinders the ability of the surgeon to maneuver precisely. As well as being difficult, heart surgery also seemed too dangerous. Any interference with the heart affects the supply of blood to the entire body. The heart has an electrical conduction system, allowing it to pump—or contract and expand—in a synchronized manner. If the surgeon inadvertently damages this system, the pumping may become uncoordinated and therefore less efficient, thus interfering with blood supply to the body. Furthermore, because the blood is pumped through the heart at high pressure, a surgical misstep could lead to rapid and fatal blood loss.

Of all the body's organs, the brain is the most sensitive to blood loss. It can withstand a loss of blood (and oxygen) for only a few minutes before it is damaged. All of these reasons combined to make doctors hesitant to operate on the heart, as the challenging operation, if it failed, could lead to death or irreversible brain damage.

Nonetheless, beginning in the 20th century, physicians began to investigate and then operate on the heart, making slow but steady progress. Werner Forssmann (1904–1979) was the first person to put a catheter into the heart, carrying out the procedure on himself in 1929.

Dwight Harken (1910–1993), a military surgeon during World War II, removed shrapnel from the hearts of wounded soldiers and then repaired stenotic (too narrow) mitral valves. (The mitral valve is a flap between the heart's left atrium and left ventricle.) His work showed that cardiac surgery was indeed possible.

The next advance in cardiac surgery was a dramatic operation at Johns Hopkins on a "blue baby," born with the tetralogy of Fallot, a congenital heart condition with four anomalies in the structure of the heart. (The anomalies include a hole in one of the heart's interior walls, narrowing of the pulmonary artery, overgrowth of the right ventricle, and the mispositioning of the aorta.) This complex set of problems interferes with the normal oxygenation of blood and leads to the babies looking cyanotic, or bluish. The condition had been described by Steno in Denmark in 1673, Fallot in Marseilles in 1888, and definitively by Maude Abbott (1869–1940) in Canada in 1936. Abbott was encouraged by William Osler (1849–1919), the great Canadian clinician and one of the founders of the Johns Hopkins medical school, to organize the specimens at the McGill Medical Museum in Montréal. She became the curator of that museum and wrote *Atlas of Congenital Heart Disease* in 1936, in which she described over a thousand cases of congenital heart disease. In this book, she linked the physical findings made during life with the findings at autopsy.

In 1944, cardiac surgeon Alfred Blalock (1899–1964), surgical technician Vivien Thomas (1910–1985), and cardiologist Helen Taussig (1898–1986) at Johns Hopkins successfully treated a baby with this condition. Using Abbott's atlas to understand the anatomy of the baby's faulty blood supply, the Johns Hopkins team joined the subclavian artery to the pulmonary artery and thus improved blood flow to the lungs, allowing the blood to become properly oxygenated.

The success of what became known as the Blalock-Thomas-Taussig shunt stimulated more cardiac investigations and surgery. Cardiologists developed clever techniques and machines to allow open-heart surgery to proceed safely, even while the heart was not pumping blood. For example, Walton Lillehei (1918–1999), a Minnesota cardiac surgeon, operated on babies while their blood supply was connected with another person's circulation. This was known as cross-circulation. Blood flow was routed from the patient to the donor's femoral vein and lungs, where it was oxygenated and then returned to the patient's carotid artery.

Wilfred Bigelow (1913–2005), a Canadian heart surgeon, then showed that cooling the body would allow the brain to survive the decreases in blood flow caused by heart surgery for longer periods of time. Bigelow established a hypothermia research unit at the Banting Institute in Toronto and performed the world's first open-heart surgery on a dog using the principle of hypothermia. (Later, he would develop the cardiac pacemaker used to control the heart's rhythm.)

Surgeons Clarence Dennis (1909–2005), John Gibbon (1903–1973), and Robert DeWall (1903–1973) worked with Lillehei and developed a series of heart-bypass machines that allowed surgeons to operate on a relatively bloodless heart while a machine nearby circulated and oxygenated the body's blood. A heart-bypass machine has to pump blood vigorously enough so that the blood reaches all parts of the body, but not so vigorously that the red blood cells are damaged. The blood must be oxygenated but cannot contain any gas bubbles that would interrupt blood flow in the smaller vessels. Some of the early machines involved membrane oxygenation; others used antifoam agents from dairies and tubing from beer and dairy plants.

Sometimes, however, the heart was so damaged that transplant, or replacement of the entire organ, seemed the only option. One of the most significant surgical advances in the history of medicine has been the ability to transplant organs from one person to another. This advance was helped by the experiments of the Nobel Prize–winning surgeon Alexis Carrel (1873–1944), who mastered the art of anastomosis (joining together) of blood vessels and who performed some early transplants in animals.

Transplantation of human hearts was difficult for many reasons, one of which was the response of the body's immune system. Peter Medawar (1915–1987), a British biologist, saw World War II soldiers with terrible burns undergo painful and ultimately unsuccessful skin grafts. He came to understand that the immune system allows the body to distinguish between its own cells and foreign, or "not-self," cells. The immune system fights off unwanted bacteria and viruses as well as the implantation of foreign organs, including skin grafts—this is known as "rejection." By 1951, Medawar's group had also shown that corticosteroids, either the hormones produced by the adrenal gland or synthetic chemicals, weakened the immune system and delayed the rejection response.

Many surgeons came to Minnesota to learn about cardiac surgery and possible approaches to transplantation from Lillehei and his team. One student was Christiaan Barnard (1922–2001), a South African cardiac surgeon, who studied at Minnesota from 1956–1958. In 1967, in Cape Town's Groote Schuur Hospital in South Africa, Barnard performed the first human heart transplant. Barnard transplanted the heart of a young woman who had died in a car accident into a 58-year-old man with serious heart disease due to coronary artery disease. Eighteen days after the transplant, the patient died of pneumonia, probably due to the immunosuppressant drugs used to combat rejection.

Barnard's work created worldwide excitement, not least among other cardiac surgeons. In 1968, cardiac surgeon Norman Shumway (1923–2006) performed the first human-to-human heart transplant in the United States. In that year, surgical teams performed over a hundred transplants.

As heart transplantation evolved and developed, so too did the definition and understanding of death. In the past, death was understood to occur when the heart stopped beating. The removal of a beating heart from a body, therefore, was considered to be murder. For physicians, the problem was that if a heart were removed from a body more than a few minutes after it stopped beating, it was less likely to be healthy enough to be transplanted into another human. But, beginning in the mid-20th century, the refinement of artificial ventilation and the development of intensive care units meant that, with the help of machines and medication, a person's heart can beat for a period of time in the absence of brain activity. If in that case the person was declared dead, the heart could be removed while it was still beating, or immediately after it had stopped, and its transplantation was thus more likely to succeed.

Henry Beecher (1904–1976), professor of anesthesiology at Harvard Medical School and an author of an influential article about medical research ethics, headed a 1968 Harvard committee consisting of 10 physicians, a lawyer, and a historian, with the goal of defining death. The Ad Hoc Committee of the Harvard Medical School to Examine the Definition of Brain Death concluded that brain death is death. The committee declared that life support could be withdrawn from patients with "irreversible coma" or "brain death" and that their organs could be removed for transplantation, with the appropriate consent. Subsequent court cases and guidelines have agreed that the earlier definition of death—the cessation of a heartbeat—be replaced by evidence of brain death. In 1980, an American Presidents Commission also agreed. But this definition of death continues to be controversial. The idea that a person can be considered dead while the heart is still beating is contrary to our intuition and often difficult for the family to accept.

The 1968 removal of a heart from a brain-dead person led to a four-year-long court case in which Richard Lower (1929–2008), a young colleague of Shumway, was accused of hastening the death of a black man so that his heart could be given to a white man. The judge began the case believing that the cessation of the heartbeat was the definition of death. But during the case, he changed his mind, influenced by the growing medical consensus, and the jury acquitted Lower in 1972.

Meanwhile, patients who had received heart transplants were not doing well. Most died of complications related to rejection within a few months, and few were able to leave the hospital. Cardiac surgeons thus reduced the number of transplants, and in 1971, only 10 were performed. Powerful immunosuppressant medications were needed to allow the recipient to accept the donor heart, but these same medications were associated with many complications, including susceptibility to infections. That same year, cyclosporine, a substance isolated from a fungus, was discovered to be an antifungal agent. In 1976, its ability to suppress the immune system without excessive toxicity was discovered. In the 1980s, solid-organ transplantation entered the cyclosporine era with better results. Worldwide, over 5,000 cardiac transplants are now performed annually.

The ability to perform cardiac transplants depended on advances in operative techniques and the development of new medications. The first transplants in humans were therapeutic experiments, in the sense that the outcome was unknown. Surgeons tried out untested or unproven procedures on people who had no expectation of survival otherwise. The experiments were designed both as a desperate last resort but also to further experience and knowledge in the transplant field. An unexpected outcome of these transplants was their contribution to the discussion surrounding the definition of death.

Frances R. Frankenburg

IRRADIATION OF PRISONERS' TESTICLES

Physicians irradiated the testes of prisoners in Oregon and Washington for a decade to investigate the effects of radiation on the male reproductive system.

One of the many concerns arising from the use of atomic bombs in the Cold War was the effect of radiation on the male reproductive system. The immediate concern of the Atomic Energy Commission (AEC) was the health of the workers in the bomb industry who were inevitably exposed to radiation. The National Aeronautic Space Agency (NASA) was also concerned because astronauts are exposed to more radiation in space than on earth. The testes are particularly sensitive to radiation, which can slow down or stop sperm cell production or increase the rate of mutations.

Carl Heller, an endocrinologist, had been conducting hormonal experiments at the Oregon state prison in Salem and submitted a proposal to the AEC to study the effects of X-rays on testicles. C. Alvin Paulsen, a student of Heller's, proposed a study of the effects of radium on testicles at the Washington state prison in Walla Walla. The AEC reviewed and approved both proposals.

Between 1963 and 1971, 67 convicts at the Oregon state prison in Salem had their testicles radiated and underwent multiple biopsies. Vasectomies were done so that the men would not pass on any radiation-caused mutations to their children. The prisoners volunteered for the experiment and were paid for each procedure. Apparently, the subjects were informed of the risks of skin burns or pain, but they were not clearly told about the increased risk of cancer that goes along with radiation—though, as the studies proceeded, Heller sometimes told prisoners that there was a chance of "tumors." Prisoners also assisted in the experiments, serving as nurses and technicians.

Officials at the Salem prison became uneasy about Heller's work, in part because Heller established close relationships with some of the prisoners—writing letters on their behalf, even taking one to live in his home. Heller irradiated his last subject in 1971. In 1973, all experiments were stopped at the Salem state prison after an administrator read an *Atlantic Monthly* article by Jessica Mitford (1917–1996) about unethical prison research.

Later, when these experiments were investigated by the Advisory Committee on Human Radiation Experiments (ACHRE), Heller's wife told the committee that he had suggested that workers and astronauts have testicular biopsies performed before they were exposed to any risk of radiation so that later on biopsies could be done to estimate how much radiation damage occurred. This suggestion was not acted upon.

Paulsen carried out similar studies in Washington State. Beginning in 1963, 64 convicts at the state prison in Walla Walla had their testicles irradiated; many were also later vasectomized. In 1969, the chief of the Research Review Committee of the Department of Institutions at Washington stopped Paulsen's research, citing troubling inconsistency between the work at Walla Walla and the principles outlined in the Nuremberg Code.

In both settings, there were no detailed protocols and a lack of informed consent. Convicts gave a variety of reasons for subjecting themselves to this radiation. In most cases, it was probably for the money, but some talked about volunteering to make amends for their crimes and to help humanity or because they did not want children. There has been no follow-up on the health of the prisoners in either study.

The ACHRE reviewed these studies and described Heller and Paulsen as showing "sensitivity to some ethical issues," but noted that the two physicians did not follow the rules of the AEC, which mandated that subjects exposed to radiation be fully informed volunteers. Nonetheless, ACHRE described the studies as "groundbreaking" and did not think that the amount of radiation to which the prisoners were exposed would lead to an increase in the risk of cancer of more than four-hundredths of 1 percent.

Frances R. Frankenburg

KATZ, JAY

Jay Katz was a psychiatrist and bioethicist who compiled an authoritative sourcebook about medical experimentation. He was a member of committees that reviewed two well-known human experiments—the Tuskegee Study of Untreated Syphilis and the Cold War human radiation experiments. In both cases, he wrote a dissenting opinion in which he emphasized the failure of the physicians to recognize the importance of voluntary and informed consent.

Jacob (Jay) Katz (1922–2008) was born in Germany. When he was 11, the Nazis came to power. At the age of 16, after being subjected to anti-Semitism at his school and after his father's arrest by the Gestapo, he escaped to Prague and eventually to New York, where he found work in an auto parts store. He attended the University of Vermont and, in 1949, received his medical degree from Harvard. He then served as a captain in the air force. In 1955, Katz began teaching psychiatry at Yale and developed an interest in the overlap between psychiatry and the law. In 1958, he became an assistant professor of psychiatry and law at Yale.

Katz rarely wrote about medical ethics without referring both to the experiments performed by Nazi doctors during World War II and the Nuremberg Code. He always emphasized the importance of the first principle of the Nuremberg Code: that consent be informed and voluntary.

In 1972, with coauthors Alexander Capron and Eleanor Glass, Katz compiled an authoritative book about medical experimentation called *Experimentation with Human Beings: The Authority of the Investigator, Subject, Professions, and State in the Human Experimentation Process*, with extensive documentation of experiments, using case studies and material reflecting the viewpoints of medicine, sociology, and law. He also included material about the formulation, administration, and review of human experimentation.

That same year, he was named to a federal panel to investigate the four-decade-long Tuskegee Study of Untreated Syphilis (TSUS), in which black men with syphilis were not treated (or were treated insufficiently). In the Final Report of the Tuskegee Syphilis Study Ad Hoc Advisory Panel, the panel described the study as "ethically unjustified" and concluded that once penicillin became available in 1943, it should have been made available to the infected participants. They also called for federal protections for medical research subjects.

Katz, however, thought that the majority report did not go far enough and wrote his own stronger statement saying that the subjects in the TSUS had been "exploited, manipulated and deceived." The committee had spent some time wondering whether the Tuskegee physicians had indeed thought that it was acceptable to withhold possibly harmful and possibly ineffective treatment from black men with syphilis. Katz wrote that instead the only relevant question was whether the subjects had been treated with dignity and as equal participants in the study: "When will we take seriously our responsibilities, particularly to the disadvantaged in our midst who so consistently throughout history have been the first to be selected for human research?"[1] A year after the Tuskegee report, Katz served on a panel of prominent academics who called for a moratorium on the use of poor people as subjects of medical experimentation.

In 1994, Katz was one of 14 members of the Advisory Committee on Human Radiation Experiments (ACHRE), established by President Bill Clinton, to review the human radiation experiments conducted between 1944 and 1974. Once again, he did not think that the committee's findings were strong enough. Katz noted that the Cold War–era physicians who conducted these studies did not think that they had to pay any attention to the principles of the Nuremberg Code for two reasons. First, from their point of view, the Nuremberg Code had been written in response to the Nazi physicians who carried out sadistic experiments on concentration camp inmates, and, second, the code only applied to nonpatients. In contrast, American physicians were not sadistic people, and they usually experimented on patients; thus, they thought (incorrectly) that the Nuremberg Code principles did not apply to their actions.

In his comments as a member of ACHRE, Katz was critical of the regulatory processes that were in effect in the 1990s. Even though consent forms and institutional review boards (committees established by institutions to review research studies) (IRBs) existed by that time, he thought that they were inadequate in protecting research subjects. He described many consent forms as so long and overly detailed that they obfuscated the essential issue, which was that research subjects were taking a risk in participating and that the likelihood that they would benefit from the experiment was usually small. Katz noted that many IRBs failed to understand the importance of consent and were often pressured by their own institutions to approve experiments. He suggested the need for a national board to oversee human experimentation.

In 2002, Katz led an investigation into the accusations against cancer researcher Cornelius "Dusty" Rhoads (1898–1959), who had been accused of deliberately giving subjects cancer in Puerto Rico while investigating hookworm and tropical sprue in 1931. Katz and the committee found no evidence of unethical experimentation. They did, however, note that Rhoads's comments about Puerto Ricans in a letter that he had written but not mailed were so offensive that the American

Association of Cancer Research should remove Rhoads's name from an award that they presented annually to a young researcher.

Since the time of Hippocrates, Katz wrote, doctors have rarely been concerned about the autonomy of patients. They have wanted to help patients, but not to involve them in treatment decisions. Katz described how difficult it was for physicians, conscious of their superior medical knowledge, to understand the importance of self-determination.

Katz was uncompromising in demanding that physicians and researchers obtain informed consent from their patients and subjects. He described how in both clinical and research situations, patients and subjects rarely understand the level of uncertainty involved in a proposed treatment. They often believe that the physician is more certain than he or she can be about the benefit of treatments. Katz argued that the physician should not perpetuate these misunderstandings, but should instead make sure that the patient fully understands the risks involved.

With respect to research, subjects often think that they will personally benefit from the experiment. Katz criticized those researchers who have been unwilling to spend the time having difficult and lengthy conversations with their subjects about what often has been hidden from them: the fact that experimental treatments or procedures are done to help physicians learn how to help people in the future, not the subject currently volunteering for the experiment.

Frances R. Frankenburg

Reference

1. Katz, in his "addenda Charge 1," in the Final Report of the Tuskegee Syphilis Study Ad Hoc Advisory Panel. In Reverby, *Tuskegee Truths*, 177.

KLIGMAN, ALBERT

Between 1951 and 1974, dermatologist Albert Kligman conducted many drug trials and experiments for pharmaceutical companies and the army on inmates at Holmesburg Prison in Pennsylvania. He helped to establish the anti-acne and anti-wrinkle effects of tretinoin (Retin-A), a form of vitamin A. His work with prisoners is now considered to be an example of unethical medical research.

Albert Kligman (1916–2010) received his medical degree from the University of Pennsylvania in 1947, and then he specialized in dermatology. A talented dermatologist, he described the hair follicle cycle and the development of acne. He was interested in fungal diseases of the skin and developed a test to differentiate between ringworm and other fungal infections. Some of this work with ringworm was done with children at the State Colonies for the Feebleminded in Vineland and Woodbine in rural New Jersey, with funds provided by the United States Public Health Service.

Because of Kligman's expertise, he was asked to investigate an outbreak of a common fungal illness, known colloquially as athlete's foot, at Holmesburg Prison in Philadelphia. When he went there, he said, "All I saw before me was acres of skin. It was like a farmer seeing a fertile field for the first time."[1] He saw the prisoners as convenient subjects for medical research—as did many others at the time—and in 1951, he began to use Holmesburg inmates in his experiments, including those performed on behalf of pharmaceutical companies. Because the Food and Drug Administration (FDA) required that new products be tested in many people with and without the condition for which the product was intended, companies needed many subjects for drug trials, and prisons offered a large, captive population to researchers. He also did experiments for companies wanting to investigate the usefulness and side effects of perfumes, deodorants, shampoos, lipstick, toothpaste, and the like.

Kligman experimented with tretinoin, or retinoic acid, a derivative of Vitamin A, as a way of softening skin. He used very high doses on patients at the University of Pennsylvania's Acne Clinic and the prisoners, both topically and by mouth, even though high doses of retinoic acid cause inflammation or irritation of the skin. Other researchers working with this drug had used lower doses to avoid this problem. But Kligman persisted with high doses for several weeks. At these elevated doses, he noted that the drug decreased acne. Plus, some of his older female patients reported that it also diminished the appearance of wrinkles and brown spots and that skin texture improved.

In other words, Kligman had discovered that high doses of retinoic acid could diminish the harmful effects of sun on the skin. Kligman was well prepared for this discovery, as he had been one of the first to describe photoaging, or the skin damage that can result from repeated exposure to ultraviolet radiation. He worked closely with the pharmaceutical company Ortho (a subsidiary of the large company Johnson & Johnson) to promote retinoic acid as an anti-aging drug, even though the FDA had only approved it as an anti-acne drug. (Ortho was later investigated by the FDA for promoting off-label uses of the drug, and was charged with obstruction of justice because they had destroyed documents during the investigation. Kligman was also involved in a patent battle between himself, Johnson & Johnson, and the University of Pennsylvania. The case was settled out of court.)

Although he was a dermatologist, Kligman also worked in other areas of medical research. For example, he worked with R. J. Reynolds, the tobacco company, to investigate the relationship between smoking and bladder cancer. He worked with both the Central Intelligence Agency (CIA) in their work with mind-altering drugs and with army physicians based at the Edgewood Arsenal in Maryland who were testing drugs to incapacitate the enemy. Holmesburg Prison, one of many sites used by the CIA and army agencies to test these drugs, provided a large number of prisoners for these experiments. The prisoners were housed in trailers separate from the rest of the prison. The army physicians complained that Kligman's work for them was carried out in a haphazard manner with insufficiently trained personnel. Not much more is known about these experiments because of their sensitive military nature and because Kligman destroyed all of his files related to these projects. Prisoners involved in these experiments experienced dizziness, perceptual illusions, and frightening hallucinations.

Between 1965 and 1966, again using his Holmesburg prisoners as subjects, Kligman studied the dermatological effects of a dioxin, tetrachlorodibenzo-p-dioxin (TCDD), a contaminant of the herbicide Agent Orange made by Dow Chemicals. This was the only study in which humans were deliberately exposed to dioxin. Dow wanted to determine the minimum amount of the drug that could cause chloracne, a type of acne, and had told Kligman to use small doses and follow the subjects carefully because dioxin is known to be very toxic. Kligman used low doses on a few subjects and saw no adverse side effects. Then he used doses far higher than what was recommended. When Dow found out, they severed their connection with him. There are no records identifying the prisoners and therefore no follow-up, so the health effects of this substance on these individuals are unknown.

In 1966, the FDA stopped him from doing more research because of problems in his data collection but later rescinded this decision, perhaps due to pressure from the university and promises from Kligman to improve the quality of his work.

Kligman's work with prisoners was complicated. Many liked the experiments because they were paid and were able to use the money to make bail, help their families, and buy toiletries in the prison. Those prisoners who acted as research associates decided which inmates would be picked as subjects and so had positions with some power. The prisoners did not take the experiments seriously and as a result did not always follow instructions. For example, when patches containing chemicals were applied to their skin, they would take the patches off once they were unobserved.

In the 1970s, the extent of his work at Holmesburg Prison became known, as did that of other prison physician-entrepreneurs, and the public became uneasy. It was just a few years after the thalidomide scare in the early 1960s in which babies with birth defects were born to women who had taken a supposedly safe drug for morning sickness; this incident had exposed what seemed like carelessness by some physicians. At the same time, the country was learning about the 40-year-long Tuskegee Study of Untreated Syphilis (TSUS), in which black Americans with syphilis were either not treated or undertreated for their condition. In 1973, Jessica Mitford wrote a book, *Kind and Usual Punishment: The Prison Business*, that exposed the abuses taking place in American prisons, including unethical medical research. Then, in January 1974, the Holmesburg Prison board of trustees voted to end experimentation at the prison. Some inmates were angry at the thought that they would no longer be receiving payment and signed a petition of support of the experimentation program.

In 1976, the National Commission for the Protection of Human Subjects of Biomedical and Behavioral Research issued a publication that effectively banned medical research in prisoners.

In summary, Kligman was an avid researcher who enthusiastically experimented on prisoners. Some were grateful for the chance to earn some money, but others claimed that they had been exploited. The prisoners may not have always been honest research participants, and Kligman may have exposed them to considerable risks. The extent of his work with prisoners appalled those who were concerned that prisoners were a vulnerable population. He worked with many substances, including mind-altering ones, but is perhaps best known for his contributions to the development of the widely used anti-acne and anti-aging topical ointment Retin-A.

Frances R. Frankenburg

Reference

1.   Quoted in Hornblum, *Acres of Skin*, 37.

LAWRENCE, ERNEST AND JOHN

Ernest Lawrence and his younger brother, John, were scientists and collaborators who were pioneers in the fields of physics and nuclear medicine. Ernest, a nuclear physicist, built the first cyclotron that produced large quantities of radioisotopes, which are used in many medical experiments. John, a physician, explored the medical uses of radiation and also arranged for their mother, who had cancer, to receive radiation, a new treatment at the time.

Ernest Lawrence (1901–1958) and his brother, John H. Lawrence (1904–1991), were born in South Dakota. Ernest completed his PhD in physics at Yale and then moved to Berkeley, California. By 1929, he had built the world's first cyclotron, also known as a particle accelerator or "atom smasher." A cyclotron accelerates subatomic charged particles along a spiral path. As the particle strikes an atom, the nucleus may either absorb it or emit another particle, or radioisotope. For the first time, large numbers of radioisotopes could be produced. (In 1939, he was awarded the Nobel Prize in Physics for the invention of the cyclotron.) Meanwhile, John had graduated from the Yale School of Medicine and realized that the radioisotopes his brother was producing could have many medical uses, including exploring the body and attacking cancer. He moved to Berkeley to work with Ernest and to develop the new field of medical physics.

In 1936, John successfully treated a leukemia patient with a radioactive isotope of phosphate. This was the first time that a radioactive isotope had been used to treat an illness in a human. The next year, he used it to treat a patient with polycythemia vera, an illness in which too many red blood cells are produced.

In 1937, Ernst and John's mother, Gertrude (or Gunda), then 67 or 68, was diagnosed with uterine cancer. The Mayo Clinic had told her that she had three months to live. With the hope of being able to do something to help her, her sons brought her from Minnesota to California, where she was treated with X-rays in San Francisco, then a new treatment for cancer. It made her ill. John, however, insisted that she continue to receive the radiation despite the side effects, and, as a result, her cancer went into remission and she was cured. She remained healthy until her death at the age of 83. In 1942, he established the Donner Laboratory within the Lawrence Radiation Laboratory (now known as the Berkeley Radiation Laboratory) to develop nuclear medicine.

During the 1930s and 1940s, the work with radiation became increasingly militarized and directed more toward national defense purposes than health care. Ernest Lawrence joined physicist J. Robert Oppenheimer (1904–1967) and other scientists on the Manhattan Project, which was established in 1942 to create an atom bomb before the Germans could.

After the war ended, the Manhattan Project announced, in 1946, a medical isotope distribution program as a top priority, partly to reassure the public that non-military advances could come from nuclear physics. This program was continued by the Atomic Energy Commission (AEC), established in 1947. The nuclear reactor at Oak Ridge National Laboratory in Oak Ridge, Tennessee, was built during World War II as part of the Manhattan Project. After the war ended, the reactor produced radioactive isotopes for peacetime scientific, medical, industrial, and agricultural uses. As well as distributing radioisotopes for medical studies or experiments, the AEC wanted to control what was done with the isotopes and insisted on reviewing all proposals. The AEC also required that the institutions establish a review process for the proposed studies.

The researchers at Berkeley were indignant. They had been the first to use isotopes (made by their own cyclotron) and argued that they did not need supervision, which they perceived as interference with their work. The AEC acquiesced. The Berkeley Radiation Laboratory thus became an independent entity, free of AEC control, and continued to be a leading institution with respect to the medical uses of radiation.

The Donner Laboratory has been called the birthplace, and John Lawrence the father, of nuclear medicine. Nuclear medicine is now a medical specialty in which radioactive substances are used both to diagnose and to treat diseases.

Frances R. Frankenburg

LEARY, TIMOTHY

Timothy Leary was a Harvard psychologist who at first approached psychedelic drugs, such as psilocybin, as a scientist, conducting experiments with these drugs in students, counterculture writers, prisoners, and theology students and professors. He later became more well-known for his less scientific enthusiasm for the mystical properties of lysergic acid diethylamide (LSD).

Timothy Leary (1920–1996) was a psychologist at Harvard University's Center for Research in Personality. In 1957, he had published an academic book about personality assessment. But his research interests took a markedly different turn after an August 1960 vacation in Cuernavaca, Mexico, where he consumed "magic mushrooms" (*Psilocybe mexicana*) containing psilocybin, a psychedelic or hallucinogenic substance that leads to euphoria, hallucinations, and a distorted sense of time. Others have described spiritual or mystical experiences after taking the mushrooms. Upon his return to Harvard, Leary gave psilocybin to friends and colleagues and then asked them to fill out personality assessments in an attempt to measure its properties. This proved difficult because many of the reported experiences with psychedelic drugs do not lend themselves to quantification. At around the same time, a large Swiss pharmaceutical company, Sandoz, began to market the active ingredient of *Psilocybe mexicana* under the trade name Indocybin, which made subsequent experimentation much easier.

Later that year, Leary initiated the Harvard Psilocybin Project to better understand the effects of psilocybin. He and his colleague Richard Alpert obtained psilocybin from Sandoz. They were interested in its effects on creativity and administered it to Harvard students and others, including writer Aldous Huxley, poet Allen Ginsberg, and writer William S. Burroughs. Most subjects reported that the experience was pleasant. However, many at Harvard felt that the project's emphasis on experience over the verbal and analytical was anti-intellectual.

To obtain rigorous data on whether psilocybin would have effects on individuals who were not necessarily interested in the arts or philosophical matters, between 1961 and 1963, Leary administered psilocybin to 32 inmates at the Massachusetts Correctional Institute in Concord, a maximum-security prison for young offenders. Leary met with the inmates for several weeks, informed them of the purpose of the study, and gave them psilocybin several times. After taking the drug, the inmates began to talk about love and ecstasy. They also showed improvement as measured by the widely used Minnesota Multiphasic Personality Inventory. Leary and colleagues reported that the recidivism (rearrest) rate in those who took the drug was 25 percent, compared to the usual recidivism rate of 80 percent. In other words, his results seemed to show that the prisoners who took psilocybin were less likely to be rearrested and returned for parole violations than those who had not taken the drug.

These experiments were not, however, as rigorous as they might have been, nor were Leary's recidivism claims quite accurate. The psilocybin group enjoyed a special status in the prison. They were given a preparole course of instruction and special assistance in obtaining housing and employment, and they maintained contact with the Harvard experimenters. Later, when the data of the original study were reviewed, Leary's mistake about the recidivism rates was discovered. Leary had compared the recidivism rates of the psilocybin group after they had been out of prison for about 10 months with the recidivism rates of control subjects who had been out of Concord prison for about 30 months. As recidivism increases over time, the comparison is not valid. When the recidivism rates for both groups at 10 months were compared, the rates were found to be the same, so there was no connection between psilocybin and recidivism.

Leary and Walter Pahnke, a Harvard theology student and physician, also experimented with psilocybin with theology students and professors at Marsh Chapel at Boston University. In 1962, they gave psilocybin to 10 subjects and a placebo (in the form of nicotinic acid, which leads to facial flushing) to 10 subjects before services on Good Friday. Nine of the 10 psilocybin subjects but only 1 of the 10 controls reported having a mystical or spiritual experience. This became known as the "Miracle at Marsh Chapel" or the "Good Friday" experiment.

Around this time, Leary was introduced to the hallucinogen lysergic acid diethylamide (LSD), which led to more dramatic experiences than psilocybin. He lost interest in the psilocybin project and became more interested in mysticism and Eastern religions. He formed the International Foundation for Internal Freedom, which promoted (unsuccessfully) the ideas that hallucinogens were like cerebral vitamins and that it was the right of everyone to take them.

Frances R. Frankenburg

LEXINGTON NARCOTIC FARM

In 1935, the United States Public Health Service established the United States Narcotic Farm in Lexington, Kentucky, to treat addicts and to conduct research. The results of some of the experiments, which led to a better understanding of substance abuse, were published in medical journals. Other experiments were done in secret to help the Central Intelligence Agency in its search for mind-control drugs to use against the enemy.

In 1935, responding to a perceived crisis of widespread addiction to narcotic drugs, the United States Public Health Service (PHS) opened the United States Narcotic Farm in Lexington, Kentucky, under the leadership of Lawrence Kolb Sr. (1881–1972), one of the country's experts in drug addiction. Until then, the PHS had typically investigated infectious illnesses, such as smallpox, yellow fever, tuberculosis, hookworm, malaria, and leprosy. The farm occupied a thousand acres in a rural setting and had a dairy and chicken coop. It was an amalgam of rural prison, hospital, and rehabilitation facility. The idea of quarantining people came naturally to the PHS, given its history of involvement with contagious diseases. Perhaps it was thought that people who started using opiates because of the stress, overcrowding, and filth of inner cities would find it easier to give up this habit in bucolic surroundings where they could work with animals and crops and be removed from their usual haunts.

Some residents were federal prisoners who were also opiate addicts, and some came voluntarily from other walks of life. The residents—sometimes termed *inhabitants*, *patients*, or *inmates*—included artists, physicians, and street hustlers. One of the most famous was William S. Burroughs, who wrote about the farm in his semiautobiographical 1953 novel *Junky*. Other residents included jazz musicians, such as Chet Baker and Sonny Rollins, and other entertainment figures, such as Peter Lorre and Sammy Davis Jr.

One part of the farm, known as the Addiction Research Center (ARC), carried out research on substance abuse. Its director from 1945 to 1963 was Harris Isbell (1910–1994), a respected medical scientist. Inmates with long histories of drug abuse were good research subjects because the researchers did not have to introduce them to drug use and also because their experience made them good reporters. In what today might be considered an act of coercion, addicts could volunteer to come to Lexington, instead of going to jail. At Lexington, they were "paid" with heroin or morphine in exchange for volunteering to be a subject in some of the drug experiments.

ARC researchers made substantial contributions to the understanding of substance abuse. They described the process of alcohol and barbiturate withdrawal. In addition, methadone, synthesized in Germany, was used first in the United States at the Lexington Narcotic Farm to help addicts overcome heroin addiction. The use of buprenorphine—an opiate with less addictive potential than other opiates—was pioneered at the farm for the treatment of heroin addiction. Isbell and his colleagues published their results in multiple papers in scientific journals, but they never divulged the identity of the subjects or the venue of the work.

In addition to the work on substance abuse, another type of research was being carried out at the farm: studies into mind control. At the time of the farm's existence, the United States government was concerned about the possible use of "brainwashing drugs" by other countries, such as China and the Soviet Union. MKULTRA, a secret program run by the Central Intelligence Agency (CIA) in the 1950s, attempted to discover ways of behavioral modification that could be used by, or against, the enemy. The program involved about 80 institutions, including universities and prisons.

MKULTRA enrolled many people, among them psychologists and psychiatrists, who experimented on the farm's residents. Drugs such as lysergic acid diethylamide (LSD) and other hallucinogens were studied for their possible use in mind control. Some subjects were given LSD for several weeks at a time, and the ARC reported that the subjects became tolerant to LSD. Isbell worked for MKULTRA and remained on the CIA payroll for over a decade. The connection between the CIA and the ARC was not publicized.

Many of the farm inmates who participated in the ARC experiments were prisoners. This was not particularly unusual at that time. Indeed, one of the greatest triumphs of the PHS had been accomplished with prisoners as subjects of medical experimentation. Physician Joseph Goldberger (1874–1929), working for the PHS in the early 1900s, had used prisoners at Mississippi's Rankin State Prison farm to discover that pellagra was caused by a nutritional deficiency, namely the lack of niacin. In other types of research, dermatologist Albert Kligman (1916–2010) tested the safety and effectiveness of many drugs, including tretinoin (Retin-A), on prisoners in Philadelphia from the 1950s to the early 1970s.

In the 1970s, however, the climate surrounding research involving governmental agencies changed. There was increasing unease about the use of prisoners in experiments and embarrassment about another PHS project, the Tuskegee Study of Untreated Syphilis (TSUS). In that four-decade-long study, black men with syphilis were not told about their illness and were either not treated or undertreated. In 1975, a U.S. Senate committee investigated intelligence gathering by the CIA and Federal Bureau of Investigation and discovered Project MKULTRA. The project was ended as a result of this investigation. The ARC itself was subsumed in 1948 by the newly established National Institutes of Mental Health (NIMH).

All of these factors, combined with a dismal recovery rate for the addicts, led to the closing of the Lexington Narcotic Farm in 1974 and its conversion back into a federal prison. Some of the experiments at the ARC would not be allowed at the present time, primarily because prisoners are now considered vulnerable subjects who cannot give voluntary consent. The practice of giving addicts heroin in exchange for their participation in experiments would also be considered questionable.

Frances R. Frankenburg

MARSHALL, BARRY

Barry Marshall, an Australian physician, swallowed *Helicobacter pylori* in 1984 and developed an inflamed stomach. This self-experiment changed the understanding of ulcers and resulted in a Nobel Prize.

In 1979, Barry Marshall (b. 1951), a resident in medicine in Perth, Australia, began to study gastritis, or stomach inflammation, and peptic ulcers with pathologist Robin Warren (b. 1937). At that time, these disorders were thought to be caused by too much stomach acid and stress. Warren had become interested in the spiral-shaped bacteria found in the stomach biopsies of people with gastritis and ulcers. These bacteria had been seen before by other pathologists, but not studied. By 1982, Marshall and Warren had developed a theory that gastritis and ulcers could be due to an infection caused by this bacterium, later to be named *Helicobacter pylori*. This possibility seemed unlikely to most researchers because the stomach is so acidic that few bacteria can live there.

Warren and Marshall had difficulty proving their theory because at first they could not grow the bacteria in culture. It turned out that technicians in the lab had been discarding the cultures after two days. But *Helicobacter* is slow-growing: once the cultures were allowed to grow for longer periods of time, the bacteria appeared. Another difficulty was that the bacteria did not seem to grow in laboratory animals, so it was not possible to have animal models of the infection.

In 1984, Marshall decided that he needed to prove his theory by deliberately infecting a healthy human with the bacterium. A colleague examined Marshall's stomach using an endoscope and declared it to be healthy. Without telling anyone, Marshall drank a culture of *H. pylori* obtained from a patient with an ulcer. A few days later, he developed nausea and began to vomit. An endoscopy showed inflammation in his stomach, and a biopsy revealed the presence of *H. pylori*. Marshall had proven the connection.

Later research showed that *H. pylori* may be one of the most common infections in humans. Anywhere from one-half to two-thirds of the world's population host this bacterium. The corkscrew-shaped bacterium burrows into the mucus layer that coats the inside of the stomach and secretes an enzyme that converts urea into ammonia; this counteracts the acidity of the stomach.

H. pylori infection does not cause illness in most infected people, but it is a major risk factor for peptic ulcer disease and is responsible for the majority of ulcers of the stomach and upper small intestine. Colonization of the stomach with *H. pylori* is also a risk factor for gastric cancer.

Marshall and Warren were awarded the Nobel Prize in Physiology or Medicine in 2005 for their work.

Frances R. Frankenburg

MARSHALL ISLANDS

During the Cold War years, the United States experimented with the detonation of nuclear devices in isolated areas such as the Marshall Islands and Nevada. Some of the detonations in the Marshall Islands were done in secret, and many involved the repeated displacement of local populations. The medical effects were investigated by the Brookhaven National Laboratory of New York. People of the Marshall Islands have claimed that they were used as guinea pigs.

In the 1940s, the nuclear bomb was a new weapon, and scientists were unsure as to the consequences of its detonation. They expected the explosion to lead to intense light, heat, and pressure waves, but they were not particularly worried about residual radioactivity. Indeed, the concept of nuclear fallout, the radioactive dust and ash produced following the explosion, was still quite new. The scientists had not expected much radiation to be emitted by the bombs dropped over Hiroshima or Nagasaki and at first denied that there had been any significant harm done to people as a consequence of radiation exposure.

The existence of the nuclear bomb also called into question the structure of the military services. For example, the possession of the bomb made the future of the navy unclear. Following the bombing of Hiroshima and Nagasaki, the army argued that the navy was obsolete. The navy argued otherwise and claimed that their ships were needed to carry the bombs; plus, their ships could not easily be sunk by bombs. In 1946, the United States began a nuclear weapons testing program in the North Pacific to answer some of these questions about the effects of radiation and the usefulness of navy ships in the atomic age.

Two chains of coral atolls, consisting of more than a thousand islands, lie just north of the equator in the North Pacific Ocean. These islands, now making up the Republic of the Marshall Islands, were the site of 66 American peacetime experimental atmospheric, ground, and underwater nuclear explosions between 1946 and 1958. The Marshall Islands were chosen as the site for these explosions because the islands were remote, had a small population, and fell under the control of the United States during World War II. This remoteness made it possible for some of the explosions to be kept secret, and the sparseness of population ensured that not very many people would be affected. The islands were not near sea-lanes or air traffic, and the winds over the islands were, for the most part, predictable.

The first set of detonations, known as Operation Crossroads, took place on Bikini Atoll, a small ring of land or coral islets just over three square miles in area that partially encircles a 230-square-mile lagoon. The plan was to detonate devices to see whether the navy's ships in the lagoon could withstand the blasts. In February 1946, Commodore Ben H. Wyatt, the military governor of the Marshalls, asked the 167 islanders living on Bikini to leave, and they agreed to do so, moving in March to Rongerik Atoll, 125 miles to the east.

In advance of the tests, the U.S. Navy blasted large channels into the reef and blew up some of the coral heads in the lagoon to allow for the placement of 95 ships in the Bikini lagoon. These ships included captured Japanese ships, such as the Japanese flagship *Nagato*, and obsolete American ships, including the *Saratoga* and the *Arkansas*. Between 3,000 and 5,000 animals were also placed on the ships to test the effects of these nuclear devices on them.

Operation Crossroads was well publicized. Observers included congressmen and journalists. On July 1, 1946, a plutonium implosion bomb called Able was dropped from a B-29 bomber and detonated in the air above the target fleet. It missed its mark by 650 meters, and five ships were sunk. Most of the radiation went into the atmosphere. Almost 20 percent of the animals died in the blast, and more than half had died five months later.

On July 25, 1946, in the second test, another plutonium implosion bomb (this one called Baker) was detonated 90 feet underwater. Two million tons of debris and water were blown a mile into the air and then fell back on Bikini and the ships in the lagoon. Ten ships were sunk. All of the target ships were contaminated by radioactive fallout. The extent of the contamination of the ships and the danger it posed to the servicemen were unexpected.

Years later, on March 1, 1954, the United States performed an initially secret test called Castle Bravo, in which the most powerful hydrogen bomb ever detonated at that time was exploded on an artificial island built off the Bikini Atoll. This bomb was 1,000 times stronger than Little Boy (the bomb dropped on Hiroshima) and Fat Man (the bomb dropped on Nagasaki). The bomb produced a much higher detonation force than had been predicted, and an unforeseen change in the winds spread the fallout to populated Marshallese islands to the east of Bikini. Almost an inch of radioactive ash was deposited on the island of Rongelap and the Utirik atolls, where 236 people lived. Most of the inhabitants of those islands experienced severe radiation sickness. Three days after the detonation, all residents of Rongelap and Utirik were evacuated. The crew of a Japanese fishing vessel a hundred miles away was contaminated as well, and one crew member died. The Bravo shot, although at first a secret, led to increased radioactivity as far away as Australia and India, and thus became an international incident.

These explosions, particularly the Bravo blast, had myriad effects on the Marshall Islanders. Many inhabitants lost their homes and were repeatedly relocated. They also lost their usual ways of life and became dependent on the United States government. The Bikinians, in particular, became "nuclear nomads." Rongerik atoll could not support the islanders, and the Bikinians were moved from Rongerik to Kwajalein Atoll and then to Kili Island. In 1969, the United States began to decontaminate the Bikini Atoll, and in 1974, some islanders were able to move back. However, researchers later found that the water and breadfruit on the island continued to contain dangerous levels of radioactivity. Urine samples from the islanders showed low levels of plutonium 239 and 240. In 1977, all those living on the island were found to have an 11-fold increase in cesium-137. In 1978, the island was deemed unsafe, and all inhabitants were evacuated again. As of 2014, only a few people live on Bikini Island. They act as caretakers and host brief diving expeditions into the lagoon.

The lives of the inhabitants of the ash-covered Rongelap were also disrupted. After being evacuated in 1954, the inhabitants returned to their island in 1957. However, in 1985, they left again because of concerns about the island continuing to have high radiation levels.

In 1954, the Atomic Energy Commission (AEC) sent an emergency medical team to the islands to assess the medical effects of the Castle Bravo operation. The government established a project, known as Project 4.1, or "Study of Response of Human Beings Accidentally Exposed to Significant Fallout Radiation." In their 1954 report, the researchers described many immediate effects, such as burns, hair loss, decreased blood counts, malaise, and nausea. Initially, it was felt that the medical effects of the bombs were limited to these immediate effects.

Two years later, the AEC requested that the Brookhaven National Laboratory (BNL) take over the medical evaluation and care of the islanders. The BNL, established on Long Island in 1947 as a research center to explore the nature of atomic energy, was part of the AEC and then transferred to the AEC's successor, the Department of Energy. This monitoring program—which entailed annual visits of the BNL to the Marshall Islands to collect of samples, such as blood, urine, and teeth—continued for over 40 years.

Marshallese Islanders not exposed to the radiation were enlisted as controls for the BNL's work so that their test results could be compared against the results of inhabitants who had been exposed to the explosions. Some Marshallese say that neither the exposed nor unexposed were ever informed about why they needed to submit to multiple (and sometimes invasive) exams. They were not asked for their permission, and there was confusion about whether the purpose of the exams was to provide medical care.

Compensation for the Marshallese has been contentious and incomplete. A Nuclear Claims Tribunal was set up in the islands to adjudicate claims and has recommended awards of several hundred million dollars to pay for environmental restoration, economic losses, and hardship and suffering. However, the fund has run out of money and has not been able to complete these payments.

The gravest complaint from the Marshallese has been the suspicion that they were moved back to their homes so that the effects of living on these contaminated islands could be studied. The U.S. government has denied this claim, and there is no clear evidence that this is the case. But other complaints are well-founded. The people of the Bikini Atoll were asked to leave without a clear explanation of what could happen to their island. In addition, the planning for the possibility of an evacuation after the Bravo detonation was insufficient. In the aftermath of the the detonations, the Brookhaven scientists did not explain their work to the Marshallese or obtain their informed consent. And at least two of the Brookhaven tests included the administration of radioactive isotopes to some islanders, which was of no therapeutic benefit.

Studies from the National Cancer Institute have shown that the bombs did result in a small increase in cancer among the Marshallese, mostly due to fallout from Bravo. Ten years after the detonation of the Castle Bravo device, thyroid nodules and thyroid cancer began to be seen in greater than expected numbers. This has been thought to be due to exposure to a broad mix of radionuclides of iodine over a short period of time. In addition, the following percentages of cancers among the Marshallese can be attributed to the bombs: 20 percent for thyroid cancers, 5 percent for leukemia, and 1 percent for other cancers. The percentages are higher for those Marshallese who were closer to the explosions. About half of all cancers suffered by the Rongelapese (those Marshallese closest to the fallout) are thought to be due to Bravo. Radiation is likely to cause particular types of cancer. For the people of the Rongelap community, the following percentages of cancers due to radiation are as follows: 95 percent for thyroid cancer, 78 percent for leukemia, 48 percent for stomach, 1 percent for colon.

Many of the details of the detonations and their consequences are still in classified documents. Some medical records were also lost in fires.

The Marshallese people were uninformed peacetime subjects in an unintended medical experiment studying the consequences of the detonation of nuclear bombs. Their displacement and medical problems were evidence of the problems and persistence of fallout.

Frances R. Frankenburg

OPERATION WHITECOAT

Operation Whitecoat was a series of medical experiments carried out by the American army between 1954 and 1973 involving Seventh-day Adventist conscientious objectors as voluntary research subjects. The goal was to enable the military to test the effects of microorganisms on human subjects.

During the period when the American draft was still in place, the followers of the Seventh-day Adventist faith were willing to be drafted and to serve in the United States military, but not to bear arms. Many Adventists chose to volunteer for biological tests as a way of satisfying their military obligations. In 1954, the Adventist hierarchy agreed to this plan, and Operation Whitecoat began. These church members were good experimental subjects, as they were young and healthy and did not abuse alcohol or drugs.

Many of the Adventists who participated in Operation Whitecoat were recruited at Fort Sam Houston, Texas, a training center for medics. The first volunteers were sent to Fort Detrick in Maryland. The scientists began their tests in January 1955. The volunteers were not required to join any experiments. They were simply asked to go to sessions in which the experiments were explained. If they did decide to take part, they were paid modest amounts of money.

A key feature of the experiments was a million-liter-capacity sphere called "the Eight Ball." Aerosols containing pathogens were released into the Eight Ball, and subjects breathed in the air through rubber hoses leading to face masks. Some of the aerosols contained microbes that led to serious, but nonfatal diseases, such as tularemia or Q fever. Once the recruits developed symptoms, they were given antibiotics, and almost all made a quick recovery.

After the first experiments, 30 recruits traveled to the Dugway Proving Ground in Utah, where they were exposed to aerosols in an outdoor setting. (A proving ground is a place where devices or theories are tested or tried out. In this case, it is a huge area of desert belonging to the U.S. Army.) In July 1955, they lined up in the desert, along with cages of monkeys and guinea pigs. About 3,000 feet away, generators sprayed an infectious mist or aerosol containing Q fever microorganisms toward them. Some of the volunteers had been vaccinated against Q fever and never got sick; others became ill. (These experiments deployed methods similar to those used by unit 731 but were far less brutal.)

The human experiments with Seventh-day Adventists continued for almost 20 years and ended in 1973, when the draft ended. In total, about 2,200 Adventists participated in Operation Whitecoat. There were no fatalities and, as far as we know, no adverse long-term results.

Because there was some secrecy about the nature of these tests, it is difficult to determine exactly what advances were made during Operation Whitecoat. The army claims that vaccines were developed against Rift Valley Fever and that methods for biological hazard containment, some still used today in laboratories and hospitals, were perfected.

Operation Whitecoat did have informed consent. Indeed, the consent form featured an unusual provision that the subject take from 24 hours to at least four weeks to think about the project and its risks and benefits before signing the consent form.

Frances R. Frankenburg

PAPPWORTH, MAURICE

Maurice Pappworth wrote a book, *Human Guinea Pigs: Experimentation on Man*, detailing hundreds of experiments performed on patients without their consent and for no therapeutic reason.

Maurice Pappworth (1910–1994), an English physician, mentored and taught postgraduate medical students in London. Beginning in the 1950s, he became increasingly troubled by his students' descriptions of medical experimentation on uninformed patients and by reports in medical journals of these experiments. He wrote letters of complaint to the journals, but few were published. In 1962, he wrote an article that detailed a few examples of what he considered to be unethical medical behavior and then he expanded this article, with additional examples, into a book. Five publishers turned the book down, fearing lawsuits. Finally, in 1967 Routledge and Kegan Paul published his book titled *Human Guinea Pigs: Experimentation on Man.* Slightly more than half of the experiments mentioned had been performed in the United States and the rest in England. The book sold primarily in England and is not particularly well known in the United States.

Human Guinea Pigs offers over 200 examples of doctors experimenting on their patients without their consent and for no therapeutic purpose. The subjects include infants, children, pregnant women, the medically and mentally ill, and the dying. Sometimes the physicians used "controls" who were patients with other illnesses. For example, if the researchers were studying the liver in those with liver disease, they would perform the same tests on patients in the hospital with other illnesses. In the experiments described in the book, the subjects never included the physicians themselves or their colleagues or family members.

Experiments were often done to allow the physicians to test new technology. For example, if there was a new type of catheter, physicians would use it, seemingly in whatever way they could. They would catheterize the right and left heart ventricles; they would catheterize the hepatic vein (the main blood vessel leaving the liver). They measured blood flow from various organs. They administered various substances to see what would happen to the patient. They x-rayed their patients. Curiosity, rather than therapeutic intent, drove the experiments.

Pappworth compiled a long list of injuries caused in these experiments: pain, puncture of arteries or bowels, fainting, loss of the use of a limb, and, in several cases, death. The physicians did not deliberately inflict harm, but they were not affected by the suffering that they caused. Pappworth also described the difficult early history of organ transplants. There was such a high failure rate among the first transplants that he considered them to be experimental.

One reason for these experiments, apart from curiosity, was that they led to publications that in turn were helpful for promotion for doctors. The clinical skills of doctors can be difficult to assess and are not in any case relevant for academic advancement. But physicians who publish research articles in well-respected journals are promoted. Pappworth was critical of the medical journals for publishing so many articles describing experiments that were carried out in unethical ways and did not advance clinical care.

Pappworth noted that most English and American physicians were not unethical researchers, and indeed, some physicians did protest the work of their colleague. However, most physicians seemed to be, in a vague way, aware of the experiments and tolerant of them. He compared this apathy to what had happened in Germany during the Nazi regime. Many German physicians were aware of the Nazi medical atrocities and did nothing to try to stop them. He described the arrogance of the English and American physicians who were amazed that their judgment or clinical practices could be questioned by others, especially by nonmedical people, or that patients should have anything to say about medical procedures carried out on them.

Pappworth's book was similar to the work of physician Henry Beecher (1904–1970), whom Pappworth often quoted with respect. Unlike Beecher, Pappworth published his book for a general readership and named names and cited articles. Perhaps because of these two reasons, his work was not well received by his English medical colleagues, and he is reported to have become a pariah within the English medical community. Some reviewers of his book were offended by the references to the Nazi physicians and felt that this alone made the book ridiculous. Many other physicians involved were incredulous that they had been criticized in public.

The Royal College of Physicians recommended that research involving human subjects undergo ethical review, and it established research ethics committees. In 1990, Pappworth wrote another article in which he described these committees as being toothless. He noted that the committees approved research in a slipshod manner and that some members approved the work of others hoping for reciprocated generosity.

Frances R. Frankenburg

PLUTONIUM EXPERIMENTS

Between April 1945 and July 1947, American nuclear scientists working for the Manhattan Project—the program that built the first nuclear bombs—organized the injection of the radioactive element plutonium into 18 people, without their knowledge, to test its effects on their health. Forty years later, a journalist wrote three articles about these experiments in the *Albuquerque Tribune*, which led to a presidential commission that uncovered thousands of similar radiation experiments from the Cold War era.

Plutonium is a radioactive, metallic element with the atomic number 94; it can be found in very small amounts in the ore pitchblende. The element was first synthesized in 1940 by American chemist Glenn Seaborg (1912–1999) and American physicist Edwin McMillan (1907–1991), working at the University of California, Berkeley. (The two of them shared the 1951 Nobel Prize in Chemistry for their discoveries of the chemistry of transuranium elements, or elements with atomic numbers greater than 92.) Using a cyclotron at the Berkeley Radiation Laboratory, they bombarded uranium with deuterons (particles composed of a proton and a neutron). Some of the neutrons released during the subsequent fission changed uranium-238 into uranium-239 that then decayed into plutonium-239, a radioactive element rarely found in nature.

In 1942, the United States established the Manhattan Project, a secret project designed to develop nuclear weapons. Plutonium was an essential part of the first nuclear bombs. The bombs used at the July 1945 Trinity nuclear test in New Mexico and in the August 1945 bombing of Nagasaki had plutonium cores, as did some of the bombs tested in the Marshall Islands.

Researchers of the time wanted to better understand the health effects of plutonium. Joseph Hamilton (1907–1957), a physician working at the University of California at San Francisco (where there were patients) and also at nearby Berkeley (where there was a cyclotron that produced radioisotopes), had experimented in a number of ways with radiation, once drinking a solution containing radioactive sodium. (This experiment did not yield much useful information.) He then turned his attention to plutonium.

Plutonium is similar in some ways to radium, another radioactive element, known to be harmful to humans because of the gamma rays that it emits. (To be more precise, it is the unstable radioactive "daughters" of radium that emit gamma rays as the nucleus loses energy, or decays.) But plutonium, unlike radium, emits no gamma rays and was therefore thought to be less dangerous. Plutonium emits alpha particles that travel a short distance and do not penetrate the skin. Hamilton administered plutonium-239 to rats and discovered that the element settled in bone, close to the bone marrow, where blood cells are formed. If inhaled, plutonium lodged in the lungs. Plutonium, unlike radium, also deposits in the liver and is excreted at a very slow rate. Researchers in Chicago injected plutonium-239 into mice, rats, rabbits, and dogs and saw that plutonium was excreted at different rates by different animals. Because it is so long-lived and deposits in such a way that, over time, can lead to malignancies of the bone marrow and lungs, plutonium turned out to be more dangerous than radium.

In August of 1944, there were two plutonium spills at Los Alamos, one of the major sites of the Manhattan Project. In that same month, a tube containing plutonium exploded in the face of a chemist. These accidents underscored the importance of understanding how the human body handled plutonium. How quickly and by what method did humans excrete plutonium, and where in the body was it deposited? Physicist J. Robert Oppenheimer (1904–1967), who headed the project's secret weapons laboratory, and others decided that a program of human experimentation would have to be carried out so that American researchers and soldiers working with this element could do so safely. The scientists involved in these experiments included those working on the bomb as well as university researchers in the Argonne National Laboratory (the "Metallurgical Laboratory" at the University of Chicago) and at the University of Rochester. Hamilton directed the plutonium injection studies into humans at the University of California, San Francisco.

Originally, the plan for the plutonium injections was to use healthy subjects because they would most likely resemble the population of workers whom the researchers wanted to protect. Later, however, physicians claimed to have selected subjects with terminal illnesses so that the plutonium injections (or injections of other radioactive materials) would not harm them, as most of the toxic effects of plutonium were thought to occur decades after exposure. However, the prognostic powers of the physicians were limited. Four of the 18 terminally ill patients lived for more than 20 years. We have some information about a number of these plutonium patients.

Ebb Cade was a healthy 53-year-old man who worked at the Oak Ridge Nuclear Facility in Tennessee. He was injured in a car accident in March 1945 and hospitalized at the Oak Ridge Hospital with non-life-threatening injuries. On April 10, 1945, Cade received an injection of almost five times the minimum amount of plutonium believed at the time to cause adverse effects. He was the first person to be injected with plutonium. He died eight years later of heart disease.

At the University of Chicago's Billings Hospital, Arthur Hubbard, a 68-year-old man with metastatic cancer, received what was described to his daughter as a "new treatment"—the second plutonium injection in the spring of 1945. He died in October of 1945, and at autopsy it was discovered that plutonium had deposited in his bone marrow and liver. It is not known whether the injection had affected his health.

The first patient in California to be injected with plutonium was Albert Stevens, a 58-year-old house painter who had been diagnosed with terminal stomach cancer. He received a mixture of plutonium isotopes on May 14, 1945. Pathology results obtained four days later showed that he did not have cancer; he had a stomach ulcer. He lived for another 20 years. During that time, he was asked to collect his urine and feces in glass bottles. He stored them in a shed behind his house, and the samples were picked up once a week. (To track the absorption and excretion of plutonium, one of the methods used was an examination of urine and feces for evidence of alpha radiation.) He died of heart disease at the age of 79.

In April 1946, Hamilton was involved with the injection of plutonium into a child. A four-year-old Australian boy, Simeon Shaw, was brought to the United States for cancer treatment and given plutonium; the parents believed that it was for therapeutic reasons. He died after his return to Australia.

In December 1946, Hamilton was instructed by his superior at the Manhattan Project to stop the plutonium injections. In January of 1947, the Atomic Energy Commission (AEC) took over the work of the Manhattan Project and issued clear rules regarding the use of humans in radiation experiments. Carroll Wilson, general manager of the AEC, wrote in a letter that human subjects had to be fully informed about the experiment and agree to it. Researchers could not perform any experiments unless they believed that there would be benefit to the patient, and the patient and the next of kin had to give complete and informed consent in writing. Wilson also noted that physicians had to be particularly scrupulous with respect to radiation tests on humans as so much of the work would be kept secret and they would not have the benefit of outside scrutiny. The AEC hid evidence of the plutonium studies that had clearly violated these guidelines.

Meanwhile, in 1946, Pullman porter Elmer Allen had broken his left leg and had been fired from his job. Still suffering from a swollen and painful leg, he went to the University of California San Francisco Free Clinic where Hamilton worked. He was diagnosed with bone cancer, and his doctors planned to amputate his leg. In July 1947—after the AEC had issued rules concerning consent—Hamilton asked Allen's physicians to delay the amputation of his leg to allow for an injection of plutonium into the calf of his leg, and then three days later for his leg to be amputated.

In 1973, scientists paid for him to go to the Argonne Laboratory in Chicago and then a lab in Rochester for tests. They said that this was because he had survived his cancer for a surprisingly long time, but in fact it was to find out how much plutonium was left in his body. Tests showed traces of plutonium throughout his body. Allen died in 1991, 44 years after the injection of plutonium. He believed that he had been used as a guinea pig but was unable to convince others of this fact. Instead, doctors diagnosed him with schizophrenia.

The plutonium experiments showed that two-thirds of the plutonium injected into subjects was deposited in the skeleton and over a fifth in the liver. It was excreted slowly, at a rate of about 0.01 percent a day. These findings led to a lowering of the maximum permissible body burden of plutonium.

These experiments had not been kept entirely secret, but the public was largely unaware of them. Reports had appeared in *Science Trends* in 1976 and in *Mother Jones* in 1981. In that same year, then-congressman Albert Gore Jr. chaired a House Subcommittee on Investigations and Oversight and asked whether patients were treated for therapeutic reasons or to gather data. Senator Ed Markey investigated 31 experiments and wrote a report, *American Nuclear Guinea Pigs: Three Decades of Radiation Experiments on U.S. Citizens*, in 1986. The investigations led to no action.

This lack of public awareness changed as a result of the investigative work of *Albuquerque Tribune* reporter Eileen Welsome (b. 1951). In the spring of 1987, Welsome noticed a report about the discovery of dumps containing radioactive animal carcasses on the Kirtland Air Force Base in Albuquerque. Over the course of her review of the report, she found a footnote referring to the injection of 18 people with plutonium.

Eventually, after much investigation, she was able to identify five of the human subjects. She published the stories of these people in a three-part series called "The Plutonium Experiments," in the *Albuquerque Tribune* in 1993, for which she was awarded a Pulitzer Prize in 1994. This time, the reports of the experiments were read by more people. Welsome showed that each person experimented on was not just a "subject" but an individual. (Welsome went on to write the 1999 book *The Plutonium Files: America's Secret Medical Experiments in the Cold War*, which described these and many other experiments carried out during the decades following World War II.)

Hazel O'Leary, then energy secretary, read the *Tribune* series and commented on it during a press conference. In response to the public uproar that followed, in 1994, President Bill Clinton established the Advisory Committee on Human Radiation Experiments to review experiments involving intentional exposure to radiation between 1944 and 1974. The committee was asked to determine whether the experiments performed in those three decades were done in accordance with the standards of the times and whether they were designed in an ethical or scientifically responsible way. During their investigations, more details about the plutonium experiments emerged.

The discovery of the plutonium experiments horrified the American public and led to larger investigations and the declassification of much previously secret material. There is, however, no clear evidence that these injections directly harmed the 18 uninformed subjects. None developed bone- or liver-related cancers, the kinds of cancers that one might expect to increase as a result of plutonium exposure. The experiments also led to useful information that allowed others to work safely in the production of nuclear weapons.

Frances R. Frankenburg

POLIO VACCINE TRIALS

The medical experiments that led to safe and effective vaccination against polio were carried out on large numbers of subjects, ranging from the families of the experimenters themselves to mentally retarded children. A large nationwide trial using schoolchildren, who were called "polio pioneers," was performed in 1954. The success of this trial helped to foster the hope that medicine in the 20th century could conquer childhood diseases.

Poliomyelitis, also known as polio or infantile paralysis, is caused by an intestinal virus, or enterovirus. Once inside the gut, the virus spreads to the lymphatic system, where it multiplies and is eventually excreted in the feces. It is then spread between people by fecal-oral contact. In most cases, the illness is mild or unrecognized, consisting perhaps of a fever and stomach upset. Sometimes, however, the poliovirus latches onto the motor neurons that control the movement of the arms, legs, and abdomen and, in more severe cases, the neurons in the brain stem controlling breathing or swallowing.

Polio epidemics began to appear in the late 1800s in Europe and the United States because of improved sanitation. More hygienic conditions meant that children were less likely to encounter the virus in infancy, when they would be protected to some extent by maternal antibodies or other factors, and would develop immunity to the illness. Young children or adults with no immunity who encountered the polio virus were more likely to become ill than those who had this early exposure. Epidemics occurred in wealthy and poor, urban and rural areas alike, but most commonly in cities during the summer months. Although not as common as other contagious illnesses such as influenza or pneumonia, polio terrified the public. People who survived were often left with varying forms of paralysis. Parents were haunted by images of children in leg braces or, worse, imprisoned in iron lungs.

Poliovirus was first identified by Austrian physician Karl Landsteiner (1868–1943) in 1908. (Landsteiner received the 1930 Nobel Prize in Physiology or Medicine, not for this work but for his work in distinguishing different blood types.) In the 1930s, physicians John Kolmer (1886–1962) and Maurice Brodie

(1903–1939) developed two kinds of polio vaccines to protect against it—live and killed.

A live polio vaccine consists of a mutated, or attenuated, form of the virus that is given by mouth and then multiplies in the gut. It leads to the production of antibodies but not to the illness itself, and, in particular, it does not lead to an infection of the nervous system. People who are treated with live virus can spread the virus to others through their feces, leading to a form of passive immunization in others—a desired consequence. However, on occasion, the live virus can revert to a form that can infect the nervous system and lead to a case of paralytic polio.

The other kind of vaccine, a killed vaccine, is prepared by exposing the virus to formaldehyde. The formaldehyde inactivates the virus, but it is still able to evoke an antibody response. This vaccine is usually given by injection.

Kolmer used an attenuated live-virus preparation in Philadelphia, and his vaccine was blamed for causing 10 cases of polio, including 5 deaths, among 10,000 subjects. Brodie's killed-virus preparation in New York sometimes led to serious allergic, or anaphylactic, reactions. These events had a chilling effect on other researchers in the field and slowed down vaccine trials for the next 20 years.

However, research did continue, thanks in part to the personal story of President Franklin Delano Roosevelt (FDR) (1882–1945). In 1921, at the age of 39 FDR's legs became paralyzed. He was diagnosed with polio, although it is now thought that he might have had Guillain-Barré syndrome, another illness that can cause a paralysis that on occasion can be permanent. In any event, he and others assumed that he had had polio, and for the rest of his life, he was associated with this illness. FDR championed funding for polio treatment and research. His law partner, Basil O'Connor (1892–1972), founded the National Foundation for Infantile Paralysis (NFIP) in 1938 and was its president for more than 30 years.

O'Connor masterminded a great deal of publicity for polio with the help of celebrities. The singer Eddie Cantor came up with the name "March of Dimes" for the organization. The actress Helen Hayes had a daughter who died of polio; she often spoke at events to raise money. A short film called *The Crippler*, starring the young Nancy Reagan, terrified people. This publicity raised awareness and money—much of which went to help those struck by polio, as few people had health insurance in those years. Meanwhile, the epidemics continued. In the United States, the worst year of the polio epidemic was 1952, when there were over 57,000 reported cases, 3,145 deaths, and about 20,000 cases of paralysis.

Much of the research to fight polio was supported by the NFIP, but some was also carried out by pharmaceutical companies. Polish physician and researcher Hilary Koprowski (1916–2013), working with the pharmaceutical company Lederle, developed a live but weakened polio virus by growing the virus in rat brain cells. He and his lab technician drank it themselves in 1948, and in 1950, he gave it to children and two adults in a New York home for the mentally disabled. He called the children "volunteers." Seventeen of the 20 children developed antibodies to polio virus—the other three apparently already had antibodies—and none developed complications. Within 10 years, Koprowski's live vaccine was being used on four continents. In 1958, he gave it to nearly a quarter of a million patients in the Belgian Congo with reported success. But his polio vaccine has never been used widely in the United States because of persistent concerns about its safety. Koprowski spent the rest of his life working with vaccines, continuing to test them on himself. (For example, he injected himself with a vaccine against Colorado tick fever and an experimental rabies vaccine in 1971.)

Physician Jonas Salk (1914–1995), who since 1947 had been the head of the Virus Research Lab at the University of Pittsburgh, had worked with influenza vaccines and had also done a great deal of work typing the polio virus. He determined that the more than 100 strains could be put into three groups. With grant support from the March of Dimes, Salk developed a formalin-treated polio vaccine.

One of the difficulties in the work with polio was that the virus could not be grown as simply as could bacteria. Bacteria grow in petri dishes on broth, but viruses need live cells to multiply. At that time, polio virus was grown in human embryonic brain tissue. It was difficult to use a vaccine from this preparation because the presence of nervous tissue made any vaccine derived from it quite dangerous as it could lead to a serious allergic reaction, encephalomyelitis, which could cause brain damage. In 1948, bacteriologist John F. Enders (1897–1985) and physicians Thomas H. Weller (1915–2008) and Frederick Robbins (1916–2003) at Harvard grew the polio virus in human embryonic skin and muscle tissue and used antibiotics to decrease the risk of bacterial superinfection. Salk used their technique to grow the virus and then kill it with formaldehyde. This killed polio virus was able to trigger the body to produce antibodies without actually causing the illness or encephalomyelitis.

In 1952, Salk injected several versions of his vaccine into children who had had polio at the D. T. Watson home for crippled children; some versions led to an increase in their antibodies. Later that year, he injected an improved version into mentally retarded residents at the Polk State School; no adverse reactions were noted. He then gave the vaccine to himself, his wife, and their children and then to 5,000 Pittsburgh-area schoolchildren, beginning in February 1954. None became ill.

Because of the rarity of polio, it was necessary to carry out even larger trials across the United States. These were done in 1954 with the help of the NFIP and a huge army of volunteers. The polio vaccine trials were one of the largest, if not the largest, medical experiments ever performed. Other polio experts disapproved of the trial, arguing that it was premature and had been rushed into operation by pressure from the NFIP. Enders and Albert Sabin (1906–1993), another physician and polio expert who thought that live vaccines were the better approach, thought that the trial was too dangerous because the safety of the vaccine had not been definitively established. Walter Winchell, the famous broadcaster, also spoke about the dangerousness of the vaccine and about "little white coffins" being prepared for the undoubtedly huge number of casualties that would result from the trials.

In addition to large numbers of subjects, the trials also needed huge quantities of vaccine. Much of this came from the Connaught laboratories at the University of Toronto, where scientists had developed the first synthetic medium in which poliovirus could be cultivated.

Thomas Francis (1900–1969), a virologist and epidemiologist from the University of Michigan in Ann Arbor, organized the trial. Francis obtained assent, consent, and approval of multiple groups of people: schoolchildren, their parents, schools, school nurses, and the state boards of health. The publicity and awareness engineered by Basil O'Connor proved its worth: more than 200,000 unpaid volunteers (including physicians, teachers, nurses, and health officers) helped to organize and carry out the trial. In a stroke of genius, or manipulation, or both, the schoolchildren and their parents were not asked to consent, as they would have been today. Instead, the parents signed papers *requesting* that their child participate in the trial.

The original plan was to conduct a double-blind placebo-controlled randomized trial, thought to be necessary because polio was occasionally difficult to diagnose and could occur unpredictably. The placebo arm and "blindness" of the trial meant that the children and the doctors involved would not know whether they had received the active vaccine and thus could not consciously or unconsciously bias the results. The randomization was also a way of ensuring that there were no differences between the active and control groups that could interfere with understanding the results. Not all agreed to this design. Some states thought that using placebo was unethical because it meant that some children would not be protected from the illness (even though the efficacy of the vaccine had not yet been established.) Other states thought that the use of placebo was essential; otherwise, the results would be impossible to interpret.

Finally, Francis and his colleagues compromised. Eleven states would enroll first, second, and third graders in a double-blind placebo trial. In 33 other states, all second graders would be vaccinated with active vaccine, with first and third graders as observational controls. All treatments—active or placebo—were given in a series of three injections. Schoolchildren in the Canadian provinces of Alberta and Manitoba, in the Canadian city of Halifax, and in Finland participated as well. In 2 percent of all cases, bloodwork was done to detect antibodies. Of the 1.8 million schoolchildren asked to participate, over 1 million, to be known as "polio pioneers," had parents who gave consent.

The trial began in April 1954. Over 600,000 schoolchildren received a series of three injections, either the vaccine or a placebo, consisting of the synthetic medium from Connaught. A six-month evaluation period followed. Almost a million other children were "observed" controls. There were, as to be expected, many problems. Some of the registrations were lost or confused. Some children got one injection of placebo and two of vaccine. Some schools did not get the vaccine in time. Some physicians may have taken the vaccine and used it for their own families. But overall it went smoothly. The trial generated huge amounts of data, all of which was sent to Ann Arbor, where statisticians and 300 college students tabulated and calculated.

Table 5.1 Polio Vaccine Trials

Double-Blind Placebo-Controlled Arm (first, second, and third grade children)—
Vaccine vs. Placebo

	Approximate number of children	Rate of polio (per 100,000)
Vaccine	200,000	28
Control (placebo injection)	200,000	71
Not participating	350,000	46

Observational Arm—Vaccine vs. Observation

	Approximate number of children	Rate of polio (per 100,000)
Second grade—vaccine	225,000	25
First and third grade—control (no injection)	725,000	54
Second grade—not participating	125,000	44

As can be seen in the table, children who received the active vaccine were less likely to develop polio, although the vaccine was not entirely effective. What is not shown is the finding that, for those children who did develop polio, the severity of polio was higher in the controls than in the ones who received the injection and yet still developed the disease. This finding extended to both arms of the study. Fifteen children died from polio; none of these children had received the vaccine. There were very few adverse reactions to the vaccine, and bloodwork showed higher antibody levels in the vaccinated.

On April 12, 1955, at the University of Michigan, Francis announced that the vaccine was effective and safe. The announcement was a huge event. Sixteen cameras were present, and some broadcast the announcement to over 50,000 physicians watching in movie theaters across the country. Salk became one of the most famous physicians of the 20th century. This large trial—an experiment in logistics as much as in medicine—had succeeded. Within a day of the announcement, the United States Department of Health and Welfare approved the vaccine, and it immediately began to be produced commercially.

The manufacturing, however, turned out to be another experiment of sorts. It was complicated to scale up vaccine production—though this fact was not fully appreciated at the time. When Salk and the people closely associated with him directed vaccine production, and when the quantities were small, it was much easier to monitor for quality. All of the pharmaceutical companies involved in the mass production of the polio vaccine, including Eli Lilly, Parke-Davis, Wyeth, and Cutter, had trouble inactivating the virus, and some children vaccinated by products from Wyeth and Cutter developed polio. Cutter, in particular, had the most trouble, and their vaccines led to 200 cases of paralysis and 11 deaths. This became known as the "Cutter Incident."

After the Cutter Incident, the rate of immunization against polio temporarily fell, but then it increased again as methods for preparing vaccine and quality control became more tightly controlled. Federal authorities increased the rigor of vaccine safety testing and surveillance after vaccinations.

Following the Cutter Incident, various governmental agencies became more involved in vaccine product and regulation. (As mentioned, the Salk polio vaccine trials had not been carried out by governmental agencies in the United States, but by the March of Dimes.) In Canada, the provincial and federal governments organized vaccinations, and using vaccine prepared by Connaught, they encountered no problems.

Another consequence of the Cutter Incident was litigation. At trial, Cutter argued that they had followed the correct procedures (this was not entirely true) and should not be penalized for something over which they had no control. The jury partially agreed, but the principle of liability without fault was established. This principle, some argue, along with large jury awards to people who may or may not have been injured by medical innovations, has discouraged those involved in vaccine production and experimental treatments in medicine.

Meanwhile, Albert Sabin produced another type of live vaccine and, in 1955, began tests of it in 47 prisoners in Chillicothe Federal Reformatory in Chillicothe, Ohio. Each man was paid $25 and received "three free days." He tested his vaccine in children's homes in Leningrad and then organized enormous vaccination programs in Russia. This work was carried out with the assistance of the Russian virologist Mikhail Chumakov, in a rare example of Cold War U.S.-Soviet collaboration.

These programs, often called trials, were not exactly trials in the rigorous sense of the word because there were no controls. Following more trials, many sponsored by the World Health Organization, Sabin's live vaccine was licensed in 1962 in the United States and is now the most widely used throughout the world. Polio has not yet been eradicated; outbreaks still occur in countries where vaccination does not take place or occasionally if the live vaccine reverts to a more virulent form.

Currently, in the United States, medical opinion has swung back to using the killed, or inactivated, polio vaccine to eliminate the risk of any vaccine-associated cases of paralytic polio. In other parts of the world, live vaccine is still used.

The 1954 Nobel Prize in Physiology or Medicine was awarded to John Enders, Thomas Weller, and Frederick Robbins for their discovery of the ability of poliovirus to grow in cultures of various types of tissue. Salk was nominated twice but did not receive it because he was not thought to have discovered anything that was new but only exploited discoveries made by others.

Frances R. Frankenburg

PORTON DOWN

During and after World War II, the British military carried out experiments in the use of and defense against chemical, biological, radiological, and nuclear warfare at Porton Down in Wiltshire, England.

As a response to the German development and use of poison gas in World War I, in 1916, the British established a research center at Porton Down, which was located in the countryside of Wiltshire, a county in southwest England. During World War II, research at Porton Down concentrated on chemical weapons such as nitrogen mustards and biological weapons, including anthrax and botulinum toxin.

During World War II, the Germans were developing a different type of poison gas using "nerve agents." Most nerve agents are organophosphates and were first synthesized as insecticides. These agents work in the following way: acetylcholine, a common neurotransmitter found throughout the nervous system, is metabolized by an enzyme called acetylcholinesterase. Nerve agents block the action of this enzyme, meaning that acetylcholine remains active. A person exposed to nerve agents will become weak, drool, sweat, and experience diarrhea. In extreme cases, the person will become paralyzed, stop breathing, and die.

After the war, the British discovered that Germany possessed large stocks of poison nerve gases, including tabun, sarin, and soman. The British military began a research program based on these newly discovered German nerve agents and other potentially militarily useful toxins and drugs.

Tests were carried out at Porton Down on British servicemen to determine the effects of toxins on human subjects. Hundreds of "volunteers" were exposed to the nerve gases. Four soldiers were hospitalized, and one became comatose. In 1953, a series of experiments involving the topical application of the nerve gases began. Ronald Maddison, a 20-year-old soldier, died 45 minutes after 200 milligrams of sarin were dripped onto a patch of uniform on his arm.

Between 1953 and 1954, some soldiers volunteered to be "guinea pigs" after being told that Porton Down scientists wanted to find a cure for the common cold. Instead of being administered benign viruses, they were given lysergic acid diethylamide (LSD) in mind-control tests, and three soldiers successfully sued the English secret intelligence agency MI6, claiming that they were deceived and had experienced terrifying hallucinations.

In subsequent investigations, some initiated by the Wiltshire police, the questions of whether the soldiers gave informed consent and whether the researchers adhered to the Nuremberg Code were reviewed. Well before World War II, the British Medical Council had often written about the necessity of informed consent, so these issues were not foreign to British researchers. The researchers at Porton Down, perhaps because of their anxiety about the poisons that the Germans had been developing and their fears of what the Russians might use in the future, did not think that their research required informed consent. Indeed, in one rebuttal to criticism, the Porton Down researchers said that it was not their responsibility to tell the servicemen too much, but that the servicemen always had the opportunity to ask questions.

Another area of work at Porton Down involved the investigation of airborne dispersion of germs. Scientists wanted to analyze how a cloud of germs (theoretically from the Soviet Union) would disperse in Britain.

On February 1, 1961, Porton Down scientists drove a Land Rover through Wedmore and to the outskirts of Bristol. The scientists wore full protective clothing and gas masks and sprayed zinc cadmium sulfide (a mixture of zinc sulfide and cadmium sulfide that fluoresces when exposed to ultraviolet light) into the air as they traveled through the English countryside. The cloud was traced at sampling stations through Somerset and Wiltshire back to Porton. Altogether, between 1953 and 1964, zinc cadmium sulfide was released in over 70 experiments to mimic biological attacks from potential communist enemies.

This work is similar to that carried out by the American military during the 1940s and 1950s, in which mock biological attacks were carried out to investigate the possibility of biological warfare aimed at American cities. Most of the work carried out at Porton Down, however, has remained secret, and only a few details have emerged.

Frances R. Frankenburg

PROJECT COAST

During the apartheid era in South Africa, Project Coast was the country's secret chemical and biological warfare project.

In the late 1970s, South Africa responded to perceived threats of chemical and biological warfare by beginning a research program into these methods of warfare. In 1983, Project Coast was formed, directed by Wouter Basson (b. 1950), a cardiologist and the personal physician of president P. W. Botha. The exact nature of the experimentation is unknown, but Basson recruited 200 researchers from other countries to help develop chemical and biological weapons.

The stated intention of Project Coast was to develop defensive equipment for the South African Defence Force (SADF) and crowd control agents for domestic use, but the project did much else besides. They gave chemical and biological warfare agents to members of the South African Police and Special Forces unit of the SADF for the purpose of assassination.

The few other details that have emerged include a 1989 project in which Project Coast tried to contaminate the water supply at Dobra, a refugee camp located in Namibia, with cholera and yellow fever organisms. They also investigated ways of sterilizing the black population and finding race-specific bacterial weapons. The researchers developed chemical and biological pathogens and may have been involved with genetic engineering.

While much of the work of Project Coast remains secret, it is known that Project Coast had contacts with British and American intelligence and the biological and chemical weapons programs of these countries. When F. W. de Klerk became president of South Africa in 1990, he ordered that lethal weapons be destroyed, and he fired Basson. The researchers at Project Coast continued their work, but they changed their interests. They investigated mind-altering nonlethal drugs, including MDMA (3,4-methylenedioxymethamphetamine, also known as ecstasy), methaqualone, cocaine, diazepam, and ketamine. In 1993, Project Coast ended.

Nelson Mandela became president in 1994, and he reappointed Basson to the SADF. In 1995, Basson was hired as the chief cardiologist and head of the heart transplant program in South Africa's main military hospital in Pretoria.

Basson's legal troubles began in 1997 when he was arrested for allegedly selling a thousand capsules of ecstasy to a police informant. Police then found two locked trunks in his house with much material about Project Coast. In 1999, Basson was put on trial and charged with involvement in 229 murders and embezzlement, drug trafficking, and possession of illegal drugs. The trial lasted until 2002. He argued that he had acted on the orders of the former South African Defence Force (SADF) when he was involved in the chemical and biological warfare program, and he was acquitted.

In 2013, the Health Professions Council of South Africa found Basson guilty of acting unprofessionally by, among other activities, supplying suicide cyanide capsules to army officers, preparing and distributing tranquilizing or disorienting substances to facilitate kidnappings, and producing large quantities of illegal psychoactive agents, ecstasy, and tear gas. As of March 2016, he has not been sentenced.

Frances R. Frankenburg

SAENGER, EUGENE

Between 1960 and 1972, physicians at the University of Cincinnati, led by radiologist Eugene Saenger and under contract from the Department of Defense, conducted total- or partial-body irradiation of 80 to 90 patients with cancer. These physicians have been accused of working in conjunction with the Department of Defense to discover the effects of high doses of radiation on the body rather than providing a form of cancer treatment.[1]

During the Cold War years, the United States Department of Defense (DoD), Manhattan Project, and the Atomic Energy Commission (AEC)—all working with and studying radiation—wanted to learn more about what would happen to American soldiers exposed to radiation. Between 1940 and 1974, they arranged at least 20 studies in about 9 institutions in which patients with malignancies or, in a few cases, healthy subjects, were exposed to total body irradiation (TBI). The exposure of these patients was thought to be justified because, for some years, there had been an expectation that irradiation might be therapeutic. (On the other hand, the healthier the subject was, the more useful the experiment could be in understanding the effects of radiation on healthy soldiers.) Studies were carried out at MD Anderson in Houston, the large cancer hospital at the University of Texas; at UCLA; and at other institutions. Many of these studies were carried out in partially secret conditions, so not all of the details are known.

The studies that received the most attention were those carried out in Cincinnati. The DoD funded work by Eugene Saenger (1917–2007), a well-respected

Cincinnati radiologist and expert in nuclear medicine. Saenger used radiation at high doses to treat patients with cancer, often irradiating their entire bodies. The experiments, carried out between 1960 and 1972, involved 80 to 90 patients; almost two-thirds were black Americans, and most were poor or working class. The patients had metastatic cancer, but not all of them were very ill. In fact, some were still able to work. To keep the study as useful as possible for the DoD, the Cincinnati patients were not given antiemetic drugs to alleviate nausea caused by the irradiation. It is doubtful that the patients had been told that they were being "used" to see whether soldiers could still fight while suffering from radiation sickness. During the time period of these experiments, TBI was falling out of favor and came to be regarded as not "standard of care."

Cincinnati physicians said that, for the first five years, they obtained verbal consent for the TBI studies. They began to obtain written informed consent in 1965. The first written form did not mention bone marrow suppression (a well-known and serious complication of radiation). The researchers did not include the side effects of nausea and vomiting either because they feared that by mentioning them, they might cause them through the power of suggestion. Later forms had more information, including the fact that the investigation was for the scientific benefit for others, but they did not mention the possibility of death. Beginning in 1968, the investigators came up with an innovation that actually made the process of obtaining informed consent somewhat more rigorous than is usual. The consent process took place over two days, allowing the patients and their representatives some time to think about what was being proposed.

The studies had been reviewed and approved by several oversight committees over the years. However, some faculty members at the University of Cincinnati had been uneasy about this study. Finally, in 1967 the National Institutes of Health rejected Saenger's plan to expand his experiment. Whether Saenger's patients were hurt by the irradiation is difficult to tell, as all had malignancies.

Saenger himself testified in 1994 that his primary purpose was to improve the well-being of his patients, that nothing he did was secret, and that DoD funds were not involved in the treatment of his patients. He did, however, admit that funding from the DoD, used to support laboratories and testing, made the irradiation possible.

Finally, a suit in federal court, presided over by Judge Sandra Beckwith, addressed the major points under dispute. Most of the details of the 1999 settlement have not been released, but a few things are known: most families received $50,000, a dozen families received $85,000, and a plaque memorializing those patients who were treated with TBI was placed on the University of Cincinnati campus.

Frances R. Frankenburg

Note

1. The terms *radiation* or *irradiation* are often used interchangeably. Irriadiation is sometimes used to refer specifically to deliberate exposure to radiation.

SEXUALLY TRANSMITTED DISEASE EXPERIMENTS IN GUATEMALA

Between 1946 and 1948, American researchers working in Guatemala inoculated prisoners, soldiers, and mental asylum inmates with syphilis and other sexually transmitted diseases in an attempt to better understand how to prevent and treat these illnesses. Few, if any, of the subjects gave consent.

In the middle of the 20th century, little could be done to prevent the spread of sexually transmitted diseases (STDs). Men were encouraged to use condoms during sexual intercourse and to rub a bactericidal ointment into their penises afterward, but compliance with these preventative procedures was not very high. The military was particularly concerned about the effects of STDs, as they diminished a soldier's fighting ability.

A major advance was made in 1943, when researchers demonstrated that the antibiotic penicillin was an effective treatment for syphilis and other STDs. Many questions remained, however, particularly regarding prophylaxis. For instance, if penicillin was given to a person after exposure to *Treponema pallidum*, the bacterium that causes syphilis, or *Neisseria gonorrhoeae*, the bacterium or gonococcus that causes gonorrhea, would that prevent the illnesses from then developing? One way to answer this question was to expose people to the infection and then test the adequacy of prophylaxis, but this would be difficult to do. Not many people would volunteer to be exposed to a sexually transmitted illness.

In 1942, the United States Public Health Service (PHS) exposed people to gonococci under controlled conditions at a federal prison in Terre Haute, Indiana, using volunteer inmates. (The Terre Haute prison was selected because it had good medical facilities.) The inmates signed informed consent forms, and at the end of the experiments, each subject received $100, a certificate of merit, and a letter of commendation to the parole board. The researchers tried to infect prisoners by depositing bacteria—sometimes gathered from prostitutes arrested by the Terre Haute police—directly on the end of the penis. But within 10 months, the experiments were abandoned because of low infection rates.

Juan Funes, a Guatemalan physician and chief of the venereal disease control division of Guatemala's Public Health Service, had worked at the PHS Venereal Disease Research Laboratory (VDRL) in Staten Island, New York, for a year and suggested to his American colleagues that work similar to the Terre Haute experiments could be carried out in Guatemala. Following his suggestion, the PHS VDRL and the National Institutes of Health, with the collaboration of the Pan-American Sanitary Bureau and other government agencies in Guatemala, exposed human subjects to STDs from 1946 to 1948 in different venues, including prisons, mental hospitals, and military facilities. (Administrators of these institutions approved the experiments.) The researchers' interest was in determining whether penicillin could be used as a prophylactic drug with respect to syphilis. They were also interested in gonorrhea and chancroid, another STD. John C. Cutler (1915–2003), a PHS VDRL physician, moved to Guatemala City to direct the studies. He was supervised by Richard Arnold and John F. Mahoney (1889–1957), one of the pioneers in the treatment of syphilis with penicillin. Funes was the primary local collaborator.

The advantage of carrying out these experiments in Guatemala was that prostitution was legal in that country, then as now. Indeed, prostitutes were allowed to visit prisoners in Guatemalan prisons. These sex workers were examined at clinics twice a week. As Funes supervised one of the main clinics, he could easily recommend infected prostitutes for experiments.

The first syphilis experiments were carried out in Guatemala's Central Penitentiary. The U.S. researchers paid infected prostitutes to have sex with prisoners. Few of the prisoners became infected. They later inoculated men directly with syphilis by rubbing bacteria onto the men's penises and on abraded areas of their forearms and faces. The researchers then began to use patients from the mental hospital. In total, 497 subjects were inoculated with live *T. pallidum*. Similar studies with gonorrhea were carried out by infecting sex workers with gonorrhea that had been cultivated in rabbit tissues. The researchers then paid the prostitutes to have sex with soldiers.

Many subjects were involved in more than one experiment. Inoculations of various STDs were administered by subcutaneous injection of infectious material into abrasions of the arm, face, cervix, or the penis, or by applying soaked cotton wads under the foreskin. In the case of seven female patients at a mental hospital, the experimenters injected syphilitic material through the back of their necks, directly into their central nervous systems. (A large collection of cerebrospinal fluid can be reached by inserting a needle into the spinal cord at the top of the neck; this is known as a cisternal puncture.) In some cases, after inoculation, different methods of postexposure prophylaxis were tried, including the use of orvus-mapharsen, a new arsenical drug.

Altogether, 1,300 subjects (prisoners, soldiers, and psychiatric patients) were exposed to STDs, either through infected sex workers or by artificial inoculations. Fewer than 700 were treated.

In addition, to improve diagnostic accuracy, the researchers performed serological tests on over 5,000 subjects, including soldiers, prisoners, psychiatric patients, children in orphanages, patients in a leprosarium, and air force personnel. These tests were designed to detect antibodies that arise after infection. Some of the tests were routine blood draws, but the researchers also punctured the spinal cord in the lumbar and cisternal (back of the skull) regions to obtain and test cerebrospinal fluid. These particular tests continued through 1953.

It is not known whether any of the subjects involved in any of these studies gave informed consent, with the possible exception of the prisoners or soldiers. Arnold wrote to Cutler in 1947: "I am a bit, in fact more than a bit, leary of the experiment with the insane people. They cannot give consent, do not know what is going on, and if some goody organization got wind of the work, they would raise a lot of smoke. I think the soldiers would be best or the prisoners for they can give consent."[1] While this passage suggests that the prisoners and soldiers did give consent, there is no evidence that it actually did happen.

As well as carrying out the experiments, the researchers and their colleagues established a venereal-disease treatment program at the military hospital and developed a prophylactic plan for the Guatemalan army. The physicians also treated some children who were ill with malaria and trained local doctors and technicians. Cutler treated 142 people who may have had venereal disease but had not been exposed to it as part of the research.

The research conditions in the prison and asylum were poor. Many records were lost. Some of the psychiatric patients were not known by name and may have been confused with other subjects. Many patients were used in multiple experiments and did not receive follow-up or treatment. Not all patients cooperated with the bloodwork.

No publications arose from the Guatemalan experiments, except for a few articles about the serological research. It is not known whether the lack of publications was because of doubts about the quality of the data or apprehension about criticism of the unethical nature of the work. In any event, it is probable that we would still know nothing of these experiments were it not for an academic researcher named Susan Reverby (b. 1946). In 2010, while researching the 40-year Tuskegee Study of Untreated Syphilis (the earlier study of undertreated syphilis in black men in the United States), Reverby examined the unpublished and archived papers of John Cutler at the University of Pittsburgh. She discovered many boxes of his correspondence and unpublished papers about these experiments in Guatemala.

Reverby discovered that these experiments were carried out with the knowledge and support of the surgeon general of the time, Thomas Parran (1892–1968). Parran had been the commissioner of health for New York and chief of PHS's Division of Venereal Diseases before being appointed surgeon general of the United States in 1936. He retained that position until 1948, when he became the first dean of public health at the University of Pittsburgh. He had taken a lead role in addressing STDs as infections that needed to be medically treated. He oversaw and funded the Guatemalan experiments. (He also had some responsibility for continuing the Tuskegee studies of syphilis.) Within the documents Reverby discovered was a letter referring to Parran's acknowledgment that the Guatemalan experiments could not have taken place in the United States. Other documents referred to the necessity of keeping these experiments hidden from the public.

In 2010, when Reverby's research was publicized, the United States officially apologized to Guatemala for its role in the studies. The Presidential Commission for the Study of Bioethical Issues investigated and concluded that "the Guatemala experiments involved gross violations of ethics as judged against both the standards of today and the researchers' own understanding of applicable contemporaneous practices."[2] The PHS looked further into the study and published a number of accounts about it. They made a deliberate decision not to use any of the data to draw any conclusions about STDs or their treatment, so it could not be said that they profited from unethical research.

Frances R. Frankenburg

References

1. Presidential Commission for the Study of Bioethical Issues, *A Study Guide to "Ethically Impossible" STD Research*, 36–38.
2. Presidential Commission for the Study of Bioethical Issues, *"Ethically Impossible" STD Research*, v.

SOUTHAM, CHESTER

Chester Southam was an immunologist affiliated with the Sloan-Kettering Institute for Cancer Research in New York. He injected live cancer cells into ill patients at the Jewish Chronic Diseases Hospital in Brooklyn without their consent, leading to adverse publicity and court action. But other doctors supported his work, and Southam proceeded to have a distinguished career.

The body's immune system can "recognize" foreign cells and then reject or kill them. This ability explains why organ transplants will not succeed unless the donor and recipient are genetically very similar or unless the recipient is treated with immunosuppressant medications. As a way of exploring immunity and rejection, physicians have at times transplanted cancer cells from one person to another, as cancer cells are, by their very nature, usually long-lived and able to survive attacks from the person's own body.

Chester Milton Southam (1909–2002) was a well-respected physician working at the Sloan-Kettering Institute for Cancer Research in New York in the areas of virology, immunology, and cancer. In a more than decade-long series of experiments investigating how the body rejects foreign tissue, Southam injected or implanted cancer cells into people at several different institutions, including hospitals and a prison.

Between February 1954 and July 1956, Southam injected cancer cells into patients already ill with cancer at Memorial Hospital, the hospital associated with the Sloan-Kettering Institute. The implanted cancer cells sometimes survived briefly and grew into a measureable nodule that within a few weeks disappeared. Occasionally, Southam would remove the nodule to examine it. The patients, even though they were ill and unable to fight off their own cancer cells, did reject the "foreign" cancer cells as was expected. In one case the implanted cancer cells spread, or metastasized, to a lymph node in the patient's armpit, but there is no evidence that this patient, or any other, sustained lasting harm from the experimental procedures.

In the mid-1950s Southam injected live cancer cells into healthy prisoners at an Ohio state penitentiary. In this case, he explained the project to the prisoners and asked for volunteers, who signed informed consent. He discovered that the healthy prisoners rejected the cancer cells faster than the Memorial Hospital patients already ill with cancer. No adverse reactions were described.

Southam continued his injections of live cancer cells into Memorial Hospital patients, but without obtaining consent or telling the patients that they were being injected with cancer cells. For two years, he injected cancer cells into all postoperative gynecology patients at the Sloan-Kettering as a way, he said, of measuring their immunologic status.

Southam wanted to know if the cancer patients were slower to reject the foreign cancer cells because of their generally debilitated or weakened state, or because they had cancer. To answer this question, he decided to inject live cancer cells into the elderly and other people debilitated by noncancerous illnesses. Would they reject the cancer cells at the rate of the healthy people or at the slower rate displayed by those ill with cancer?

To find out, in July 1963, he approached Emanuel Mandel, director of medicine at the Jewish Chronic Disease Hospital (JCDH) in Brooklyn, to obtain his permission to use JCDH patients who were ill but did not have cancer. By that time, he had injected or implanted live cancer cells into over 300 patients with cancer and over 300 healthy subjects. Southam reassured Mandel and the JCDH that he had successfully carried out some of these experiments at the Sloan-Kettering Institute and that he received some funding from the United States Public Health Service and the American Cancer Society. He told the JCDH that he did not explain the nature of the injection to the patients because there was no risk that these implants would cause any cancer, and it was not necessary to do so in this case either. The JCDH agreed to help Southam with his research.

Mandel asked physicians at the JCDH to participate in this experiment. Three refused, feeling uneasy about the experiment. A fourth physician agreed, and chose 19 JCDH patients to be subjects for Southam's study. (Inexplicably, Mandel chose another 3 patients with cancer to be subjects.) On the morning of July 16, Southam injected into three patients a suspension of human cancer cells, grown in tissue culture, just under the skin on two places on the front of the thigh. Then the JCDH physician carried out a similar procedure in the remaining 19 patients. The patients rejected the cancer implants at a rate similar to that shown by the healthy prisoner volunteers and once again displayed no adverse effects.

The next month, in August, the three physicians who had refused to participate resigned their positions to avoid the appearance of condoning the research. They told a lawyer, William Hyman—who was also one of the hospital's directors—about what they considered to be unethical behavior on the part of Southam and Mandel. Hyman was outraged, partly because he misunderstood the experiment and believed that the researchers were trying to cause cancer. He asked to review the records of the patients, but the hospital would not allow him to do so. So, in December 1963, Hyman went to the Kings County Supreme Court in Brooklyn to obtain access to the patients' records.

A great deal of publicity ensued, and some of the discussions became personal. The lawyer and physicians who objected to the research were accused of having a personal animus toward Mandel. The physicians were also accused of being untruthful, poor doctors, and of being interested in monetary profit and career advancement from the dispute. Southam, on the other hand, made things worse for himself when a reporter for the journal *Science* asked if he had injected himself with live cancer cells. He answered,

I would not have hesitated if it would have served a useful purpose. But to me it seemed like false heroism, like the old question whether the General should march behind or in front of his troops. I do not regard myself as indispensable—if I were not doing this work someone else would be—and I did not regard the experiment as dangerous. But, let's face it, there are relatively few skilled cancer researchers, and it seemed stupid to take even the little risk.[1]

In a second lawsuit, in a hearing before the Board of Regents of the University of the State of New York, the state attorney general tried to revoke the medical licenses of Southam and Mandel because of the lack of informed consent from the patients. At trial, Southam and Mandel defended themselves by saying that doctors often did not use the word "cancer," even when talking to patients who had the disease. They believed that a person's reaction to the word "cancer" was so extreme as to make the individual unable to understand that no risk was involved in the implantation of cancer cells. The two physicians claimed that the cancerous origin of the cells was irrelevant because there was no risk of harm—no chance that the implanted cells could survive or cause cancer. Southam and Mandel also said that each of the 22 patients did receive a general explanation of the procedure—that it was a measurement of their immune response. They said that the patients gave oral consent. Many physicians and cancer researchers defended Southam and Mandel, saying that they worked in similar ways and that the work of Southam was both safe and important.

Critics of Southam and Mandel noted that they did not review their project with the research committee of the hospital nor with the doctors responsible for the clinical care of the affected patients. There was no documentation of informed consent in the patients' charts, and the difficulty of explaining the risks and benefits of this unusual experiment to the ill patients meant that the researchers were almost certainly experimenting without any sort of consent. They also did not inform the families or ask for their permission. As Southam had previously obtained written consent in his Ohio prison study, he could not have claimed ignorance of this concept.

Although he said that the procedure entailed no risk, Southam's own refusal to volunteer for the experiment shed some doubt on his claims of its complete safety. In his interview with *Science*, he modified the statement of "no risk" to a "little risk" for a hypothetical procedure involving himself. In addition, although there was no evidence of harm at the time, the researchers had not followed the patients for very long. As cancer cells are known to be long-lived and cancer can reappear some years after remission, perhaps the claims of safety were premature. Southam himself might have thought this, as he wrote an article describing a late recurrence of cancer at the site of a (presumably excisional) biopsy of a nodule.

Thus, the researchers deceived the patients by telling them that they were measuring their immune response instead of sharing the true nature of the study. This statement, probably incomprehensible to many of the patients, carried with it the implication that they were undergoing a test relevant to their clinical condition and treatment.

In sum, Southam and Mandel acted too quickly, without reviewing their experiment with the hospital at large, and without asking for informed permission from the patients or their families. It is difficult not to think that the illness of the patients—what made Southam and Mandel deem them appropriate subjects—was also the very thing that made their lives less important to the researchers. Had the patients or their families fully understood the procedure, they might have refused to allow it. The secrecy and the speed of the experiment are consistent with the criticism that the experiments involved some risk that the researchers wanted to hide.

The United States Public Health Service was asked by the New York attorney general to comment. It replied that ethical research practices could most clearly be safeguarded by the involvement of the researchers' peers and not by regulation.

In 1964, both Southam and Mandel were put on probation for a year by the Board of Regents of the University of the State of New York. Southam proceeded to have a successful career and, in 1968, was elected president of the American Association for Cancer Research.

Frances R. Frankenburg

Reference

1. Quoted in Langer, "Human Experimentation," 551.

STANLEY, JAMES

While serving in the U.S. Army in 1958, Master Sergeant James Stanley was given lysergic acid diethylamide (LSD) without his knowledge. He blamed LSD for his subsequent emotional problems and filed a lawsuit against the United States that reached the Supreme Court. His suit failed because the Supreme Court argued that it was part of his military duty to participate in an experiment.

In February 1958, Master Sergeant James B. Stanley was stationed at Fort Knox in Kentucky. He volunteered to be a test subject in a chemical weapons study and was transferred to the study location, the Edgewood Arsenal in Aberdeen, Maryland. At first, he thought that he was volunteering to test protective clothing for the army. Instead, he was given a clear liquid to drink that, unbeknownst to him, contained lysergic acid diethylamide (LSD). Stanley subsequently developed emotional problems and he and his wife divorced in 1970.

In 1975, the army asked him to go to the Walter Reed Army Medical Center in Washington, D.C., to participate in a follow-up study of people who had taken LSD. Before this request, Stanley had not been told that he had been given LSD.

After learning the news, he blamed his emotional problems on the LSD and filed suit against the United States for injuries sustained as a result of the Edgewood experiment. The case went all of the way to the U.S. Supreme Court, and in 1987, the Supreme Court found against him, 5-4, arguing that his injuries were "incident to service" and that he could not therefore sue the United States. The majority invoked the Feres Doctrine, which states that a member of the armed forces cannot bring a claim against the federal government for injuries caused by activity related to his or her military service. The dissenting justices noted that Stanley had been an involuntary and uninformed subject and that the experiment violated the Nuremberg Code.

Stanley then testified before Congress. As a result of his testimony, the Department of Defense awarded him $625,000 in damages.

Frances R. Frankenburg

STREPTOMYCIN CLINICAL TRIAL

Medicine's first major randomized clinical trial tested the usefulness of the drug streptomycin against tuberculosis. In this study, there was an element of uncertainty as to the value of streptomycin. The trial organizers used an experimental design to allot treatment.

Tuberculosis, an illness caused by a bacterium called *Mycobacterium tuberculosis*, is usually an illness of the lungs, but the bacteria can also infect the kidney, spine, and brain. Once the leading cause of death in the United States, tuberculosis remained a serious illness without effective treatment until the middle of the 20th century. Because tuberculosis had a high mortality rate and an unpredictable course, finding an effective treatment was both important and difficult.

Soil microbiologist Selman Waksman (1888–1973) at Rutgers University in New Jersey had been analyzing microorganisms in the soil, many of which killed other microorganisms. He became interested in a type of bacterium known as *actinomycetes*. He organized a methodical screening program to see which variety of actinomycetes could produce substances toxic to other bacteria, specifically those that caused human illnesses. Albert Schatz (1920–2005), a PhD student working with Waksman, found a type of actinomycetes in a chicken's throat, presumably picked up while the chicken was pecking in the dirt. This microorganism produced a substance, that would become known as streptomycin, that was toxic to other microbes but not to larger organisms, such as chickens or humans. In 1952, Waksman won a Nobel Prize in Physiology or Medicine for this discovery. (Some thought that the prize should have been shared with Schatz.)

Streptomycin was tested at the Mayo Clinic in Minnesota and thought to be active against tuberculosis. But production was difficult, so it was both scarce and expensive. In England, in the aftermath of World War II, patients and doctors had no money to buy adequate supplies of the new tuberculosis treatment. As the available amounts were only sufficient for a few patients and there was no definitive evidence that streptomycin was effective and safe, the English Medical Research Council (MRC) designed a research project in which streptomycin would be assigned to patients in a random manner. Otherwise, selection of patients for this promising but unproven treatment could have been difficult.

The trial was carried out at the MRC Tuberculosis Research Unit under the direction of the eminent British physician Sir Geoffrey Marshall (1887–1982) in 1947.

Tuberculosis patients thought to be eligible for the trial were randomly assigned to either active drug or control. Before this trial, there had been a few randomized trials in which patients were allotted to groups by alternation, meaning that the first patient was assigned to the active group, the second to the control group, the third to the active group, and so on. This method was possibly flawed, as physicians could on occasion know to which group the last patient had been assigned, which might affect their decision about how to "time" the selection of their next patient. Austin Bradford Hill (1897–1991), professor of medical statistics at the London School of Hygiene and Tropical Medicine (later to become more famous for his work on the unexpected dangers of tobacco smoking), had been writing about experimental design for 10 years. He suggested a new scheme of randomization that safeguarded against any selection bias by using random numbers and concealing the allocation schedule.

After a physician identified a potentially eligible subject, information about that subject was sent to the national coordinating center of the trial. If the subject met the eligibility criteria, he or she was admitted to the closest next available hospital bed. Each gender in each center was allotted a numbered series of envelopes, bearing only the name of the hospital. Each envelope contained a card indicating "S(treptomycin)" or "C(ontrol)." The numerical order of the envelopes was based on a series of random numbers. After a subject was accepted into the trial, the next envelope for that center and gender was opened. Control treatment consisted of bedrest.

This trial was, by modern standards, unusual, in that neither group of patients knew that they were in a trial and no consent was obtained. Bradford Hill saw no need for informed consent, and the trial remained secret throughout its 15-month duration. All patients received monthly chest X-rays, which were graded by radiologists who were "blind"; that is, they were unaware of whether or not the patient was receiving streptomycin. Somewhat weakening the element of equipoise in this study was the decision by the MRC to treat a senior physician with streptomycin obtained outside the study.

The study design was innovative, and the results of the study were both disappointing and important. Patients treated with streptomycin did improve, but only briefly before the tuberculosis bacteria gained resistance to the drug. The discovery of the rapid acquisition of drug resistance was unwelcome but essential in learning the limitations of antibiotics. Another important result was the demonstration that, in studies of new treatments in medicine, patients could be enrolled in multiple sites, and their allocation to study groups could be done in a randomized manner applied by a central office. The "blindness" of the radiologists was an important advance in trial methodology, as this meant that their readings of the chest X-ray could not be biased by their particular beliefs about whether streptomycin was effective. By later standards, the secrecy of the study and absence of informed consent were problematic.

Frances R. Frankenburg

THALIDOMIDE

In the late 1950s and early 1960s, the drug thalidomide, originally marketed as a safe sedative, led to birth defects in the children of thousands of women who took it while pregnant. One of the results of this international tragedy was the realization by the American public that more testing was needed before drugs are issued to the public; this realization in turn eased the passage of the Kefauver-Harris Amendments to the Federal Food, Drug, and Cosmetic Act. While not strictly related to experiments, the amendments' requirement for increased caution when new products are given to humans was a harbinger of increased regulation of research to come. The amendments also led to a requirement that new drugs be tested on more subjects before they could be marketed, a form of experimentation in itself.

In the 1950s, there were no safe sedative drugs on the market. Barbiturates were used to help people sleep, but these were lethal in overdose and highly addicting. The German pharmaceutical firm Chemie Grunenthal introduced the drug thalidomide as a safe over-the-counter sleeping pill and advertised that it was even safe for pregnant women, who also used it to treat morning sickness. By 1960, it was being sold in much of Europe, Canada, and Australia.

In December of 1960, the *British Medical Journal* (*BMJ*) published a letter from A. Leslie Florence, a Scottish general practitioner, who had prescribed thalidomide to his patients and seen four cases of peripheral neuritis, a painful tingling of the arms and feet, in patients who had taken the drug for periods ranging from 18 months to 2 years. The problem diminished but persisted even after the drug was stopped.

Meanwhile, in the United States, Frances Kelsey (1914–2015), a physician and pharmacologist working at the Food and Drug Administration (FDA), was hesitant to approve of the distribution of thalidomide. Kelsey, who had just started working at the FDA that year, after two years of investigating the posterior pituitary gland of the armadillo, had had some experience with the unexpected complications of drugs. In the fall of 1937, a new preparation of the antibiotic sulfanilamide was released. The antibiotic was dissolved in diethylene glycol (antifreeze), and this preparation was responsible for the deaths of over a hundred children. Kelsey investigated this tragedy in the laboratory and wrote later that she vividly remembered seeing rats develop renal failure and die after exposure to diethylene glycol. While working with antimalarial drugs during World War II, she observed that rabbit embryos, quite different from adult rabbits, could not break down quinine. When she joined the FDA, she already understood that new drugs or preparations could be dangerous and that there could be differences between adults and embryos in how drugs are metabolized.

Kelsey thought that the toxicology testing that the pharmaceutical company submitted about thalidomide was not very extensive and that the clinical reports were poor. As well, at the time of the introduction of thalidomide, the FDA was becoming more careful about the effects of drugs on the human embryo. She was aware of the BMJ letter and was concerned that a drug that could damage nerves, possibly irreversibly, could also affect a developing fetus if the pregnant mother with insomnia took it throughout her pregnancy. It turned out later that there had been European cases of peripheral neuritis, but this side effect had not been well publicized or relayed to the FDA.

Kelsey did not authorize thalidomide to be marketed in the United States. At the time, she was criticized for her caution, and the pharmaceutical company Merrell-Richardson, working with Chemie Grunenthal, exerted a great deal of pressure on her to change her mind. While awaiting FDA approval, Merrell sent out 2.5 million thalidomide "samples" to physicians in the United States. As many as 20,000 patients—including 207 pregnant women—took the drug without being informed that, at least in the United States, it was still investigational.

In 1961, William McBride, an obstetrician in Australia, saw an increase in birth defects in children born to women who had taken the drug. Some children were born with phocomelia, or the absence of fully developed limbs. These children had short limbs, with digits sprouting from hips and shoulders. He reported this finding in a letter to the English medical journal *Lancet* in December 1961, and by March 1962, as reports of birth defects accumulated, the drug was banned from most countries. In total, more than 10,000 children in 46 countries were born with deformities as a consequence of thalidomide use.

One of the first American physicians to observe the effects of thalidomide on children was the renowned Johns Hopkins pediatric cardiologist Helen Taussig (1898–1996). She had trained a German physician who informed her that many of the German thalidomide babies also had heart defects. Taussig spent six weeks in Germany talking to physicians and parents and examining the babies. She came back to the United States with photographs and case histories and spoke to the American College of Physicians and a House Committee about the connection between thalidomide and birth defects. Her accounts helped American physicians and politicians to understand the extent of the tragedy and the need to impose more regulations on the pharmaceutical industry.

In the United States, 17 children were born with thalidomide-associated deformities. The FDA never did approve thalidomide for use in the United States, and the number of affected American children would have been much higher had it not been for Kelsey's caution, experience with drug toxicity, and her ability to withstand pressure from the pharmaceutical companies.

The news of the thalidomide tragedy changed the attitude of the public toward the pharmaceutical companies, making it easier for U.S. senator Estes Kefauver of Tennessee to amend the Federal Food, Drug, and Cosmetic (FD&C) Act, despite opposition from the pharmaceutical industry and the American Medical Association. In 1962, Kefauver and U.S. representative Oren Harris of Arkansas were able to push through what came to be known as the Kefauver-Harris Amendments to the FD&C Act. These amendments authorized the FDA to demand evidence from animal testing and "adequate and well-controlled investigations" that drugs are safe and effective before their release. In addition, people who took investigational drugs would be required to sign informed consent. Before this act, patients were often not informed that they were taking investigational drugs. The drug companies would also be required to report serious postmarketing side effects to the FDA.

One unanticipated consequence of these amendments was that the new burden of proof made the process of drug development both more expensive and time-consuming because pharmaceutical research now focuses on the placebo-controlled, randomized, controlled trial. These trials are difficult and costly. Preventing another tragedy such as the thalidomide tragedy turns out to be a challenging undertaking.

Frances R. Frankenburg

URANIUM MINERS

Between 1948 and 1971, the Atomic Energy Commission agreed to buy all the uranium that could be mined in the United States, leading to a mining boom. Uranium mining was already known to be dangerous, and the United States Public Health Service monitored the environment and health of the miners. The miners were not deliberately exposed to the unsafe conditions, but they were not clearly told of or protected from these hazards until the 1960s. Without their consent or knowledge, they were experimental subjects.

During the Cold War, the United States needed a domestic supply of uranium for the manufacture of nuclear bombs. In 1948, the newly established Atomic Energy Commission (AEC) announced that it would pay a guaranteed price for uranium mined in the United States. This set off a mining boom, particularly in the Southwest, as uranium is predominantly found in Utah, Colorado, New Mexico, and Arizona. Private companies did much of the actual mining. Because much of the uranium was on or close to Navajo lands, many of the workers in the mines were Navajo.

Uranium had been mined in Europe since the 16th century, and the high rate of lung diseases among uranium miners was well known. By the 1930s, the harm was so well documented that Germany and Czechoslovakia had declared that lung cancer in uranium miners was an occupational disease that warranted compensation. The harm comes from the radon gas that is emitted as uranium-bearing rock is broken up. As radon gas decays, it leads to "radon daughters," solid particles that can attach to other airborne particles and be inhaled. The radon daughters emit alpha radiation that harms lung tissue. Both radon gas and radon daughters are invisible and odorless. It was also known that the harm could be mitigated by improving ventilation in the mines.

After exposure to radon, there is a latency period of about 10 to 20 years before its health effects can be seen. The U.S. Public Health Service (PHS), aware of the probable long-term harm, conducted a prospective observational study of the mining environment and the health of the miners from 1949 to 1960. The miners received periodic physical exams and chest X-rays until 1960.

In 1952, the PHS and Colorado Health Department distributed a report recommending that uranium mines be ventilated to lower the very high radon levels. The recommendation was repeated later in different ways and in different venues. There were some mine inspections, but mine operators took little or no action to make mining conditions safer.

In 1954, the PHS teamed up with the AEC to study the uranium miners. The AEC, interested in the risks run by researchers who were exposed to radiation, welcomed the chance to work with the PHS. The AEC provided staff, vehicles, and help getting access to the miners. In 1954, the joint team of researchers examined 1,319 miners in a more organized manner than the PHS had managed to do earlier on its own.

To maintain access to the mines and miners, the PHS promised the mine owners that they would not inform the miners of the known dangers—of which the miners were generally not aware. During these examinations, the miners were therefore not routinely nor officially told about the dangers of their work or purpose of the study. However, it is possible that some examiners did try to let the miners know of the risks, and in late 1959, a warning pamphlet was given to the miners.

Federal officials met several times with mine operators and state officials about the dangerous conditions of the mines. The states began to adopt guidelines for lowering radon levels, but there was little enforcement of these regulations until the 1960s. The AEC did not insist on ventilation, believing that the states or the mining companies were responsible for the health of the miners.

The safety concerns in this situation were similar to those regarding exposure to beryllium, another mined substance used in the nuclear industry. With respect to beryllium, the AEC insisted in 1949 that miners not be exposed to high levels of the substance. However, when later work showed that even the accepted levels were too high, the Department of Energy did not pursue the matter, unwilling to interfere with production.

In 1967, the secretary of the Department of Labor, Willard Wirtz (1912–2010), became aware of the health and safety issues in mining. Using the Public Contracts Act of 1936—which required companies supplying products to the federal government to ensure safe working conditions for their employees—the Department of Labor put mining safety regulations into place and enforced them. Finally, working conditions in the mines became safer.

Meanwhile, evidence of the harm to American miners caused by exposure to uranium was growing. In 1962, the PHS documented high rates of lung cancer, tuberculosis, and other respiratory diseases. In 1964, a tenfold excess of lung cancer was found among underground uranium miners. Later analyses showed that Navajo uranium mine workers were almost 30 times more likely to develop lung cancer than those Navajos who had not worked in the mines. Few of the Navajos smoked, and before they worked in the uranium mines, lung cancer was rare in this population.

By 1974, from a group of 3,500 miners, 144 cancer deaths had occurred, about 114 more than would have been expected. By 1990, in a group of 4,100 Colorado

Plateau miners, 410 miners had died from lung cancer. Without this exposure in mines, researchers calculated that there would have only been about 75 deaths from lung cancer.

In 1979, the Navajo miners and their survivors sued the U.S. government, claiming that safety standards had not been established early enough and that they had not been warned of known dangers. In 1984, a federal court found that the PHS had acted in a way consistent with the standards of the 1940s and 1950s. The court believed that it was reasonable not to inform the miners of the risks that they faced because this could have interfered with their willingness to work in the mines. During the case and the subsequent appeal, government lawyers testified that the government had studied the miners to establish what a safe level of exposure to radon would be.

The miners were a vulnerable population. Many were poorly educated and eager to work. The Navajos in particular had high rates of unemployment before this opportunity to work in the mines. Few spoke English, had telephones, or had any background in science or politics. They had difficulty understanding the issues around radiation or how to change the situation.

The scientific questions posed by the PHS epidemiologic study were not pressing. The risks and ill effects of uranium mining were already well-known. There was uncertainty as to the exact causes of the illnesses, but no uncertainty as to the value of ventilation in reducing this risk. The reports emerging from this natural experiment were done at the predictable expense of the health of the miners. The miners had never agreed to be research subjects and were not told clearly that risks could have been mitigated. While they were not deliberately harmed or duped by medical researchers, the medical researchers were working with people, such as the mine operators, who could have protected the miners. The researchers used the miners to prove the ill effects of uranium mining—although these effects were already known. For two decades they collected data about the deteriorating health of the miners while taking little action to protect it. Their work may have helped future miners, but at the expense of the health and, in some cases, lives of the workers of that time.

Frances R. Frankenburg

VANDERBILT UNIVERSITY NUTRITION EXPERIMENTS

In the 1940s, researchers at Vanderbilt University gave lemonade containing radioactive iron to almost 200 children between the ages of 7 and 10 to track iron absorption. They also gave radioactive iron to over 800 pregnant women to study the absorption of iron during pregnancy. These studies were not done in secret, but the children, their parents, and the pregnant women involved were not informed of the radioactive tracers used in these experiments. There is, however, little evidence of harm resulting from the studies.

In the 1940s, radioisotopes became widely available to medical researchers. Isotopes of a chemical element differ from the element only in their mass number, or the number of protons in the nucleus. This difference does not affect their chemical reactions. If the atomic nucleus of an isotope is unstable, the nucleus decays—making it radioactive. Radioisotopes of elements such as iron can serve as tracers because they emit radiation that can be detected outside the body. Because a radioactive isotope of iron is chemically identical to the nonradioactive form of the element, following radioactive iron in the body yields much information about how the body handles iron.

Beginning in 1945, researchers at Vanderbilt University in Nashville, Tennessee, started to investigate iron absorption using radiotracers. Iron is an important mineral to study because it is an essential ingredient of hemoglobin, and hemoglobin is the molecule in the red blood cell that carries oxygen. Radiation chemist Paul Hahn (1908–1963), who already had five years of experience with radiotracers, came to Vanderbilt in 1943, where he initiated studies on absorption of iron in childhood and pregnancy. He worked with William Darby (1913–2001), an expert in nutrition.

In 1945, with permission from the local school board, Hahn and Darby gave lemonade containing a heavy isotope of iron, Fe 59, also known as radioiron, to 188 Nashville schoolchildren between the ages of 7 and 10. The goal was to measure the amount of iron absorbed by growing children. They explained their study as an important investigation of nutrition, but they did not mention that they would be using radioactive iron. The permission of the parents was not obtained, nor was there follow-up of the students.

In another project, the Vanderbilt researchers were interested in iron absorption during pregnancy because of the common problem of iron-deficiency anemia. When pregnant, a woman's need for iron increases along with the volume of her blood, and she also has to supply iron so the fetus can make his or her own hemoglobin. If she does not consume enough iron (either as a supplement or in foods) or does not absorb it properly, she can develop an iron-deficiency anemia.

Between 1946 and 1949, the researchers enrolled all women attending the Vanderbilt University Hospital Prenatal Clinic who were more than three weeks away from their delivery date into the iron study. These women were all poor and white. At their first visit, they were asked to complete dietary questionnaires and submit to some blood tests. They were given B vitamins, and their urine was collected to measure their B vitamin levels. On their second prenatal visit, they were given a dose of iron tagged with Fe 59. On the third visit, a blood sample was drawn so that the percentage of absorbed iron could be studied. The blood of the baby at birth was then tested for radioactivity. The study was not explained to the women, nor were they asked for their consent, though some of them might have been told that they were being given a "vitamin cocktail." The study was funded in part by national organizations such as the United States Public Health Service and the Rockefeller Foundation. Altogether, 829 pregnant women were given radioactive iron.

At the time, Vanderbilt issued press releases about this pioneering experimental work with pregnant women and explained that the radioactive iron came from the cyclotron at Massachusetts Institute of Technology and from the nearby Oak Ridge reactor. At least two articles describing the project were published in the Nashville press, and many others were published in the medical literature. However, none of the women in the pregnancy study seem to have been aware that they were given radioiron, or indeed even know that they were subjects in a study.

Twenty years later, another Vanderbilt medical team, interested in any long-term effects of the radioactivity on the women or their fetuses, contacted these women and asked them multiple questions about their health and the health of their children. They did not explain to the women the real purpose of their questions, not wanting to alarm them. These researchers found a small, but possibly significant, increase in cancer rates. There were three cancers in the children of the study subjects and none in a comparison group. (There were actually four cancers in the study group, but the fourth cancer was thought unlikely to have been caused by the radioactive iron.) The finding was published in a medical journal but not shared with the women or children.

In 1993, following revelations about the large number of radiation experiments carried out in the United States during the Cold War period, reports about the Vanderbilt experiments appeared in the Nashville press. Litigators contacted some of the women involved in the original study. At the class-action trial that followed, experts called by both sides disagreed about the amount of radioactivity to which the women and their children had been exposed and whether there was a significant increase in cancer in the fetuses exposed to the radioiron. Vanderbilt attorneys argued that the researchers were behaving like all researchers at the time and should not be judged by standards of 40 years later. The case was settled out of court. Vanderbilt agreed to pay the women $10 million and to apologize.

Unlike some of the other studies involving radiation, these studies used the radiation as a tool and not as the subject of the study itself. Nonetheless, they are often included with the other radiation studies of the time, such as the plutonium studies.

The Vanderbilt studies increased our understanding of iron absorption. While it is impossible to determine whether they caused any harm to the subjects, it is certain that they offered no benefit to the schoolchildren, pregnant women, or their fetuses. The studies were not a secret in the medical community or even in the community at large, but the children, their parents, their school board, and the pregnant women involved were never informed that they were being exposed to radioactivity, nor of the possible risks they might have incurred through exposure.

Frances R. Frankenburg

VIPEHOLM HOSPITAL EXPERIMENT

Between 1945 and 1953, Swedish dentists investigated the relationship between dental cavities and sugar in the diet in a group of mentally ill patients at the Vipeholm hospital and found that between-meal consumption of sticky sweets was most likely to lead to cavities. None of the patients gave consent to participate in the study.

In the 1940s, dental health was poor in Sweden, as it was in much of the developed world. In 1945, the Swedish Medical Board began to investigate the cause of cavities. Dietary deficiency of some nutrients and the consumption of sugar were suspected to be at least some of the causes, but neither link was proven. In a study at the Vipeholm hospital, the country's largest facility for "uneducable retards," Swedish dental researchers supplemented the institutional diet with vitamins, fluoride, and bone meal, but dental decay did not decrease.

Then, from 1947 to 1949, the researchers fed 436 patients varying amounts and types of sugar, including sugary drinks, sweetened bread at meals, or specially prepared toffees between meals. Between 1949 and 1951, the trials were changed to test a more normal carbohydrate-rich diet. Controls were fed higher quantities of fats, such as margarine, so that their diets contained the same number of calories. The researchers examined the teeth, blood, urine, and saliva of the subjects.

The study found that subjects who were fed a higher carbohydrate diet developed more tooth decay than the controls. Sticky sweets, such as toffee and caramels, eaten throughout the day were more likely to lead to dental decay than sugar eaten with meals. Results of studies of saliva showed that children with large numbers of lactobacilli (a type of bacteria found throughout the body) in their saliva were particularly likely to develop cavities as a result of eating carbohydrates.

The study has become a classic, but it also caused much unease in Sweden as none of the patients gave consent.

Frances R. Frankenburg

WILLOWBROOK HEPATITIS EXPERIMENTS

Between 1956 and 1971, physicians gave mentally retarded children at the Willowbrook State School in New York milkshakes containing feces infected by hepatitis virus or injected them with a hepatitis-infected serum with the goal of better understanding the illness. The Willowbrook studies were one of the examples of unethical experimentation described by physician Henry Beecher in his influential 1966 article "Ethics and Clinical Research." These controversial trials also led to advances in our understanding of hepatitis and contributed to the formation of effective life-saving hepatitis vaccines. The experimenters have been both reviled and praised for their work.

Willowbrook State School was established in 1942 on Staten Island as a facility to care for disabled children in the greater metropolitan area of New York. It was converted into an army hospital for soldiers wounded in World War II and then converted back into a facility for children in 1947. Two years later, children at the facility began to become ill with infectious hepatitis. This situation set the stage for the notorious Willowbrook experiments.

Hepatitis is an inflammation of the liver and can be caused by excessive alcohol consumption, toxins, or by the body's own defenses. However, the most common cause is infection by a virus. There are several types of hepatitis viruses, each assigned a letter of the alphabet. Symptoms of all types of hepatitis include general discomfort, fever, nausea and vomiting, and general aches. In more severe cases, the person can lose his or her appetite and develop a swollen liver. If there is sufficient disruption of the functions of the liver, the blood levels of bilirubin (a yellow waste product resulting from the normal breakdown of red blood cells) can become high and lead to jaundice, a condition that causes the skin or whites of the eyes to look yellow. Hepatitis with jaundice is known as icteric hepatitis and is more serious than nonicteric hepatitis.

Children can be infected with hepatitis and be able to infect others, yet remain free of symptoms. In cases where the person seems to be well but hepatitis is suspected, it can be diagnosed by checking blood levels of liver enzymes and other markers of liver dysfunction. The illness is more serious in adults.

At the time that the Willowbrook experiments began, physicians thought that there were two types of hepatitis—infectious and serum. Infectious hepatitis, now known as hepatitis A, is generally spread by eating or drinking food contaminated by infected feces. Infectious hepatitis was common in crowded institutions such as Willowbrook and military barracks. (For this reason, the army was also interested in hepatitis research.) Serum hepatitis, now known as hepatitis B, is a more serious illness that is generally spread by contaminated needles or by sexual contact. It can become chronic and lead to cirrhosis of the liver or liver cancer.

In the overcrowded setting of Willowbrook, where many children were incontinent and hygiene was difficult to maintain, infectious hepatitis was common. Indeed, the children sometimes spread it to the adult attendants. In the early 1950s, the school asked Saul Krugman (1911–1995), a respected pediatrician and immunologist from New York University, to consult on the school's hepatitis problem. Krugman was chosen because he had worked in the army with a variety of illnesses and was also familiar with a measles vaccine developed by John Enders (1897–1985). Measles then had a fatality rate of nearly 10 percent, and Krugman was one of the first to use Enders's vaccine at Willowbrook. He used it experimentally, before it was licensed, and rid Willowbrook of this illness.

Clinical researcher Joseph Stokes Jr. (1916–1972) and others had already demonstrated the utility of injections of gamma globulin in temporarily preventing hepatitis. Gamma globulin is a concentrated solution of antibodies obtained from pooled human plasma. It provides passive immunity—the "loaning" of antibodies to a vulnerable person. While passive immunity acts quickly, it usually lasts only for a few weeks. Some of Stokes's work was done in institutions housing mentally retarded children, and some of it was supported by the Armed Forces Epidemiological Board. The optimal dosing of gamma globulin was not then known.

In 1956, Krugman began a series of experiments at Willowbrook to understand more about hepatitis. Many experiments involved the administration of different types of hepatitis virus to the children in varying strengths and by different methods, such as by mouth or by injection. Gamma globulin in different strengths was sometimes used. Hepatitis was diagnosed either by clinical symptoms, the appearance of jaundice, or abnormal bloodwork. The Willowbrook experiments also included the first prototype of a hepatitis B vaccine. The experiments lasted until 1971.

The first experiments were carried out between 1956 and 1967 to establish the optimal dose of gamma globulin. In June 1956, Krugman's group inoculated one-third of the children at Willowbrook with gamma globulin at a dose of 0.01 milliliters per pound of body weight; this decreased the incidence of new cases of icteric hepatitis by about two-and-a-half fold when compared to the uninoculated controls. In January 1957, the group inoculated one-half of those children who had just been admitted and one-half of the uninoculated children from the earlier experiment with gamma globulin at a dose of 0.06 milliliters per pound of body weight. This higher dose worked better and decreased the incidence of new cases of icteric hepatitis by tenfold. The immunity lasted for 39 weeks—longer than expected. Krugman suspected that this might have been due to the fact that the children were becoming infected with the virus at the same time that they were getting the globulin. The infection with the actual virus meant that the person's own immune cells formed a long-lasting memory of the illness, so protection against the illness also lasted for a longer time.

Stokes had suggested that concomitant injection of virus and gamma globulin could lead to so-called passive-active immunity, which would be longer-lasting than that produced by gamma globulin alone. In other words, the person would become ill and thus develop a long-lasting immunity, but not at the price of suffering the symptoms of illness, as the gamma globulin prevented the symptoms from becoming severe.

To test this way of providing immunity without causing symptomatic illness, in one set of experiments, all children newly admitted to the school were inoculated with gamma globulin and then some were deliberately fed the strain of hepatitis virus common at Willowbrook, known as Willowbrook virus, a particularly mild variant of hepatitis, in gradually increasing strengths. The virus was taken from the feces of children with icteric hepatitis. The stool was suspended in water and then centrifuged. The supernatant (the part that rose to the top) was treated with penicillin and chloramphenicol to kill any bacteria. This material had been tested for safety by first injecting it into monkeys and mice. No ill effects in the animals were noted. This was the well-known "milkshake" that was fed to some of the children.

In another set of experiments, in December 1956, newly admitted children were brought to an isolation unit. The researchers administered what was known as pooled Willowbrook serum to the children, either by mouth or intramuscular injection. Some children were also treated with gamma globulin.

Several other similar experiments were carried out. Researchers noted that children who became ill had incubation periods ranging from 39 to 71 days. Some control subjects, who were not fed the virus but housed with the others who were, also developed jaundice, presumably picking it up from the ill children. In a few cases, a child developed hepatitis twice, which was initially confusing because, in most cases, one case of hepatitis conferred immunity.

In seven trials between 1964 and 1967, Krugman and his group examined the effects of using the serum from one boy who had contracted hepatitis twice from being administered pooled serum. The serum from his first attack of hepatitis was known as MS-1, and from the second attack MS-2. The researchers injected or fed MS-1 and MS-2 serum into other children. Children infected with MS-1 virus developed hepatitis in about 30 days; those infected with MS-2 developed hepatitis in about 50 days.

Other work being done at about the same time clarified what was happening. In 1964, American physician and researcher Baruch Blumberg (1925–2011) discovered a surface antigen in the blood of an Australian aborigine, which turned out be a marker for hepatitis B. He then discovered the actual virus in 1967. (Blumberg received the 1976 Nobel Prize in Physiology or Medicine, largely for this work.) Krugman and his colleague Joan Giles had kept frozen samples of serum and, in 1969, were able to show, by testing the sera for the Australia antigen, that MS-1 was hepatitis A and that MS-2 was hepatitis B. When compared to hepatitis B, the incubation period of hepatitis A was shorter, and the ill child experienced a shorter period of elevated liver enzymes.

To the surprise of the researchers, many children at Willowbrook had both hepatitis A and hepatitis B. This explained the puzzling finding that some children had hepatitis twice. Hepatitis B infection could be transferred by intimate physical contact and exposure to body fluids: sexual contact or contaminated needles were not always required as had originally been thought. There was no cross-immunity between the two types of hepatitis virus.

In 1971, Krugman took blood from patients with hepatitis B and injected it into 25 children, 24 of whom became ill. Then he took serum infected with hepatitis B, diluted it, heated it for a minute, and injected it into other children. Then he injected these children with *untreated* infectious serum and 70 percent stayed well. The heating had destroyed the infectivity but left the Australia antigen—the molecule that involved the protective immune response—intact. This was the first hepatitis B vaccination.

In many ways, Krugman's work was a paradigm of excellent and ethical research. Hepatitis does not affect many laboratory animals and the virus could not at that time be grown in culture. It was therefore necessary to perform hepatitis research in human subjects. Krugman argued that because most children who came to Willowbrook would develop hepatitis anyway and it was usually a mild illness, he was not harming them. Moreover, he was working on a way to prevent the illness and was acting with the knowledge of others. His experiments were sponsored or approved by the New York University School of Medicine, the New York State Department of Health, the Armed Forces Epidemiological Board, the Office of the Surgeon General, the U.S. Army, and the New York State Department of Mental Hygiene.

He explained that he had used children at Willowbrook because hepatitis was so common there, not because the children were mentally retarded. He only included children who had parents who consented to these trials and did not enroll children who were wards of the state. The method of consent evolved over the years and came to include tours of the facility and group presentations with time for questions. Group presentations allowed the more thoughtful or articulate parents to pose questions that the less articulate or shy might not have asked. Parents were encouraged to review the research with their own physicians. Parents signed written consents and were told that they could withdraw their consent at any time. Although his work was unpleasant, Krugman was not the first researcher to transmit hepatitis to others by injection or by using feces.

However, there were some troubling and controversial aspects of the research. Although he did obtain consent from the parents, the letter Willowbrook sent to the parents did not make it entirely clear that the children would be deliberately infected with hepatitis—or how this would happen. The letter made it seem as though the children were being helped by the experiment, by referring to it as "prevention," and by deliberately fostering a therapeutic misperception—the idea that the experiment was for the subject's direct benefit. Indeed, the letter almost suggested that the parents would be remiss in not consenting.

Another problem was that in 1964, the facility was so crowded that Willowbrook no longer was able to accept new admissions. Exceptions were made, however, if the parents agreed to have their children admitted to an experimental wing. The researchers argued that this was not unusual: people who agree to participate in experiments are admitted to experimental units. Others argued it was coercion.

Willowbrook was later the subject of adverse publicity. In 1965, Robert Francis Kennedy, then the senator from New York, visited and described it as a "snake pit." In 1972, reporter Geraldo Rivera made it the subject of a television exposé. The children at Willowbrook were provided with no diagnosis, education, or treatment. The institution was overcrowded. Water fountains and toilets did not always work. Visitors to the wards described partially clothed or naked children—often filthy, scratched, or bruised—who were watched by a few overwhelmed, unsupervised, and untrained staff. Lawsuits were brought against Willowbrook (not because of the hepatitis experiments, but because of the generally inadequate conditions, and as part of the anti-institutional movement of the 1970s and 1980s), and the institution was closed in 1987.

An unexpected consequence of the hepatitis experiments was that the children faced additional stigma. One of the goals when Willowbrook closed was to reintegrate these children into society. But some of the children were known to be hepatitis B carriers and therefore were potentially contagious for prolonged periods of time. Parents of other children were afraid that their children would become infected by Willowbrook children and protested the reintegration.

The Willowbrook experiments have become an example of unethical research and indeed were described as such in Henry Beecher's influential 1966 article "Ethics and Clinical Research" in the *New England Journal of Medicine*. The fact that these children, already so poorly treated, were used in experiments was disturbing to many. Feeding children a virus from feces or injecting them with pooled serum to test a theory seemed grotesque. Parents may not have known exactly was being done to their children, and most of the children could not have understood their illnesses or the repeated bloodwork.

Yet, Krugman himself was a highly admired physician who was honored for his work with pediatric illnesses. In 1983, he won the Lasker Award, which is given to people who have made major contributions to medical science, and is sometimes known as the American Nobel Prize. His ingenuity, perseverance, and thoughtfulness yielded much information about hepatitis. However, his argument that most of the children would have become ill anyway with hepatitis has been debated, and, in any event, sounded disingenuous. The Willowbrook children were a vulnerable population, and their parents may have signed consent without being fully informed of the experiments and while feeling anxious about finding a place for their children to live.

Frances R. Frankenburg

DOCUMENTS

VENEREAL DISEASE EXPERIMENTATION IN GUATEMALA (1947)

Researchers sometimes take advantage of vulnerable populations, such as children, prisoners, or third-world populations. The documentation of the studies on the transmission of venereal illnesses in Guatemala illustrates this painfully well. Researcher Susan Reverby uncovered this correspondence between American scientists while investigating the Tuskegee study. Robert Coatney was a well-respected malariologist offering to help John Cutler, one of the organizers of the Guatemala study, to treat malaria in Guatemala. This seems laudable. At the same time, Coatney makes it clear that he, Thomas Parran, a highly respected venereologist, and Cutler can agree that the basic experiments that Parran and Cutler are carrying out would be disapproved of in the United States and that it is somehow amusing that they can nonetheless do these experiments on Guatemalan subjects.

17 February 1947

Dr. John C. Cutler
Caribbean Sector
Pan-American Sanitary Bureau
Apartado No. 383
Guatemala City, Guatemala

Dear Doctor Cutler:

We are sending you 500 0.3 gram (base) tablets of chloroquine (SN-7618) (aralen) and if you should need an additional supply, I shall be glad to send it along.

The Bureau of Prisons has agreed to send you some current literature, I hope it has already gone, and to put you on the mailing list for monthly publications.

I saw Doctor Parran on Friday and he wanted to know if I had had a chance to visit your project. Since the answer was yes, he asked me to tell him about it and I did so to the best of my ability. He was familiar with all the arrangements and wanted to be brought up to date on what progress had been made. As you well know, he is very much interested in the project and a merry twinkle came into his eye when he said, "You know, we couldn't do such an experiment in this country."

I really enjoyed my short stay in Guatemala and wish to say thanks to you for taking so much time toward trying to educate a malariologist. I was so taken by the chances for investigative work in that country that I find it hard to get down to work here again. As Fred Brady would say, "I'm looking over the fence."

Cordial regards to you and Mrs. Cutler.

Sincerely yours,

G. Robert Coatney

Sc. (Malariologist)

Source: Correspondence. Records of John C. Cutler, CDC, Record Group 442, Hollinger Box 1a, Folder 11. National Archives.

PARENTAL NOTIFICATION OF NUTRITION EXPERIMENTS AT THE FERNALD STATE SCHOOL (1953)

Nutrition researchers from the Massachusetts Institute of Technology, in collaboration with Quaker Oats and the Atomic Energy Commission, tagged the calcium and iron in the food of children at the Fernald State School with radioisotopes to measure the absorption of these elements. These children had a variety of problems, ranging from mental retardation to difficult-to-control behavior. Parents and guardians were asked for their permission or consent but were not given complete information about the studies. The use of radioisotopes was not mentioned. This letter is particularly troubling because the lack of response from a parent or guardian is assumed to mean consent. There is no evidence that the children were harmed by the small amount of radioactivity, but, as many have noted, the researchers did not choose to tell the children or parents about what exactly they were doing, nor did they choose the students of private schools as subjects.

Parental Authorization

The Massachusetts Task Force found two letters sent to parents describing the nutrition studies and seeking their permission. The first letter, a form letter signed by the superintendent of the school, is dated November 1949. The letter refers to a project in which children at the school will receive a special diet "rich" in various cereals, iron, and vitamins and for which "it will be necessary to make some blood tests at stated intervals, similar to those to which our patients are already accustomed, and which will cause no discomfort or change in their physical condition other than possibly improvement." The letter makes no mention of any risks or the use of a radioisotope. Parents or guardians are asked to indicate that they have no objection to their son's participation in the project by signing an enclosed form.

The second letter, dated May 1953, we quote in its entirety:

Dear Parent:

In previous years we have done some examinations in connection with the nutritional department of the Massachusetts Institute of Technology, with the purposes of helping to improve the nutrition of our children and to help them in general more efficiently than before.

For the checking up of the children, we occasionally need to take some blood samples, which are then analyzed. The blood samples are taken after one test meal which consists of a special breakfast meal containing a certain amount of calcium. We have asked for volunteers to give a sample of blood once a month for three months, and your son has agreed to volunteer because the boys who belong to the Science Club have many additional privileges. They get a quart of milk daily during that time, and are taken to a baseball game, to the beach and to some outside dinners and they enjoy it greatly.

I hope that you have no objection that your son is voluntarily participating in this study. The first study will start on Monday, June 8th, and if you have not expressed any objections we will assume that your son may participate.

Sincerely yours,

Clemens E. Benda, M.D.
[Fernald] Clinical Director

Approved:_____.

Malcom J. Farrell, M.D.
[Fernald] Superintendent

Source: *Advisory Committee on Human Radiation Experiments: Final Report* (Washington, D.C.: Government Printing Office, October 1995), 342–343.

WILLOWBROOK VACCINATION EXPERIMENT LETTER FOR PARENTAL CONSENT (1958)

Saul Krugman and colleagues developed several vaccines and did much to diminish the burden of pediatric infectious diseases. They were also criticized for what seemed like the exploitation of disabled children. In this letter, the director of Willowbrook State School in Staten Island, New York, is disingenuous in his description of the Krugman hepatitis study. The overarching goal of the study was to learn how to prevent hepatitis, but this particular experiment put the children at risk for becoming ill without clearly saying so—indeed, suggesting the opposite by implying that the parents were depriving their children of "prevention" if they did not sign. Not all the children received gamma globulin, but all were fed live hepatitis virus.

November 15, 1958

Dear Mrs. _____

We are studying the possibility of preventing epidemics of hepatitis on a new principle. Virus is introduced and gamma globulin given later to some, so that either no attack or only a mild attack of hepatitis is expected to follow. This may give the children immunity against this disease for life. We should like to give your child this new form of prevention with the hope that it will afford protection.

Permission form is enclosed for your consideration. If you wish to have your child given the benefit of this new preventive, will you so signify by signing the form.

Source: Willowbrook Review Panel Records, Special Collections & Archives, University at Albany, SUNY.

Further Reading

Allen, Arthur. 2007. *Vaccine: The Controversial Story of Medicine's Greatest Lifesaver*. New York: W. W. Norton.

Altman, Lawrence K. 1987. *Who Goes First?: The Story of Self-Experimentation in Medicine*. New York: Random House.

Annas, George J., and Michael A. Grodin. 1992. *The Nazi Doctors and the Nuremberg Code: Human Rights in Human Experimentation*. New York: Oxford University Press.

Beecher, Henry K. 1968. "Ethical Problems Created by the Hopelessly Unconscious Patient." *New England Journal of Medicine* 278 (26): 1425–1430. doi:10.1056/NEJM196806272782605.

Beecher, Henry K. 1966. "Ethics and Clinical Research." *New England Journal of Medicine* 274 (24): 1,354–1,360.

Beecher, Henry K. 1955. "The Powerful Placebo." *Journal of the American Association* 159 (17): 1,602–1,606.

Bell, Terry. 2003. *Unfinished Business: South Africa, Apartheid and Truth*. London: Verso.

Brugge, Doug, and Rob Goble. 2002. "The History of Uranium Mining and the Navajo People." *American Journal of Public Health* 92 (9) (September): 1,410–1,419. doi:10.2105/AJPH.92.9.1410.

Cameron, D. E. 1956. "Psychic Driving." *American Journal of Psychiatry* 112 (7) (January): 502–509.

Campbell, Nancy D., J. P. Olsen, and Luke Corydon Walden. 2008. *The Narcotic Farm*. New York: Abrams.

Carlton, Jim. 2001. "Of Microbes and Mock Attacks: Years Ago, the Military Sprayed Germs on U.S. Cities." *Wall Street Journal*, October 22.

Cleghorn, Robert A. 1990. "The McGill Experience of Robert A. Cleghorn, MD: Recollections of D. Ewen Cameron." *Canadian Bulletin of Medical History* 7: 53–76.

Cohen, Sidney. 1964. *The Beyond Within: The LSD Story*. New York: Atheneum.

Collins, Anne. 1988. *In the Sleep Room: The Story of the CIA Brainwashing Experiments in Canada.* Toronto, Canada: Lester & Orpen Dennys.

Creager, Angela N. H. 2013. *Life Atomic: A History of Radioisotopes in Science and Medicine.* Chicago: University of Chicago Press.

Crofton, J. 2006. "The MRC Randomized Trial of Streptomycin and Its Legacy: A View from the Clinical Front Line." *Journal of the Royal Society of Medicine* 99 (10): 531–534. doi:10.1258/jrsm.99.10.531.

Doblin, Rick. 1998. "Dr. Leary's Concord Prison Experiment: A 34-Year Follow-Up Study." *Journal of Psychoactive Drugs* 30 (4) (Fall): 419–426. doi:10.1080/02791072.1998 .10399715.

Eisenberg, Mickey S. 1997. *Life in the Balance: Emergency Medicine and the Quest to Reverse Sudden Death.* New York: Oxford University Press.

Elliott, P. J., C. J. Phillips, B. Clayton, and P. J. Lachmann. 2002. "The Risk to the United Kingdom Population of Zinc Cadmium Sulfide Dispersion by the Ministry of Defence during the 'Cold War.'" *Occupational and Environmental Medicine* 59: 13–17. doi:10.1136/oem.59.1.13.

Emanuel, Ezekiel J. 2011. *The Oxford Textbook of Clinical Research Ethics.* Oxford: Oxford University Press.

Florence, A. L. 1960. "Is Thalidomide to Blame?" *British Medical Journal* 2 (5217) (December): 1954. doi:10.1136/bmj.2.5217.1954.

Frankenburg, Frances R. 2014. *Brain-Robbers: How Alcohol, Cocaine, Nicotine, and Opiates Have Changed Human History.* Santa Barbara, CA: Praeger/ABC-CLIO.

Frankenburg, Frances R., and Ross J. Baldessarini. 2008. "Neurosyphilis, Malaria, and the Discovery of Antipsychotic Agents." *Harvard Review of Psychiatry* 16 (5): 299–307.

Gilliland, Frank D., William C. Hunt, Marla Pardilla, and Charles R. Key. 2000. "Uranium Mining and Lung Cancer among Navajo Men in New Mexico and Arizona, 1969 to 1993." *Journal of Occupational and Environmental Medicine* 42 (3) (March): 278–283. doi:10.1097/00043764-200003000-00008.

Goodman, Jordan, Anthony McElligott, and Lara Marks. 2003. *Useful Bodies: Humans in the Service of Medical Science in the Twentieth Century.* Baltimore: Johns Hopkins University Press.

Gordon, Archer S., Charles W. Frye, Lloyd Gittelson, Max S. Sadove, and Edward J. Beattie. 1958. "Mouth-to-Mouth versus Manual Artificial Respiration for Children and Adults." *Journal of the American Medical Association* 167 (3) (May): 320–328. doi:10.1001/jama .1958.72990200011008a.

Gostin, Lawrence O. 2008. "Biomedical Research Involving Prisoners." *Journal of the American Medical Association* 297 (7): 737–740.

Harken, Dwight E., Laurence B. Ellis, Paul F. Ware, and Leona R. Norman. 1948. "The Surgical Treatment of Mitral Stenosis." *New England Journal of Medicine* 239 (22): 801–809.

Harkness, Jon, Susan E. Lederer, and Daniel Wikler. 2001. "Laying Ethical Foundations for Clinical Research." *Bulletin of the World Health Organization* 79 (4): 365–372.

Hill, Austin B. 1990. "Suspended Judgment. Memories of the British Streptomycin Trial in Tuberculosis. The First Randomized Clinical Trial." *Controlled Clinical Trials* 11: 77–79.

Hornblum, Allen M. 1998. *Acres of Skin: Human Experiments at Holmesburg Prison: A Story of Abuse and Exploitation in the Name of Medical Science.* New York: Routledge.

Hornblum, Allen M. 1997. "They Were Cheap and Available: Prisoners as Research Subjects in Twentieth Century America." *British Medical Journal* 3215: 1,437–1,441.

Hornblum, Allen M., Judith L. Newman, and Gregory J. Dober. 2013. *Against Their Will: The Secret History of Medical Experimentation on Children in Cold War America*.

Johnston, Barbara Rose. 2007. *Half-Lives and Half-Truths: Confronting the Radioactive Legacies of the Cold War*. Santa Fe, NM: School for Advanced Research Press.

Jones, James H. 1981. *Bad Blood: The Tuskegee Syphilis Experiment*. New York: Free Press.

Jonsen, Albert R., Robert M. Veatch, and LeRoy Walters. 1998. *Source Book in Bioethics*. Washington, D.C.: Georgetown University Press.

Katz, Jay. 1984. *The Silent World of Doctor and Patient*. New York: Free Press.

Katz, Jay, Alexander Morgan Capron, and Eleanor Swift Glass. 1972. *Experimentation with Human Beings; The Authority of the Investigator, Subject, Professions, and State in the Human Experimentation Process*. New York: Russell Sage Foundation.

Kelsey, Frances O. *Autobiographical Reflections*. n.d. Accessed May 30, 2016. http://www .fda.gov/downloads/AboutFDA/WhatWeDo/History/OralHistories/SelectedOral HistoryTranscripts/UCM406132.pdf.

Krasse, Bo. 2001. "The Vipeholm Dental Caries Study: Recollections and Reflections 50 Years Later." *Journal of Dental Research* 80 (9): 1,785–1,788. doi:10.1177/002203450 10800090201.

Krugman, Saul. 1986. "The Willowbrook Hepatitis Studies Revisited: Ethical Aspects." *Reviews of Infectious Diseases* 8 (1): 157–162.

Land, Charles E., Andre Bouville, Iulian Apostoaei, and Steven L. Simon. 2010. "Projected Lifetime Cancer Risks from Exposure to Regional Radioactive Fallout in the Marshall Islands." *Health Physics* 99 (2) (August): 201–215.

Langer, Elinor. 1964. "Human Experimentation: Cancer Studies at Sloan-Kettering Stir Public Debate on Medical Ethics." *Science* 143 (3606) (February): 551–553. doi:10.1126 /science.143.3606.551.

Lee, Martin A., and Bruce Shlain. 1992. *Acid Dreams: The Complete Social History of LSD: The CIA, the Sixties, and Beyond*. New York: Grove Weidenfeld.

Lerner, Barron H. 2007. "Subjects or Objects? Prisoners and Human Experimentation." *New England Journal of Medicine* 356 (18): 1,806–1,807.

Marks, John. 1978. *The Search for the "Manchurian Candidate": The CIA and Mind Control: The Secret History of the Behavioral Sciences*. New York: Times Books.

Mashour, George A. 2005. "Altered States: LSD and the Anesthesia Laboratory of Henry Knowles Beecher." *Journal of Anesthsia History* 23 (3) (July): 11–14.

Masterson, Karen M. 2014. *The Malaria Project: The U.S. Government's Secret Mission to Find a Miracle Cure*. New York: New American Library.

Mcbride, W. G. 1961. "Thalidomide and Congenital Abnormalities." *The Lancet* 278 (7216) (December): 1,358. doi:10.1016/s0140-6736(61)90927-8.

McCoy, Alfred W. 2007. "Science in Dachau's Shadow: Hebb, Beecher, and the Development of CIA Psychological Torture and Modern Medical Ethics." *Journal of the History of the Behavioral Sciences* 43 (4) (Fall): 401–417. doi:10.1002/jhbs.20271.

Mitford, Jessica. 1973. *Kind and Usual Punishment: The Prison Business*. New York: Knopf (distributed by Random House).

Moore, Francis D. 1995. *A Miracle and a Privilege: Recounting a Half Century of Surgical Advance*. Washington, D.C.: Joseph Henry Press.

Moreno, Jonathan D. 2000. *Undue Risk: Secret State Experiments on Humans*. New York: W. H. Freeman.

Niedenthal, Jack. 2001. *For the Good of Mankind: A History of the People of Bikini and Their Islands*. Majuro, Marshall Islands: Bravo Publishers.

Nuland, Sherwin B. 1988. *Doctors: The Biography of Medicine*. New York: Knopf.

Offit, Paul A. 2005. *The Cutter Incident: How America's First Polio Vaccine Led to the Growing Vaccine Crisis*. New Haven: Yale University Press.

Offit, Paul A. 2007. *Vaccinated: One Man's Quest to Defeat the World's Deadliest Diseases*. Washington, D.C.: Smithsonian Books.

Oshinsky, David M. 2005. *Polio: An American Story*. Oxford: Oxford University Press.

Pappworth, M. H. 1990. "'Human Guinea Pigs'—A History." *British Medical Journal* 301: 1, 456–1,460. doi:10.1136/bmj.301.6766.1456.

Pappworth, Maurice H. 1967. *Human Guinea Pigs: Experimentation on Man*. London: Routledge and Kegan Paul.

PBS. n.d. "Operation Whitecoat." http://www.pbs.org/wgbh/americanexperience/features/general-article/weapon-operation-whitecoat.

Porter, Roy. 1997. *The Greatest Benefit to Mankind: A Medical History of Humanity*. New York: W. W. Norton.

Preminger, Beth A. 2002. "The Case of Chester M. Southam: Research Ethics and the Limits of Professional Responsibility." *Pharos* (Spring): 4–9.

Presidential Commission for the Study of Bioethical Issues. 2011. *"Ethically Impossible" STD Research in Guatemala from 1946 to 1948*. Washington, D.C.

Presidential Commission for the Study of Bioethical Issues. 2012. *A Study Guide to "Ethically Impossible" STD Research in Guatemala from 1946 to 1948*. Washington, D.C. http://bioethics.gov.

Regas-Riewerts, Jennifer L. 2011. "A Reexamination of William J. Darby's Radio Iron Tracer Studies." Master's thesis, Vanderbilt University.

Reverby, Susan, ed. 2000. *Tuskegee's Truths: Rethinking the Tuskegee Syphilis Study*. Chapel Hill: University of North Carolina Press.

Reverby, Susan M. 2012. "Ethical Failures and History Lessons." *Public Health Reviews* 34 (1): 1–18.

Rothman, David J. 1987. "Ethics and Human Experimentation: Henry Beecher Revisited." *New England Journal of Medicine* 317 (19): 1,195–1,199.

Rothman, David J., and Sheila M. Rothman. 2006. *Trust Is Not Enough: Bringing Human Rights to Medicine*. New York: New York Review Books.

Rothman, David J., and Sheila M. Rothman. 1984. *The Willowbrook Wars*. New York: Harper & Row.

Safar, Peter, ed. 1975. *Advances in Cardiopulmonary Resuscitation*. New York: Springer-Verlag.

Safar, Peter, Lourdes A. Escarraga, and James O. Elam. 1958. "A Comparison of the Mouth-to-Mouth and Mouth-to-Airway Methods of Artificial Respiration with the Chest-Pressure Arm-Lift Methods." *New England Journal of Medicine* 258 (14) (April): 671–677. doi:10.1056/NEJM195804032581401.

Schmidt, Ulf. 2006. "Cold War at Porton Down: Informed Consent in Britain's Biological and Chemical Warfare Experiments." *Cambridge Quarterly of Healthcare Ethics* 15 (4) (Fall): 366–380. doi:10.1017/S0963180106060488.

Shuster, E. 1997. "Fifty Years Later: The Significance of the Nuremberg Code." *New England Journal of Medicine* 337: 1,436–1,440.

Simon, Steven, Andre Bouville, Charles E. Land, and Harold L. Beck. 2010. "Radiation Doses and Cancer Risks in the Marshall Islands Associated with Exposure to Radioactive Fallout from Bikini and Enewetak Nuclear Weapons Tests: Summary." *Health Physics* 99 (2) (August): 105–123.

Smith, Jane S. 1990. *Patenting the Sun: Polio and the Salk Vaccine*. New York: W. Morrow.

Smith, Krista Thompson. 1996. "Adventists and Biological Warfare." *Spectrum* 25 (3): 35–50.

Starzl, Thomas E. 1992. *The Puzzle People: Memoirs of a Transplant Surgeon.* Pittsburgh: University of Pittsburgh Press.

Stephenson, Jeffrey E., and Arthur O. Anderson. 2007. "Ethical and Legal Dilemmas in Biodefense Research." In *Medical Aspects of Biological Warfare*, edited by Zygmunt F. Dembek, 559–577. Washington, D.C.: Borden Institute, Walter Reed Army Medical Center.

Stevens, Jay. 1987. *Storming Heaven: LSD and the American Dream.* New York: Atlantic Monthly Press.

Streatfeild, Dominic. 2007. *Brainwash: The Secret History of Mind Control.* New York: St. Martin's Press.

Swazey, Judith P. 1974. *Chlorpromazine in Psychiatry; A Study of Therapeutic Innovation.* Cambridge, Mass: MIT Press.

Taussig, Helen B. 1962. "A Study of the German Outbreak of Phocomelia." *Journal of the American Medical Association* 180 (13) (June): 1,106–1,114.

Thuillier, Jean. 1999. *Ten Years That Changed the Face of Mental Illness.* London: Martin Dunitz.

United States. 1977. *Project MKULTRA, the CIA's Program of Research in Behavioral Modification Joint Hearing Before the Select Committee on Intelligence and the Subcommittee on Health and Scientific Research of the Committee on Human Resources, United States Senate, Ninety-Fifth Congress, First Session, August 3, 1977.* Washington, D.C.: Government Printing Office.

United States. 1996. *Final Report of the Advisory Committee on Human Radiation Experiments.* New York: Oxford University Press.

United States. 2008. *Intelligence Activities and the Rights of Americans: 1976 U.S. Senate Report on Illegal Wiretaps and Domestic Spying by the FBI, CIA and NSA: Church Committee (US Senate Select Committee on Intelligence Activities within the United States).* St Petersburg, FL: Red and Black Publishers.

Weisgall, Jonathan M. 1994. *Operation Crossroads: The Atomic Tests at Bikini Atoll.* Annapolis, MD: Naval Institute Press.

Welsome, Eileen. 1999. *The Plutonium Files: America's Secret Medical Experiments in the Cold War.* New York, NY: Dial Press.

Yoshioka, Alan. 1998. "Use of Randomisation in the Medical Research Council's Clinical Trial of Streptomycin in Pulmonary Tuberculosis in the 1940s." *British Medical Journal* 317 (October): 1,220–1,223.

Era 6: Post–Cold War to the Present

INTRODUCTION

The experiments that took place during the Cold War era, particularly those with radiation, continued to influence medical research throughout the post–Cold War period. One notorious set of Cold War experiments, in which 18 Americans were injected with plutonium without their knowledge or consent, was first brought to widespread American attention in 1993 by journalist Eileen Welsome (b. 1951), in a series of articles in the *Albuquerque Tribune* (and later a 1999 book, *The Plutonium Files: America's Secret Medical Experiments in the Cold War*). The secretary of energy, Hazel O'Leary, mentioned the articles at a press conference, and President Bill Clinton, in response to the subsequent public pressure, chartered the Advisory Committee on Human Radiation Experiments (ACHRE). ACHRE's published report and the declassification of many government reports revealed the extent of experimentation.

Yet, the conclusions of ACHRE were, in the view of many, rather mild. The committee—with the exception of bioethicist Jay Katz (1922–2008)—did not blame the researchers, feeling that it was improper to use standards that were not applicable at the time of the actual research. They did, however, suggest that government officials and investigators should write policies to protect the rights and interests of human subjects.

Following this 1996 report, there has been ever-increasing interest in the protection of human subjects, with the regulations governing clinical trials becoming more complex and onerous. Tragedies stemming from new medications, such as sulfanilamide and thalidomide, and new therapies, such as gene therapy have added to the pressure to increase the rigor of the regulations.

As some researchers have started shifting toward the third-world for research subjects, institutions have begun to face new issues. The number of people needed for clinical trials has increased, and some argue that the practice of using people living in developing countries as subjects is similar to the practice of using prisoners and other vulnerable populations in the past. People in third-world countries may be more anxious for medical attention and less aware of the risks inherent in a clinical trial. But others argue that clinical trials offer people in poor countries much-needed medical attention and the opportunity to be treated with medications that they might otherwise not be able to afford. Short trials of AZT compared with placebo in pregnant women with HIV in poor countries highlighted these issues. (In the developed world, women were treated with longer courses of AZT, and placebo was not used.)

In 1990, the International Conference on Harmonisation of Technical Requirements for Registration of Pharmaceuticals for Human Use (ICH) began the process of coordinating regulations between different countries with respect to research. The ICH created Good Clinical Practice (GCP) guidelines to guide clinical trials involving human subjects. The FDA requires that foreign studies conducted in foreign countries follow the GCP guidelines.

Another relatively new group of subjects is the professional guinea pig—the person who makes a living out of being a subject in a clinical trial.

In a different set of human experiments, researchers worked on the Twins Study with the National Aeronautics and Space Administration (NASA) to investigate whether astronauts could survive the possible six- to eight-month trip to Mars and back. The experiment will also ultimately yield clues about human physiology and aging. It reflects the scope of experimentation on humans, using perhaps the most advanced technology available—travel to outer space and genome collection, while relying on time-honored and venerable practices—the comparison of twins. The subjects are NASA astronauts and twins Scott and Mark Kelly (b. 1964). Scott traveled to the International Space Station (ISS), circling 200 miles above the earth for a year, beginning in March 2015, while Mark stayed behind in Tucson, Arizona.

Twelve universities and the NASA biomedical laboratories collected many types of samples from the twins. One area of interest was the possibility of changes to the genome, or epigenetic changes. The basic component of the genome is deoxyribonucleic acid (DNA), the hereditary material that makes up the genes in the chromosomes. Epigenetics refers to the way that genes are expressed rather than a change in the DNA itself and is influenced by many factors in the environment. Identical twins, for example, are born with the same genome, but there is some epigenetic "drift" as they age. Nonetheless, the Kelly twins probably have as close to identical genomes as any other two adults, and that will make it easier to examine any differences between their genomes that have accrued after Scott's year on board the ISS.

Research in the post–Cold War era is becoming ever more complicated. Subjects, including people in third-world countries, who may or may not be exploited, and people who have made careers out of being research subjects are protected—perhaps—by increasingly rigorous and complex regulations. The gene is replacing the body as the subject of research in many areas. Yet, the human is still at risk, and experimental gene therapy has led to the death of one subject. Finally, research is leaving the confines of the earth as scientists are studying the epigenetic effects of space travel.

TIMELINE

1993	Eileen Welsome (b. 1951) publishes a three-part series about plutonium experiments, "The Plutonium Experiment," in the *Albuquerque Tribune*, for which she receives a Pulitzer Prize in 1994. The

series prompts the further investigation of these and related experiments.

1994   The results of the AIDS Clinical Trial Group (ACTG) 076 study demonstrate that a long course and complicated regiment of AZT lowers mother to child transmission of HIV. Researchers subsequently begin clinical trials of short-course AZT in third-world countries. Some women receive a placebo. These decisions lead to much criticism.

1994–1996   The Advisory Committee on Human Radiation Experiments (ACHRE), created by President Bill Clinton in 1994, releases its results in 1995 and publishes its report in 1996.

1995   President Clinton establishes the National Bioethics Advisory Committee in response to suggestions made by ACHRE.

1996   An epidemic of meningitis strikes the northern state of Kano in Nigeria, and a hundred children are given an experimental oral antibiotic called Trovan, while another hundred received ceftriaxone, the usual treatment. Patients and their families sue Pfizer, claiming that there was not proper consent.

1996   Hoiyan Wan, a 19-year-old student, dies after undergoing a bronchoscopy during an experiment at the University of Rochester.

1999   Welsome publishes a book, *The Plutonium Files: America's Secret Medical Experiments in the Cold War*, with more details about experimentation in the United States carried out without proper consent.

1999   Jesse Gelsinger (1981–1999), a 19-year-old student, dies after volunteering to be a subject in a gene transfer experiment at the University of Pennsylvania.

2001   Ellen Roche, a 24-year-old research assistant, dies after volunteering to be a subject in an asthma experiment at Johns Hopkins.

March 2015–March 2016   Scott Kelly (b. 1964) spends a year in space as commander of the International Space Station, while his identical twin brother, Mark, stays on earth so that the effects of space on the human body can be studied.

REFERENCE ENTRIES

ADVISORY COMMITTEE ON HUMAN RADIATION EXPERIMENTS

In 1994, President Bill Clinton established the Advisory Committee on Human Radiation Experiments to review federally funded experiments that intentionally exposed people to radiation between 1944 and 1974. Most of these experiments had been kept hidden from the public.

In 1942, the United States, with the help of Great Britain and Canada, established the Manhattan Project to build a nuclear weapon before Germany did. In the course of this effort, scientists worked with radioactive materials that were then poorly understood. Two years later, after some accidents involving the highly radioactive plutonium, J. Robert Oppenheimer (1904–1967), the scientific director of the Manhattan Project, and others decided that a program of human experimentation was necessary to better appreciate the hazards of this work. Between 1944 and 1974, physicians and scientists conducted thousands of largely secret experiments involving radiation, many funded directly or indirectly by the United States government.

People involved were rarely told that they were the subjects of experiments. In 1974, following the publicity around the Tuskegee Study of Untreated Syphilis—in which black Americans with syphilis were the unwitting subjects of a study assessing the course of untreated or undertreated syphilis—the U.S. Department of Health, Education, and Welfare issued rules for the protection of subjects of federally sponsored research. In that same year, Congress also passed the National Research Act establishing the National Commission for the Protection of Human Subjects of Biomedical and Behavioral Research. This commission, known as the National Commission, produced the influential 1979 Belmont Report, which outlined the basic ethical principles that must guide all research involving humans.

These experiments over three decades were known to some, but only came to public awareness when journalist Eileen Welsome (b. 1951) wrote a three-part series for the *Albuquerque Tribune* about 18 people injected with plutonium without their knowledge. The series, "The Plutonium Experiment," won Welsome a Pulitzer Prize in 1994. Hazel O'Leary (b. 1937), the secretary of energy, mentioned the series in a press conference. President Bill Clinton, reacting to the concerns raised by Welsome and O'Leary, established the Advisory Committee on Human Radiation Experiments (ACHRE) to review these experiments. He asked the committee to determine whether the federally funded experiments were done in accord with the standards of those times and whether the experiments were designed in an ethical or scientifically responsible way.

Ruth Faden (b. 1949), a bioethicist from Johns Hopkins University, chaired the 14-member committee, which was composed of a retired banker, two lawyers, three experts in radiation, three bioethicists, one historian, one physician with an interest in international health, one biostatistician, and one president of a medical school. During the next 18 months, they conducted over 1,900 interviews and held public meetings in Washington, D.C., Cincinnati, Knoxville, San Francisco,

Santa Fe, and Spokane. President Clinton ordered the declassification of much documentation, and the committee and its staff reconstructed and reviewed hundreds of thousands of pages of it.

The committee found that several thousand experiments concerning radiation had been carried out, but despite the declassification, very little information was available about most of these experiments: it had been either lost or destroyed. In total, they were able to review about 4,000 studies, but there may well have been more. Many of the experiments were carried out in secret out of concern for national security. The researchers disclosed few details about their work because they were also hesitant to alarm the public or put the government at risk of being sued. One exception was the radioisotope program. These experiments were described both to the public and to the medical community at large. Even here, however, there was no disclosure to the actual subjects themselves.

The committee released its report to the White House in 1995 and issued a final report in 1996. This more than 600-page book reviewed bioethics and summarized the radiation experiments, concluding with 19 findings and 39 recommendations that emphasize the following: In most of the experiments, the radioactivity probably did not harm the subjects. In particular, the experiments involving radioisotopes as radiotracers, designed to study metabolic processes in the body, were probably relatively safe. These radiotracer experiments, ACHRE concluded, had significantly advanced medical knowledge.

ACHRE concluded that much of the other experimentation had been wrong but were reluctant to assign any blame. They accepted the argument that, by criticizing the researchers, they were applying standards that were not used at the time of the actual research. They wrote, "Even where a wrong was done, it does not follow that anyone should be blamed for the wrong."[1] ACHRE did, however, note that "government officials and investigators are blameworthy for not having had policies and practices in place to protect the rights and interests of human subjects who were used in research from which the subjects could not possibly derive medical benefits. . . (but) . . . to the extent that research was thought to pose little or no risk, government officials and biomedical professionals are less blameworthy."[2] They noted the improvements that had taken place since the governmental actions of 1974.

One member of the committee, bioethicist Jay Katz (1922–2008), dissented. Katz did not think that the regulations and policies of 1974 had led to much improvement, and he argued that research continued to be carried out in ethically troubling ways. He explained that many consent forms were so long and overly detailed that they hid the essential issue: the subject was taking a risk and was not likely to be helped by participating in the study. Katz noted that many institutional review boards—institutional committees established to safeguard the safety of subjects—failed to understand the importance of consent and were often pressured by their own institutions to approve experiments. He suggested the establishment of a national board to oversee human experimentation. (This suggestion has not been acted upon.)

Following the release of the report of ACHRE, President Clinton apologized to the subjects of these experiments and to their families. His administration arranged financial compensation for many of them. At the same time the Clinton administration recognized that some human experimentation would, by necessity, continue to be classified and that there would continue to be dangers from these experiments because of the lack of outside scrutiny. Therefore, Clinton directed all federal agencies to keep all records related to classified human experiments and to ensure that all such research involves informed consent. At the suggestion of ACHRE, the National Bioethics Advisory Committee was established in 1995 to continue investigations and suggestions to do with the ethics of medical research in the United States.

Frances R. Frankenburg

References

1.   United States. *Final Report,* 123.
2.   Ibid., 503–504.

ASTHMA EXPERIMENTS AT JOHNS HOPKINS

In 2001, a healthy 24-year-old woman participated in a Johns Hopkins University asthma drug study and died a month later. During the ensuing investigation, many research studies at Hopkins were temporarily suspended, and the university increased its supervision of research.

Asthma is a chronic disease sometimes known as *reactive airway disease.* The airways, or passages, through which air moves from the nose or mouth to the lungs can constrict or expand in response to various triggers. A healthy person's airways will constrict when exposed to certain irritants, such as pollen, pollutants, or some drugs; then, after some deep breaths, the airways will relax and then expand again. But the airways of the asthmatic person tighten and will not relax again, and the person then has difficulty breathing and feels chest tightness. This complicated set of activities, controlled to at least some extent by the nervous system, has been difficult to understand.

Researchers at Johns Hopkins University, in Baltimore, Maryland, investigated airway relaxation to understand why it does not happen in asthmatics. In one study, "Mechanisms of Deep Inspiration-Induced Relaxation," funded by the National Institutes of Health (NIH), healthy volunteers inhaled various substances, including hexamethonium, a substance that blocks the actions of some neurotransmitters, or messengers, in the nervous system. Hexamethonium was used to temporarily paralyze some of the nerves in the airways as a way of exploring the role of the nervous system in causing the airways to expand after a deep breath.

Ellen Roche was a 24-year-old woman working as a technician at the Johns Hopkins Asthma and Allergy Center. She often volunteered for research studies, and in 2001, she volunteered for this study. The first subject in the study developed a mild cough for nine days following exposure to hexamethonium. The second subject suffered no symptoms. Roche, the third subject, was exposed to hexamethonium on May 2, 2001, and the next day developed a cough. It worsened, and a few days later, she was hospitalized. Her lungs became increasingly stiff, and her breathing deteriorated. She was transferred to an intensive care unit, where she died on June 2.

On July 19, the United States Office for Human Research Protections (OHRP)—established in 2000 after the death of a subject in a gene-therapy experiment—suspended nearly all of the federally funded medical research involving human subjects at Johns Hopkins University and all of the projects of the principal investigator of the study in which Roche died. The initial response from Johns Hopkins was that the suspension was "unwarranted, unnecessary, paralyzing, and precipitous."[1]

The OHRP discovered a number of problems with the Hopkins research. The principal investigator had made the determination that hexamethonium was safe by reviewing the literature that he found using three online search engines and also by consulting textbooks on pulmonary pharmacology. Older reports of the danger of inhaled hexamethonium existed, but he had not found them.

In the informed consent, hexamethonium was incorrectly referred to as a medication. Hexamethonium had been used in the past as a medication to control high blood pressure but the Food and Drug Administration (FDA) withdrew it from the market in the 1970s. Therefore, the use of hexamethonium by inhalation was experimental and had only been used in this way in 20 human subjects in earlier studies at the University of California in San Francisco.

In those earlier studies, the events were somewhat similar to those that had occurred in Baltimore, but the Johns Hopkins researchers were not aware that two San Francisco subjects had adverse reactions because these reactions had never been reported. Officials at the University of California in San Francisco said that they did not report the adverse reactions because they did not believe that the problems were caused by hexamethonium. Still, following Roche's death, they reviewed their earlier work. A researcher involved in the earlier studies noted that three of the five members of the original research team inhaled hexamethonium themselves, with no ill effects, before giving it to six subjects. One subject complained of a headache and general malaise and withdrew from the study, but researchers blamed it on another medication. Another subject went to an emergency room because of chest tightness and shortness of breath. Physicians not involved in the research diagnosed this subject with viral pneumonia, and he improved.

The principal investigator of the Hopkins study had not reported the symptoms of the first participant to the Johns Hopkins Institutional Review Board (IRB), thinking that they were related to a mild cold. The similarity to the situation in the California study is striking and, in retrospect, possibly significant. The symptoms suffered by the San Francisco subjects and the first Hopkins participant, in light of the terrible events suffered by Roche, could have been indications that inhaled hexamethonium was not safe.

Finally, many questions were raised about the Johns Hopkins IRB itself. There was a consensus that the members of the IRB at Johns Hopkins were overworked and that the processes that they had devised to cope with the work were inadequate. Sometimes only a subcommittee of the IRB reviewed a study before approving it.

The FDA also investigated Roche's death and made a series of criticisms. They noted that the researchers had not sought or received FDA approval to use hexamethonium, an unlicensed drug, in the experiment. They also noted that the principal researcher would have known that he needed FDA approval because he had sought FDA approval for a drug for a similar experiment a few years earlier and his request had been turned down. However, it was not entirely clear whose responsibility it was to obtain approval. The Johns Hopkins IRB had previously asked the FDA if they needed to be involved in the use of experimental agents that were not drugs, and the FDA had replied that the issue was complicated and was being investigated. The researcher trusted the IRB to tell him whether he needed FDA approval for hexamethonium; the IRB relied on the experience of the researcher and continued to wait for guidance from the FDA. (Another criticism of the research was that the investigators had changed the protocol somewhat during the study and had not informed the IRB. But it is doubtful that these changes had anything to do with Roche's death.)

In response to Roche's death and the criticisms from the OHRP and FDA, Johns Hopkins instituted a number of changes. The principal investigator received more training in research ethics, and his research was supervised for a period of time. The university created additional IRBs and improved IRB training for the faculty. They arranged for more extensive review of all protocols and full-group IRB reviews of all protocols. They also developed standards to improve searches into the safety of drugs and required investigators to provide more evidence for the safety of drugs in human use. The chief executive officer of Johns Hopkins Medicine talked about changing the culture of the university, emphasizing that the safety of the research subject needed to be the first priority. Investigators were required to report all adverse effects to the IRB—whether or not the effect was thought to be due to the experiment.

Frances R. Frankenburg

Reference

1.   Savulescu and Spriggs, "The Hexamethonium Asthma Study," 3.

AZT TRIALS IN THE THIRD WORLD

In several trials in third-world countries, drugs that had been shown to reduce the transmission of Acquired Immunodeficiency Syndrome (AIDS) from mother to child were compared to a placebo. Critics compared these studies to the Tuskegee Study of Untreated Syphilis, while others said that the trials were ethical.

At the end of the 20th century, there was much concern about the transmission of Human Immunodeficiency Virus/Acquired Immunodeficiency Syndrome (HIV/AIDS) from mother to unborn child. In 1994, the Pediatric AIDS Clinical Trials Group (PACTG), a group of academic medical investigators funded by the National Institutes of Health (NIH), published the results of a study known as Protocol 076, or PACTG 076. The study showed that treating pregnant women who were ill with AIDS with the antiretroviral agent azidothymidine (AZT, or zidovudine) decreased the transmission of AIDS to the child by about two-thirds—from 23 percent to 8 percent.

Treating pregnant women who had AIDS with AZT became the standard of care in the United States. The protocol involved the administration of the drug by mouth five times a day at or after 14 weeks of gestation, then as an intravenous infusion during labor, and then by mouth to the newborn for 6 weeks. The women were not allowed to breastfeed (HIV can be passed from mother to child via breast milk), and both mother and child had to be monitored carefully for toxicity. The protocol cost about $800 for mother and child.

An important question was whether a simpler, shorter, and cheaper course of therapy, given only toward the end of the pregnancy, could be as effective in reducing the transmission of AIDS, particularly in the third world, where the toll of AIDS was very high. Administration of the drug at the end of pregnancy would decrease the expense and any possible toxicity to the fetus while providing protection at the time when transmission was most likely—during delivery. In response to direction from the World Health Organization (WHO), 16 clinical trials were organized in a dozen developing countries in which other approaches (such as vitamin A or vaginal disinfection during labor) or shorter courses of AZT or other antiretroviral drugs, usually comparing active treatment to placebo, had been tried. Nine studies were conducted under the sponsorship of the National Institutes of Health (NIH) or Centers for Disease Control (CDC).

Three studies, one from Thailand and two from Africa (Côte d'Ivoire and Burkina Faso), compared an abbreviated course of AZT to placebo and showed that the shorter course reduced transmission. In the study from Thailand, the mothers did not breastfeed, and there was about a 50 percent reduction in HIV transmission compared to placebo. In the two African studies, where most women breastfed, there was about a 38 percent reduction of HIV transmission. The shorter course of AZT was not as effective as the longer course had been in earlier trials, but it was better than placebo.

The American Public Citizen's Health Research Group criticized the use of placebo in these trials. Marcia Angell, then the executive editor of the influential *New England Journal of Medicine* (NEJM), wrote that the use of placebo was not consistent with the Declaration of Helsinki that stated that control groups should receive the "best proven diagnostic and therapeutic method."[1] The critics compared the researchers with those who had run the Tuskegee Study of Untreated Syphilis, in which the U.S. Public Health Service had either not treated or inadequately treated black Americans who had syphilis.

Other researchers argued the reverse, claiming that the host countries should be allowed to approve studies that they thought ethical. Indeed, two members of the editorial board of the NEJM resigned in protest against Angell's editorial. They noted that the subjects in the AZT studies were told that some would get placebo. The directors of the NIH and CDC defended their sponsorship of the trials. They argued that they were following the principles of the 1979 Belmont Report—which outlined the basic ethical principles that must guide all research involving humans—in particular those of beneficence and justice, by attempting to find treatments that could be used by developing nations.

The host countries argued that conditions there were different. Many pregnant women were anemic, which made AZT more difficult to tolerate. Plus, the first AZT regimens used in pregnancy were too complicated to be administered in these countries. Many women lived too far from medical centers to be able to receive the necessary monitoring, and five times a day medication administration was not always practical for women coping with multiple other burdens. In addition, without the research studies, none of the pregnant women would have received any treatment. Researchers have suggested that the Helsinki standards be amended to recognize that the best therapy is not available to every potential research subject and that therefore, in some cases, providing placebo treatment is acceptable. "Best therapy" is legitimately dependent on place and circumstances. Placebo-controlled studies were required to establish the safety of AZT in countries where conditions were so different that its safety could not be assumed. The idea that American scientists should decide that researchers in the third world were not capable of designing and carrying out ethical trials reeked of imperialism.

Experiments in medicine have often been controversial, but these trials in particular led to an unusual degree of disagreement. Well-respected scientists accused each other of violating basic ethical codes. Eventually, placebo trials were stopped, but neither side conceded victory in the ethical argument.

Frances R. Frankenburg

Reference

1.   Declaration of Helsinki II, 29th World Medical Assembly, Tokyo, Japan, October 1975. In Annas and Grodin, *The Nazi Doctors*, 333–336.

CLINICAL TRIALS

Both experiments and clinical trials expose humans to imperfectly understood treatments and investigations. Clinical trials are now large, statistically complex, and closely regulated in most countries and an important part of evidence-based medicine.

Knowledge of the human body and therapeutics is advanced by many scientific activities, including both experiments and clinical trials. An experiment addresses competing models or hypotheses or tests an existing theory to verify or refute it.

With respect to medicine, an experiment tests a theory about how the body works, what causes an illness, or whether a treatment works. A clinical trial, in contrast, is usually designed to determine whether a new treatment works as well or better than another treatment or placebo. The elements of novelty and uncertainty are greater in experiments, while the goal of improving treatment is more important in a clinical trial. A clinical trial can answer specific questions raised by an earlier observation or experiment. Clinical trials should come from a position of equipoise, where the investigators do not know whether the new drug, dose, or delivery is better than the accepted one.

Many activities can be considered as either an experiment or a clinical trial. Physician James Lind's 1747 experiment with treatments for scurvy is sometimes known as the first clinical trial, in that it was designed to answer the question of which of various options was the best treatment for scurvy. It was "controlled," meaning that similar groups of men were exposed to different treatments for scurvy. Lind was not sure which of the six treatments, if any, would be effective.

Another early clinical trial was conducted by Ignaz Semmelweis (1818–1865) in the infamous First Division hospital in Vienna, a maternity hospital with a high mortality rate due to puerperal, or childbed, fever. After reviewing many cases and seeing the different death rates in different parts of the hospital, Semmelweis correctly linked the deaths to the doctors and medical students themselves, who often would examine a cadaver and then a woman in labor. Semmelweis insisted that medical students wash their hands in a solution of chloride of lime between the two activities. This handwashing decreased the transmission of beta hemolytic streptococcus and other organisms that caused the fever, and the death rate fell. Semmelweis did not entirely understand why the handwashing worked. This great trial was controversial at the time, but it is now difficult to believe that there was ever any need to test the hypothesis that cleanliness would cut down on infections.

The clinical trial matured as statistics developed. Sir Ronald Fisher (1890–1962), a Cambridge-trained mathematician who worked at an agricultural research center, emphasized the importance of randomization, the allocation of subjects to different treatments by chance. The goal is to eliminate any bias by ensuring that the treatment, not the treatment group, is the only variable that is not constant.

Clinicians often distrust statisticians, experiments, and trials, feeling that their primary duty is to the welfare of their individual patient and being reluctant to have their work assessed, evaluated, or questioned. Semmelweis, for example, was personally attacked by his colleagues for daring to suggest that they were harming their patients by not washing their hands. Austin Bradford Hill (1897–1991), a leading British medical statistician, who knew Fisher well, and conscious of clinicians' uneasiness with trials and statistics, wrote about the importance of the clinical trial, making explicit the connection with experimentation:

The physician's first duty is to his patient—to do all in his power to save the patient's life and restore him, as rapidly as possible, to health. That fundamental and ethical duty must never be overlooked—though with the introduction of better, brighter and ever more toxic drugs, and with the wide prevalence of surgical procedures such as tonsillectomy, the onlooker may perhaps with good reason sometimes ask the clinician "are you sure you know where that duty lies?" It seems to me sometimes to be unethical *not* to experiment, not to carry out a controlled clinical trial.[1]

In the 20th century, three large and important clinical trials were those involving streptomycin, the Salk vaccine against poliomyelitis, and the oral contraceptive pill. (The first two trials are described briefly here and in full detail elsewhere.)

In 1947, the British Medical Council organized the first large randomized clinical trial when it decided to test the use of streptomycin in treating tuberculosis. In this study, there was an insufficient supply of streptomycin to treat all who might benefit, but also, somewhat confusingly, an element of uncertainty as to the value of streptomycin. The organizers of the trial, including Hill, also used a new experimental design, randomized numbers, to allot treatment.

The 1954 polio trials used an unusual dual-protocol design in which there were two arms. In one arm, children participated in a double-blind placebo-controlled trial and either received Jonas Salk's (1914–1995) killed-polio vaccine or a placebo, and in the other arm, children either received the killed-polio vaccine or were "observational controls." This design was successful in that it allowed the participation of a huge number of children, which was necessary to assess the usefulness of the vaccine. Over 600,000 schoolchildren were injected with the vaccine or a placebo, and over a million other children were observed either as controls or nonparticipants. The awkward compromise was due to the need to design a trial that would be acceptable to as many people as possible. The trial ended up being "a scientific demonstration, political statement, and mass participation event."[2]

The development of the oral contraceptive is associated with scientist Gregory Pincus (1903–1967), who was fascinated by the human reproductive cycle, and gynecologist John Rock (1890–1984). To test the efficacy and side effects of the medication, they experimented on three groups of patients: infertile women, patients at a state hospital, and poor women, mostly in Puerto Rico.

Pincus had been working as a scientist in Shrewsbury, Massachusetts, giving synthetic versions of the hormone progesterone to rabbits and rats to stop ovulation. Rock used the same hormone to stop ovulation in his infertile patients for several months, hoping that the body would "rebound" after the hormone was stopped, allowing the women to conceive.

In 1954, Rock treated 50 infertile women with synthetic oral progesterone, and none ovulated. (How much his patients knew about the medication is difficult to determine.) The team also tested the oral contraceptive on 12 or 16 female and 16 male psychiatric patients at Worcester State Hospital, not far from Shrewsbury. Apparently, Pincus received permission from the patients' relatives, but little is known of what was told to the patients. The study's goal was to test the long-term effects of the drug on the reproductive system in males and females. The results were inconclusive.

It was difficult for the team to carry out large-scale trials of a contraceptive in Massachusetts where, as in many other states, there were strict anti–birth control laws. They therefore decided to move the trials to Puerto Rico, which was close enough to Boston for the researchers, yet far enough away from the mainland press and unwanted publicity. The island, a U.S. territory, was densely populated and had no anti–birth control laws; indeed, 67 birth control clinics already in place on the island dispensed birth control advice. Sterilization and abortions were common.

In April 1956, the trials with a synthetic form of progesterone, norethynodrel (Enovid) (now known as the "pill"), began in Rio Piedras, Puerto Rico. Many of the women who participated were poor, not all spoke English, and some were illiterate. They were told that they would be taking a drug that would prevent pregnancy, but they were not told that this was a clinical trial, nor that the pill was still somewhat experimental, nor that there was a chance of potentially dangerous side effects. In one of the trials, 100 women were given the pill, and another 125 women who were not given the pill were told that they were taking part in a survey of family size. Then, more women were recruited from rural parts of Puerto Rico and Haiti. Altogether, 20,000 women participated.

Edris Rice-Wray, a faculty member of the Puerto Rico Medical School and medical director of the Puerto Rico Family Planning Association, was in charge of the trials. She found that the pill was 100 percent effective when taken properly, but that side effects were common: 17 percent of the women complained of nausea, dizziness, headaches, stomach pain, and vomiting. Three women died while participating in the trials. No investigation was conducted to see if the pill had caused the young women's deaths. (The early formulation of the pill contained 10 milligrams of norethynodrel; later formulations had lower doses of the synthetic progesterone and contained estrogen to make the pill safer and more tolerable.)

Rock and Pincus believed many of the complaints were psychosomatic and, in any event, minor compared to the contraceptive benefits of the drug. In 1955, physician Henry Beecher (1904–1976) had written an influential review about "placebo reactors" and suggested that clinical trials include a placebo-treated arm to account for the presence of "placebo reactors." Beecher also described "noxious" responses to placebo in which people described adverse events such as nausea and dizziness, even though they were not given an active drug. To differentiate the placebo reactions from the "real" ones, Pincus designed a study. He gave one group of women Enovid with a description of side effects, one group Enovid with no description of side effects, and one group placebo with a warning about side effects. The rate of unpleasant side effects was similar in the groups given the warnings—whether or not they were on the active drug. Confident in the safety of the pill, Pincus and Rock did not assess the side effects further.

After the trials in Puerto Rico and Haiti, the drug was approved in the United States in 1957 as a medication to treat menstrual side effects. In 1960, it was approved as a female oral contraceptive. The team developing the oral contraceptive compared themselves to the National Foundation for Infantile Paralysis, the organization that had done such a masterful job in the Salk vaccine trials. But the trials were quite different. One of the strengths of the polio trial was the inclusion of ordinary American schoolchildren. Vulnerable children, although they had been used in earlier trials of the vaccine when the safety was not so certain, were not preferentially selected in the famous 1954 trial. There was a great deal of publicity and openness about the polio vaccine trial, and the schoolchildren were given pins and certificates and praised for being "polio pioneers." In comparison, there was less publicity about the oral contraceptive trials, and Rock and Pincus have been accused, correctly or not, of using vulnerable subjects and of exploiting the women. The introduction of the oral contraceptive pill, strongly opposed by the Catholic Church, allowed women to be sexually active without having children and was more complicated with far-reaching sociocultural implications than the introduction of the polio vaccine.

The polio vaccine trial, now a milestone in trials, was nonetheless criticized at the time for putting people at risk from an insufficiently tested substance. Salk's vaccine turned out to be safe, but other substances were indeed introduced prematurely.

One example had to do with the antibiotic sulfanilamide. In 1937, the drug company Massengill discovered that sulfanilamide could be dissolved in diethylene glycol, resulting in a liquid that was easy to swallow and had a pleasant appearance and taste. The company sent shipments throughout the country, unaware that the diethylene glycol was toxic. This new preparation of the antibiotic led to the deaths of more than a hundred people in 15 states. The public outrage at this led, in part, to the passage of the 1938 Food, Drug, and Cosmetic Act (FD&C), which increased the authority of the Food and Drug Administration (FDA) to regulate drugs.

In one of the most well-known and tragic cases of a hasty drug introduction, the drug thalidomide was marketed in the late 1950s as a sleeping pill, safe even in pregnancy. As is well-known, it caused birth defects in the children of women who took the drug while pregnant, even though the effects in the women themselves were minor. As a consequence, the American public demanded more testing before drugs can be issued to the public. In 1962, the Kefauver-Harris Amendments to the FD&C were passed, authorizing the FDA to request pharmaceutical companies to provide evidence from animal testing and clinical trials that drugs were safe and effective. One result was that new drugs had to be given to a large number of subjects before they could be marketed. Toward the end of the 20th century, there was also increasing concern about varying requirements for clinical trials in different countries, and the possible exploitation of subjects in developing countries.

In 1990, the International Conference on Harmonisation of Technical Requirements for Registration of Pharmaceuticals for Human Use (ICH) was created to coordinate the work of the regulatory authorities and pharmaceutical industry in Japan, the European Union, and the United States. The purpose was to eliminate the duplication of testing by "harmonizing" work done in different countries, while maintaining strict guidelines to protect the health of the public.

The ICH created Good Clinical Practice (GCP) Guidelines, one of which was the protection of subjects. The ICH issued 13 principles, the third of which states that the rights, safety, and well-being of the trial subject are more important than the general interests of science and society. Another goal is the achievement of scientific rigor of these studies.

Clinical trials in many countries are now conducted in a number of phases, each designed to answer a question about the new drug. In Phase 0, which is not always carried out, a small number of people are briefly exposed to a low dose of the drug to examine how the drug is handled by the human body. In Phase 1, researchers test the drug or treatment in 20 to 80 healthy people to evaluate its safety, dosage range, and side effects. This is, in a way, the most experimental part of the trial because, until this point, the drug has usually only been used in animals. Occasionally, Phase 1 subjects will have the illness that is of interest. In Phase 2, to test the drug's safety and effectiveness, the drug is given to 100 to 300 patients who have the disease or condition that the drug is supposed to treat. In Phase 3, the drug is given to 1,000 to 3,000 people while comparing its effectiveness to other drugs. And in Phase 4, information, particularly to do with side effects, is gathered about the drug after it has been marketed.

In the United States, the National Institutes of Health requires that clinical trials be monitored in a way appropriate to the risks involved in the study. For most Phase 3 trials, research centers are required to form a Data and Safety Monitoring Board (DSMB) composed of experts knowledgeable in the area, including at least one statistician. None of the members of DSMB should be directly involved in the study. The DSMB regularly assesses the trial and offers recommendations concerning its continuation.

Despite these advances and precautions, problems remain. Researchers complain about the burden of paperwork required by regulations and what they see as the stultifying effect of regulation on innovation. As a result, some pharmaceutical companies carry out clinical trials in countries where regulation is less intense or, from a different point of view, less intrusive. The FDA does require that foreign studies be conducted in accordance with GCP guidelines.

Clinical trials, when conducted rigorously, are an important part of evidence-based medicine (EBM). David Sackett (1934–2015), who has been described as the father of evidence-based medicine, said that EBM is the "conscientious, explicit, and judicious use of current best evidence in making decisions about the care of individual patients."[3]

One of the most important contributors to EBM was Archibald Cochrane (1909–1988). Cochrane conducted a clinical trial, an experiment of sorts, while a physician and prisoner of war in Salonika, in Greece, in 1941. An epidemic of lower leg edema (swollen legs) developed among the prisoners. Cochrane thought that the edema might be due to wet beriberi, an illness caused by a thiamine deficiency. He chose 20 young men with edema and divided them into two groups. He gave one group yeast, which is rich in thiamine, and one group vitamin C. While Cochrane was carrying out this experiment, he himself was jaundiced, malnourished, and starving. The men treated with yeast got better, and Cochrane used this to convince the German prison administrators to give all of the prisoners yeast. The health of the prisoners improved.

Cochrane described the experiment as his "first, worst, and most successful trial."[4] He later decided that he had not done the study rigorously and that the edema was not beriberi. He thought that the general protein content of the yeast (not the thiamine) was what improved the health of the prisoners. His original concern about beriberi was not however unreasonable. Beriberi did occur in prisoner-of-war camps. Indeed, R. C. Burgess, a physician and prisoner of war at the infamous Changi prison in Singapore, described beriberi in the prisoners and did what he could to increase the thiamine content of the food.

After the war, Cochrane studied with Hill and became further convinced of the necessity of clinical investigations. He lamented the unscientific state of medicine in which practitioners followed authorities or their own instincts rather than being guided by the evidence and became a staunch advocate of randomized control trials.

Inspired by his work, obstetrician Iain Chalmers (b. 1943) established the Cochrane Collaborative in 1993 to present to clinicians the results of studies examining interventions in illnesses, with randomized control trials being considered the highest level of evidence. Chalmers has also established a library documenting trials and treatments in medicine and named it after James Lind (1716–1794), who performed one of the earliest controlled trials to discover the cure for scurvy.

Frances R. Frankenburg

References
1. Hill, "The Clinical Trial," 113.
2. Meldrum, "'A Calculated Risk,'" 1,235.
3. Sackett, "Evidence Based Medicine," 71.
4. Cochrane, "Sickness in Salonica," 1,726.

COMMISSIONS TO REVIEW ETHICAL ISSUES IN RESEARCH

Since the 1990s, the federal government has set up several advisory bodies to review ethical issues in research. The best known are the National Bioethics Advisory Commission (NBAC) and the Presidential Commission for the Study of Bioethical Issues (also known as the Bioethics Commission).

Human experimentation has become increasingly complex because of new discoveries allowing manipulation of the genome, ongoing questions about consent, and revelations of misdeeds from the past. In response to these issues, advisory panels that include bioethicists, physicians, lawyers, and other experts are established from time to time to give advice to the government about what actions might need to be taken to redress any problematic areas.

In 1995, the National Bioethics Advisory Commission (NBAC) was established at the suggestion of the Advisory Committee on Human Radiation

Experiments—which itself was set up after revelations that American citizens were exposed to radiation without their knowledge or consent—to review bioethical issues regarding research on humans. Eighteen members were appointed in 1996. During the commission's five-year life, it submitted six reports to the White House that contained 120 recommendations concerning ethical questions, including the cloning of human beings, research involving persons who might not have the ability to give informed consent, stem cell research, clinical trials in developing countries, and protection of human research participants. Agencies responsible for much of the federally funded research involving human participants, particularly the National Institutes of Health, have adopted several of NBAC's recommendations and issued research guidelines based on those recommendations.

The Presidential Commission for the Study of Bioethical Issues (known as the Bioethics Commission), an advisory panel of American experts in medicine, science, ethics, religion, law, and engineering, was established in 2009. The Bioethics Commission was asked to give advice to the administration on questions relevant to ethical problems arising from human experimentation and research. The commission has issued a number of reports, one of which reviewed the medical experimentation with sexually transmitted diseases (STDs) in Guatemala: *"Ethically Impossible" STD Research in Guatemala from 1946 to 1948.*

Frances R. Frankenburg

COMMON RULE

Beginning in the 1960s, many American agencies issued regulations with respect to ensuring safe medical experiments involving humans. In 1991, to bring some uniformity to the field, the federal government issued the "Common Rule," which has become the primary mechanism for protecting human subjects. It has been adopted by most federal agencies that sponsor research.

The foundation for the United States government's approach toward ensuring the safety of subjects of medical experimentation is the Belmont Report and its three principles of respect for the person, beneficence, and justice. These principles have led to a plethora of recommendations and regulations from different agencies. In 1981, the Department of Health and Human Services (DHHS) and Food and Drug Administration revised their existing regulations for human subjects and made them as consistent as possible. The DHHS regulations were revised several times. The June 18, 1991, revision (codified as Title 45, Part 46 of the Code of Federal Regulations) involved the adoption of the Federal Policy for the Protection of Human Subjects. The Federal Policy, or "Common Rule," as it is often called, was adopted by the 16 federal agencies that conduct, support, or otherwise regulate research involving human subjects. The Department of Veterans Affairs adopted this same rule as 38 CFR Part 16. Today, the 1991 federal policy is shared by 17 departments and agencies, representing most, but not all, of the federal bodies sponsoring this kind of research.

The Federal Policy for the Protection of Human Subjects has four subparts. Subpart A is the section known as the "Common Rule," and its main elements include requirements for assuring compliance by research institutions; researchers obtaining and documenting informed consent; and institutional review board (IRB) membership, function, operations, review of research, and record keeping. Subpart B offers additional protections for pregnant women, human fetuses, and neonates. Subpart C provides additional protections for prisoners. And Subpart D has additional protections for children. Not all agencies have adopted these subparts.

Frances R. Frankenburg

GELSINGER, JESSE

Jesse Gelsinger (1981–1999) had a mild form of a rare but serious genetic illness. In 1999, he agreed to an experimental gene transfer at the University of Pennsylvania and died four days after the experiment. His death led to much adverse publicity about research in gene therapy and calls for increased research regulations.

Ornithine transcarbamylase deficiency (OTCD) is a rare genetic illness caused by a deficient gene carried on the X chromosome. The normal gene codes for an enzyme, ornithine transcarbamylase, which breaks down ammonia, a metabolic waste product and itself a breakdown product of protein. Females, who carry two X chromosomes, can have one normal gene and one abnormal gene and be only mildly ill, as they will produce a sufficient amount of the ornithine transcarbamylase. Because males carry only one X chromosome, when they have the deficient gene, they have no counterbalancing normal gene and become very ill. In most cases, the person with OTCD dies soon after birth as a result of high ammonia levels in the brain. The disease could theoretically be treated if the "correct" gene, and thus the correct enzyme, could somehow be inserted into the person's liver, where metabolism of ammonia takes place.

At the University of Pennsylvania (Penn), researchers at the Institute for Human Gene Therapy (IHGT) were experimenting with exactly that process, known as gene therapy. Penn researchers at Children's Hospital of Philadelphia interested in OTCD and the researchers at IHGT devised a new way of treating the illness. The first step was to infect a common virus with the correct gene for the enzyme ornithine transcarbamylase. The researchers used the adenovirus, a virus that causes mild infections such as the common cold, as a "vector" for the gene. The goal was to introduce the virus with the gene into the person with OTCD in the hope that the gene would be inserted into the liver cells of the ill person.

The IHGT research team at Penn performed experiments on mice, monkeys, and baboons to test the efficacy and safety of the procedure. They discussed trying to transfer the correct gene to babies with OTCD. Arthur Caplan, Penn's resident bioethicist and consultant to the IHGT, said that experimentation on ill babies would be unethical because desperate parents, faced with a dying child, could not make a voluntary or informed decision about whether to allow their infant to participate in the study. Instead, Caplan proposed, it would be more ethical to conduct the experiment on healthy adults with mild forms of OTCD.

This experiment was approved by the Penn institutional review board (IRB) and funded by the National Institutes of Health (NIH). Before it was carried out, the experiment was also reviewed by a federal committee, the Recombinant DNA Advisory Committee, which, after some hesitation, approved the study. The Food and Drug Administration (FDA) also reviewed and approved the experiment.

The experiments started as a form of Phase 1 dose escalation clinical trials. At this stage, a new treatment is tried on a small number of healthy adults. Although Phase 1 clinical trials are not primarily designed to test how well a new treatment works, investigational treatments in this phase are sometimes used on ill people. In this case, the experiment was first tried on 17 adults, all with mild forms of OTCD. There were three groups, and each group received a higher "dose" of the vector than the previous group. The 2nd subject in the highest dose cohort and the 18th subject was Jesse Gelsinger.

Gelsinger had a mild case of OTCD. He was a "mosaic" in that some of his cells produced the correct enzyme and some did not. By following a very low-protein diet and taking medication, he remained well for the most part. At the age of 17, he volunteered for the gene-therapy experiment, wanting to help newborns afflicted with OTCD, but he was not old enough to participate. When he turned 18, and thus was old enough to participate, he and his father went to Penn to meet the research team. A member reviewed the protocol and consent form with Gelsinger and his father. Gelsinger signed an 11-page informed consent document. The consent stated that other subjects had been injected with the adenovirus without serious complications. The consent form did mention the possibility of death and also stated that Gelsinger would be informed of any adverse effects suffered by other subjects. Penn did some laboratory tests, and several weeks later, Gelsinger was approved as a participant in the study.

The adenovirus carrying the gene was injected into his liver on September 13, 1999. Within a few hours, he became sick to his stomach and developed a fever. His ammonia levels increased. He became increasingly ill and was put on a ventilator. He became comatose. His family removed him from life support, and on September 17, 1999, four days after the injection, at the age of 18, Gelsinger died.

In the investigation that followed, several facts emerged. First, experimental animals had become ill and two monkeys had died after receiving the virus. This information about the deaths of the monkeys appeared on the consent form submitted to the NIH review board, but it did not appear on the form Gelsinger signed. The monkeys had died from a blood-clotting disorder and severe liver inflammation. Gelsinger did not have exactly the same symptoms. The monkeys had received "first generation" vector; Gelsinger received a "third generation" vector. The doses of vector were much higher in the monkeys. It is not clear if the deaths of the monkeys were related to Gelsinger's death, or, if he had known about them, that he would not have agreed to participate.

Second, some of the earlier research subjects had become mildly ill after the injections. This information was not given to Gelsinger, and, again, it is not clear how much it would have influenced his decision to join the trial.

Third, the lead scientist and Penn had a financial interest in the development of the adenovirus vector being used in the OTC gene-therapy trial. Although he had not been involved directly in the trial, the lead scientist was in a position to make a great deal of money if the therapy was successful because he could patent the way of delivering the gene. Penn was aware of his conflict of interest, had reviewed it extensively, and ensured that the lead scientist had no personal involvement with the selection of Gelsinger or the actual trial. This information about the conflict of interest was in the informed consent that Gelsinger had signed. However, the extent of the connection with both the scientist and Penn came as a surprise to Gelsinger's family.

Fourth, Gelsinger had mildly elevated ammonia levels at the time of injection of the adenovirus. The protocol was not entirely clear about whether this elevation was high enough to exclude him from the trial.

Fifth, this was a Phase 1 trial. The purpose of the trial was to test the safety of the injection of the vector at increasing doses when administered to healthy subjects, with no expectation of benefit to Gelsinger. This was stated clearly in the consent form. However, one of the investigators had told Gelsinger (incorrectly) that another subject, also with mild OTCD, had benefited from the injection. This information might have contributed to a "therapeutic misperception"—that is, Gelsinger could have thought that he would benefit, at least temporarily, from the treatment.

Sixth, the research team had originally planned to inject the adenovirus into the subjects' veins. After much discussion with the FDA, they decided to inject it directly into the liver, the target organ, to minimize the risks of exposing the adenovirus to the rest of the body. The team did not inform the Recombinant DNA Advisory Committee of this change. Again, whether this change had anything to do with Gelsinger's death is not known. The cause of Gelsinger's death remains unclear, although it is assumed to be due to an immune reaction to the adenovirus.

The ensuing lawsuits and publicity highlighted the importance of scrupulously accurate paperwork and clear protocols, but many issues remain unresolved. Financial conflicts of interest were discussed at length, but perhaps at the risk of underestimating other forces driving research. The wish to achieve fame, or to be "the first," or to help people can also lead researchers to take shortcuts or make mistakes. In addition, the lead scientist and other people working on the project may have been overworked.

These problems were not unique to this case. Gelsinger's death led to a review of other gene-transfer experiments and revealed the failure of many other groups to report adverse events.

All of these revelations did lead to some changes. Congress moved the Office for Protection from Research Risks from NIH to the Department of Health and Human Services, renaming it the Office for Human Research Protections. Many new regulations were introduced, involving closer oversight of experiments and more education for all involved.

Frances R. Frankenburg

INFORMED CONSENT

Carried away by ambition or other considerations, researchers can lose sight of the importance of obtaining the agreement of a subject to participate in an experiment. While the details of consent are complicated, and become more so as medicine advances, it remains the case that all subjects of medical research should give informed consent.

The decision to participate in a medical experiment should be left to the individual, and that person should understand both the details of the experiment and its risks and benefits. This basic principle of informed consent in clinical research has often been ignored. The egregious cases, of course, are those experiments done in concentration camps by the Nazi physicians and the somewhat lesser-known Japanese Unit 731 during the 1930s and 1940s, but medical history is replete with other examples. Prisoners, indigenous people, children, and ill people have often been subjected to experiments without their consent.

The conflict between physician and patient or researcher and subject is not new. In the past, even when researchers knew little more about their area of research than their subjects, they did not always think that they should disclose the details of a medical experiment to the subject, let alone get that person's consent. Lack of knowledge did not confer humility on the experimenter or make him consider his subject as his equal. Nonetheless, on rare occasions in the past, some researchers understood that they should ask the subject to agree to the experiment before proceeding. Often, however, nonscientists, particularly lawyers, understood this principle of consent better than the physicians.

Some form of consent may have been obtained as early as 1666, as English physicians were trying to compete with their French colleagues in inventing new medical procedures. In one example, doctors in England explained the concept of blood transfusion to a man named Arthur Coga, an eccentric but educated person. Coga agreed to the experiment and received a transfusion of lamb's blood. This is an example of physicians seeming to understand that the subject of an experiment should give consent. But, at the same time, Coga was also described as having some mental instability, and he was also paid for his participation, so it is not clear that he gave voluntary and informed consent or—in modern terms—that he necessarily had the capacity to give informed consent or that it was not coerced.

In another later instance, the court was more attentive than the physicians to the importance of consent. In 1767, an Englishman broke his leg. A surgeon set the leg, but nine weeks later, the leg was crooked. Two doctors decided to break the patient's leg and reset it. In so doing, they used a new instrument. The patient sued, claiming that the second surgery had only taken place to allow the physicians to practice with the new instrument and that he had not agreed to the procedure. The patient thought that he was the subject of an experiment and objected. The court found the doctors guilty of acting without the patient's consent.

As the gap in knowledge between physicians and their patients grew, physicians became increasingly comfortable acting without explaining themselves to their patients. In the late 19th century, doctors often practiced a "benevolent" deception and told their patients little that might upset them. This disinclination to inform others was also common among medical researchers, and concerns began to be raised. Charles Francis Withington (1852–1897), an American physician at Boston City Hospital, was concerned about the rapidly increasing number of experiments on humans. In 1886, he wrote in a pamphlet, "The Relation of Hospitals to Medical Education," that there should be a "Bill of Rights" to "secure patients against any injustice from the votaries of science" because researchers "had no right to make any man the unwilling victim of such an experiment."[1]

At the beginning of the 20th century, the importance of informed consent began to be recognized by researchers and governments and perhaps first, and most surprisingly, in Germany. In 1900, the Prussian minister of religious, educational, and medical affairs prohibited medical interventions other than for therapeutic purposes without informing the subject of potential adverse consequences and obtaining consent. The experiment had to be clearly explained in writing, and the medical director of the institution had to take responsibility for the experiment.

One of the great achievements of the Yellow Fever Commission established by George Sternberg (1838–1915) and headed by Walter Reed (1851–1902) at the beginning of the 20th century was the researchers' realization that they could not expose people to yellow fever without their permission. They might have been helped by being aware of the uproar caused by Giuseppe Sanarelli (1864–1940), an Italian physician who infected several people with a bacterial toxin, a suspected cause of yellow fever, without their consent. Subjects in Reed's Cuban yellow fever experiments signed papers, written in English or Spanish (depending on their nationality), in which they agreed to the experiments. (They were paid for their participation—more so if they developed the illness.) These agreements are one of the first examples of signed consent.

Written informed consent also took place in the Philippines in the early 20th century. In 1906, Richard Pearson Strong (1872–1948) experimented with cholera while working at Bilibid Prison in the Philippines. Some prisoners died, and Strong was criticized for not having obtained their consent. Having learned a difficult lesson, in his later experiments with beriberi, also at Bilibid, he obtained written consent. Around the same time at Bilibid, Ernest Linwood Walker (1870–1952) and Andrew Sellards (1884–1941) were investigating amoebic dysentery. After obtaining written consent from the prisoners, they fed them amoebic organisms. The researchers in both cases used the native dialect in their consent forms.

Justice Benjamin Cardozo (1870–1938) of the New York Court of Appeals issued a legal opinion in 1914 that has often been cited as the foundation for the right to self-determination for medical procedures of all types. This came about in response to an operation, rather than an experiment. A woman had agreed to have an abdominal examination under anesthesia. During the examination, the surgeon found and then removed a tumor. The woman sued, not having agreed beforehand to any actual operation, and Cardozo ruled in her favor, stating, "Every human being of adult years and sound mind has a right to determine what shall be done with his own body."[2] This has become an oft-quoted statement in discussions of informed consent.

In 1931, in Germany, the Reich Regulation Concerning New Therapy and Human Experimentation expanded upon the earlier Prussian directive. The new regulation stated that "innovative therapy may be carried out only after the subject or his legal representative has unambiguously consented to the procedure in the light of relevant information provided in advance."[3] Once again, a written report was required, and the final responsibility for the experiment rested with the medical director of the institution.

Despite the examples of recognition for the need for consent from the subject from Cuba, the Philippines, Germany, and Justice Cardozo, during the 1930s to 1950s, many vaccine trials were carried out on American children in institutions with little concern for informed consent. Consent was usually obtained in a perfunctory manner from the head of the institution or, on occasion, from the parents.

In 1936, the Scientific Medical Council of the Peoples Commissariat of Health Care in Russia established rules regarding the development of new drugs and procedures with human research subjects, addressing issues of risk, harm, consent and assent, and prior animal studies. These rules were not widely known outside of Russia.

In December 1946, the Judicial Council of the American Medical Association (AMA) wrote that before humans could be experimented on, (1) researchers first had to try the experiment on animals, (2) the subject of medical experimentation should give consent, and (3) there must be proper medical protection and management.

Some of the worst examples of experimentation without informed consent happened in the 1930s and 1940s in Germany and Japan. In response to the sadistic experiments of the Nazi physicians, American physicians and jurists wrote the Nuremberg Code in 1947, the first principle of which states that the subject has to understand the experiment and willingly consent.

One of the first groups of scientists to describe the importance of informed consent was the Atomic Energy Commission (AEC). In January 1947, the AEC took over responsibility for medical research involving radiation and radioisotopes, which formerly had been carried out by the Manhattan Project. The AEC, aware of the events in Nuremberg and the public nervousness about radiation, issued strict rules limiting the use of human subjects. In April 1947, Carroll Wilson, general manager of the AEC, became concerned about the ethics of experimenting on people without their permission and the possible harm such experiments might cause. To express his concern, he wrote a letter to the head of the Interim Medical Advisory Committee, indicating that there must be a possibility that a patient participating in an experiment could be helped and that two doctors had to document that the patient understood the experiment and agreed to participate. In November 1947, Wilson repeated and elaborated on these themes in a second letter, noting that the consent should be in writing, and could be revoked. He used the term "informed consent," perhaps for the first time. These letters were not widely read.

Meanwhile, the AEC found itself in an embarrassing situation because it had, in a sense, "inherited" the plutonium injection experiments that had started in April 1945 and were not to end until July 1947. In these experiments, the patients were not informed that they were being exposed to the radioactive material or that the experiments were of no benefit to them. The AEC decided not to allow any papers to be published about these injections, fearing lawsuits.

Another American document addressing informed consent was issued a few years later, but its influence was likely blunted by its classified status. In 1953, Charles Wilson, the secretary of defense, issued a memorandum known as the Wilson Memorandum. Wilson wrote that subjects of research that involved atomic, biological, or chemical warfare had to sign consent, the signature had to be witnessed, and the research had to be approved of by the secretary of defense. Prisoners of war could not be used. Because this memorandum was kept secret—as was the case with Wilson's earlier letters—these documents, along with the AMA report, were either not known about, not taken seriously, or ignored.

Change came slowly. In 1962, the thalidomide tragedy struck and had a major impact on public opinion. Across the world, women who had taken the sedative drug during pregnancy gave birth to babies with musculoskeletal deformities. The ensuing outrage made it easier for Congress to pass the Kefauver-Harris amendments to the Food, Drug, and Cosmetic Act, which mandated that subjects who took investigational drugs had to sign informed consent.

Concerned physicians on both sides of the Atlantic began calling attention to what they saw as abuses and harms caused by ethically questionable medical experiments. In England, Maurice Pappworth (1910–1994) wrote *Human Guinea Pigs: Experimentation on Man* in 1962 about experiments carried out by English and American physicians in which consent was either not obtained or was obtained in an incomplete way. In a supplement to his book, Pappworth noted that physicians had explained to him that they would get consent for cardiac or liver catheterizations by telling the patients that they would insert a tube or catheter into a leg or arm blood vessel, without telling them that the catheter would go into the heart or liver. He also noted the importance of documenting the informed consent:

> The vast majority of published accounts of experiments on patients, including most of the reports quoted in this book, do not mention whether or not consent has been asked or obtained. . . . This ambiguity may cause injustice to experimenters who have obtained genuine valid consent. The fault lies with the writers themselves and the editors of medical articles, who should always not only state but give unequivocal evidence of having obtained genuine and legally valid consent.[4]

In 1966, in the United States, Henry Beecher (1904–1976) published an influential study, "Ethics and Clinical Research," in which he described 22 examples of unethical studies. This study made many aware that physicians were carrying out procedures without telling the subjects what they were doing. Beecher, however, did not come to the conclusion that others did. He wrote about how difficult it was to obtain informed consent, although the researcher should always strive to do so. He thought it unlikely that lay people could understand medical experiments, and he emphasized, instead, the responsibility of the physicians to behave ethically.

An example of an experiment without informed consent was the British Medical Research Council's post–World War II trial of streptomycin for the treatment of tuberculosis. None of the patients knew that they were in a trial, and no consent was obtained. Sir Austin Bradford Hill (1897–1991), one of the lead researchers in that trial, saw no need for informed consent, thinking that the patients had no need to know any of the details of the medical procedures. He, like Beecher, believed that it was incumbent on the physicians to take responsibility and that regulations could not substitute for a physician's moral sense.

In the mid- to late 20th and early 21st centuries, as more information about the sometimes irresponsible behavior of researchers and physicians emerged, and perhaps as respect for authority became tempered, many people came to think that the physician should discuss the details of treatments or procedures with patients and that, in a similar way, the experimenter should fully disclose all the relevant information to the research subject so that the subject could come to his or her own decision. (Physicians and those who perform experiments still sometimes find this concept difficult to put into practice.)

In 1974, Congress passed the National Research Act, which required that research projects funded by the Department of Health, Education, and Welfare (DHEW) have committees known as institutional review boards (IRBs) to ensure, among other issues, that all subjects provide adequate informed consent before the research can receive DHEW funding. In 1978, this requirement was extended to all institutions receiving federal funding.

The Department of Health and Human Services (DHHS, formerly DHEW) and the Food and Drug Administration have revised their regulations on human subjects several times. The June 18, 1991, revision involved the adoption of the Federal Policy for the Protection of Human Subjects. The federal policy (or "Common Rule," as it is sometimes called) has been adopted by 17 departments and agencies, representing most, but not all, of the federal departments and agencies sponsoring human-subjects research. One of the main elements of the Common Rule is that there must be an IRB at each institution involved in research that ensures that proper informed consent has been obtained.

According to the Common Rule, the patient or his or her legal representative must be told, at the very least, a number of elements. The consent must include an explanation of (1) the investigational nature of the study and what it is intended to do; (2) the procedures that will take place and their duration for the subject; (3) the foreseeable risks and benefits; (4) reasonable alternatives; (5) any issues concerning confidentiality; (6) compensation if injury occurs; (7) how the subject can get answers to research-related questions; (8) and a reminder that participation is voluntary and that the subject can withdraw if he or she so desires. The consent form has to be approved by the IRB, and then read, initialled, and signed by the subject (or their representative).

The principle of informed consent is simple in theory but difficult in execution. Many questions remain and continue to be addressed in ever-changing declarations from regulatory bodies. Some have argued that informed consent from subjects is not enough and that this assigns too passive a role to the subject in research. The AIDS Coalition to Unleash Power (ACT-UP) movement of the 1990s highlighted the importance of researchers collaborating with the subjects. In those years, the treatment for Human Immunodeficiency Virus/Acquired Immunodeficiency Syndrome (HIV-AIDS) was inadequate, and many people with the illness, desperate for new treatments, were impatient with the slowness of the National Institutes of Health and the Federal Drug Administration in developing new therapies. They insisted on working directly with the scientists, regulatory agencies, and pharmaceutical companies to lessen the imbalance between subject and those entities.

The ACT-UP movement pioneered the use of parallel track experiments, in which unproven treatments are given to people who have not responded to other treatments, and probably led to a faster introduction of new HIV-AIDS treatments than otherwise would have happened. Ill patients were, it turns out, more ready to consent to unproven therapies than perhaps researchers would have thought.

Another consequence of the ACT-UP movement was the broadening of the definition of who could be a research subject. Some groups of people, such as the ill, the poor, children, minority populations, and pregnant women, have often been considered vulnerable, and regulations have been established to protect them. But at the same time, if they are left out of studies, they are less likely to reap the benefits of research.

One of the thorniest problems with informed consent is assessing the competency of the person to understand and sign the consent. Doctors overestimate the competency of their patients, particularly if the patient is agreeing with them; this overestimation also applies to signing consent forms. The problem is at its most difficult when the experimentation has to do with psychiatric illnesses because the illness itself at times interferes with comprehension.

Another complication is what has come to be known as therapeutic misperception. Research participants, particularly if they are ill, may incorrectly believe that the research project is designed to help them. The medically ill are sometimes considered as vulnerable because they are not always thinking clearly and perhaps so anxious and desperate for help that they might be susceptible to therapeutic misperception. In other words, the medically ill may not always be able to give informed consent. However, not to include the ill in research is to deprive them of new treatments.

Many other issues remain controversial: Who, if anyone, should give consent for children or the mentally ill? Can someone give informed consent for an ill-designed or unethical experiment? How much oversight should nonclinical people have over experiments and the nature of the consent? How can the quality of the consent be confirmed? Should the results of experiments without consent be published? Can payment or a reduction of a prison sentence be considered a form of coercion? If the experiment is a therapeutic experiment, should insurance pay for it? Are clinical trials of new or unproven treatments experimental? How often do patients who participate in clinical trials or therapeutic experiments give informed consent? Is consent different in third-world countries where subjects may feel that the only way they can get medical treatment is to participate in research? Does the experimenter need informed consent if he (or she) experiments on himself (or herself)? What about experiments on our own biological products, such as our cells or genes? The questions are complicated and have no easy answers.

The advice of Pappworth—that informed consent must not only be obtained but documented—has been heeded by regulatory bodies. Documentation of informed consent is required. Informed consents are now written, witnessed, and kept by the researchers, and the subject should get a copy of the form. It is now usually suggested that the language used on the consent form be understandable by those with a sixth to eighth grade education. But some problems have emerged. The consents are becoming lengthy and sometimes so full of legal boilerplate that they are difficult for a layperson to understand. The purpose of the informed consent sometimes seems more designed to protect the researcher from lawsuits rather than to explain the nature of the research to the subject.

As medicine becomes more complicated, it becomes increasingly difficult for the subject to understand the experiment, and therefore the quality of the informed consent becomes more important. At the same time, patient advocacy groups, beginning with ACT-UP, emphasize the importance of subjects and patients being not just consenting or passive subjects but also full or equal partners in treatment or experimentation.

Frances R. Frankenburg

References

1. Jonsen, *The Birth of Bioethics*, 131–132.
2. Lederer, *Subjected to Science*, 16.
3. Annas and Grodin, *The Nazi Doctors*, 130.
4. Pappworth, *Human Guinea Pigs*, 194.

INSTITUTIONAL REVIEW BOARDS

As numerous examples of unethical human experimentation throughout history have demonstrated, researchers do not always consider the safety of their subjects. To ensure the quality and safety of human experimentation, institutions are now required to have committees, often known as institutional review boards (IRBs), to review research using human subjects and, in particular, to ensure the safety of the subject and the quality of the informed consent. However, IRBs have always been controversial.

The researcher who designs a study does not always welcome supervision or review by others. But as early as 1900, in Germany, and later again in 1931, regulations were issued that stated that a researcher had to obtain permission from the medical director of his or her institution before experimenting on humans. In other words, the director of an institution had to be aware of and approve all potentially problematic activities taking place in the institution because he or she would have to take responsibility for such serious and potentially harmful activity as human experimentation.

Following the sadistic experiments of the Nazi physicians before and during World War II (and many have commented on the irony that these shameful acts took place in the very country that had the first regulations designed, in part, to prevent abuse of subjects), American physicians and judges formulated the Nuremberg Code, the first principle of which states that the subject has to understand the experiment and willingly consent to it. Although the code says nothing about external reviews, it is one of the first documents to outline the requirements for ethical experimentation. Subsequent work has clarified and expanded on the details of how to ensure that consent for experiments is obtained and that the other principles outlined by the Nuremberg Code ensuring safety for the subjects are honored.

In 1947, the Atomic Energy Commission (AEC) took over responsibility for medical research being carried out by the Manhattan Project and became one of the first groups of scientists to regulate the use of human subjects. In April 1947, Carroll Wilson, the general manager of the AEC, in two letters about research, wrote that subjects should consent to research. He made the important point that, because so many experiments of the AEC were kept secret, physicians had to be particularly careful because they would not be able to benefit from external review.

The AEC had not previously insisted on reviews of research projects, but it began to do so with a series of radioisotope experiments that were not secret, unlike the earlier experiments. The AEC encouraged experiments with radioisotopes, hoping to show that there were medical benefits to be obtained from radioactive substances. The AEC distributed radioisotopes to researchers and insisted that its own and local committees review the research projects. In 1949, after facing some opposition, the AEC reiterated that they would review and approve all allocations of radioisotopes. However, the AEC did not follow their own mandate and, for example, allowed researchers at the Berkeley Radiation Laboratory to carry out their own experiments without AEC oversight.

The injection of uranium into comatose patients in Boston, carried out at the Massachusetts General Hospital (MGH) between 1953 and 1957 with the active involvement of the AEC, was another problematic series of experiments. The MGH use of uranium was not seen as coming under the purview of the AEC's Subcommittee on Human Applications, as the AEC's particular interest in this set of studies was the occupational hazards of the uranium.

The plutonium experiments and much of the AEC's work was kept from the public until the investigations of journalist Eileen Welsome (b. 1951) in Albuquerque in 1993 and then the 1995 release of a report by the Advisory Committee on Human Radiation Experiments. But by then, other more public examples of mishaps in the medical field had already led to the formation of review committees.

The thalidomide tragedy, much worse in other parts of the world than in the United States, was one of the incidents that led to increasing recognition that external review (and delay) of physicians trying out new treatments is needed. In 1961, some American physicians gave thalidomide, a sedative, to patients without telling them that it was somewhat experimental. Some of these patients were pregnant and gave birth to infants with deformities, including absent legs or arms. A few years later, in 1971, the Food and Drug Administration (FDA) began to require review committees for investigational drugs.

In 1964, after publicity about Keith Reemtsma's (1925–2000) transplant of a chimpanzee kidney into a woman and experiments at the Jewish Chronic Diseases Hospital in New York in which cancer cells were injected into elderly patients without their consent, the director of the National Institutes of Health (NIH), James Shannon (1900–1994), appointed a committee to review issues in human experimentation, headed by Associate Director Robert B. Livingston (1918–2002). The Livingston Committee concluded that the investigator's judgment did not suffice to reach conclusions about the ethics of experiments. The committee did not recommend any particular code of standards and indeed advised against the NIH becoming too involved in overseeing clinical research.

Shannon disagreed with his committee. He worked with Surgeon General Luther Terry (1911–1985) and the United States Public Health Services (PHS), and in February 1966, the Research Grants Division of the PHS issued a memorandum saying that all clinical research projects of the PHS had to be reviewed by a "committee of his institutional associates" to ensure that the rights and welfare of the subjects were being respected and that the subjects (and patients) were giving appropriate consent. In other words, peer review was mandated as a check of the investigator's own judgment with respect to the welfare of the subjects. In 1969, this memorandum was modified so that the committee would include nonscientific members, and in 1971, the use of community standards was added.

Meanwhile, in 1966, Henry Beecher (1904–1976) had published a study, "Ethics and Clinical Research," describing 22 examples of studies of questionable ethics. This exposé, along with the earlier publication of the English book *Human Guinea Pigs: Experimentation on Man* by Maurice Pappworth (1910–1994) in 1962, once again brought more publicity to the problems surrounding human experimentation. The two authors, both physicians, outlined examples of researchers so absorbed by their research that they were oblivious to the humanity of those on whom they experimented. The researchers may not have intended to hurt their subjects, but they did—and with no compunction.

Following these and other revelations, Congress passed the National Research Act in 1974 that required that research projects funded by the Department of

Health, Education, and Welfare (DHEW) have "institutional review boards." This was the first time that the term *institutional review board*, now known as IRB, was officially used. In other words, the institution had to assure that the research complied with federal requirements and, in particular, that human participants faced minimal risks and gave adequate informed consent before the research could receive DHEW funding, modifying the 1966 PHS policy.

In 1978, the National Commission for the Protection of Human Subjects of Biomedical and Behavioral Research (established by the 1974 National Research Act) issued a report on institutional review boards. In this report, they recommended that all institutions receiving federal funds should follow regulations established by the DHEW with respect to IRBs. In other words, the requirement for an IRB was not restricted to those carrying out DHEW-funded research.

In 1981, in response to the commission's reports and recommendations, both the Department of Health and Human Services (DHHS, formerly DHEW) and the FDA revised their regulations on human subjects. The DHHS regulations were codified and revised several times. The June 18, 1991, revision involved the adoption of the Federal Policy for the Protection of Human Subjects. The federal policy (or "Common Rule," as it is sometimes called) is shared by 17 departments and agencies, representing most, but not all, of the federal departments and agencies sponsoring research on human subjects.

One of the main elements of the Common Rule is that there must be an IRB involved in research. The IRB must have at least five members, be multidisciplinary, have no conflicts of interest, and have at least one member with no scientific background and one member not affiliated with the institution. IRB membership should not be limited to one gender or profession and should reflect community attitudes. The IRB can approve, comment on, or deny projects involving human research projects.

Perhaps unsurprisingly, tension between researchers and the idea of external review has existed for years. For example, Beecher, whose 1966 article is sometimes given credit for leading to the formation of IRBs, did not recommend anything resembling a committee to approve research. Instead, he wanted the editors of medical journals to review studies, and he implored researchers to be more aware of rights of the subjects. Pappworth, in comparison, suggested that hospitals establish committees of doctors to review the medical research projects and that one member should be a nonphysician.

Physicians take exception to the idea of nonphysicians being involved in their work. For example, Senator Walter Mondale, concerned about the rapid progress in organ transplantation, held hearings in 1968 about issues in medical ethics. Organ transplantation, then in its infancy, was experimental, and most of the first recipients of transplanted organs died soon after receiving the transplant. Mondale argued that people other than physicians should be involved with the issues that these advances raised. Owen Wangensteen (1898–1991), chief of surgery at the University of Minnesota and mentor to Christiaan Barnard (1922–2001) and Norman Shumway (1923–2006), the two surgeons who performed the first human heart transplants, strongly objected. Wangensteen scoffed at the idea of multi-disciplinary review and testified that medical innovators "would be manacled by well-intentioned but meddlesome intruders. . . . I would urge you with all the strength I can muster, to leave this subject to conscionable people in the profession who are struggling valiantly to advance medicine. . . . If we are to retain a place of eminence in medicine, let us take care not to shackle the investigator with unnecessary strictures, which will dry up untapped resources of creativity." When asked about input from nonphysicians, he said, "If you are thinking of theologians, lawyers, philosophers and others to give some direction . . . I cannot see how they could help. . . . The fellow who holds the apple can peel it best."[1]

At another conference in 1975, ethicists continued to insist that external committees were needed. At this meeting, Francis Moore (1913–2001), a pioneer in organ transplants, argued that "nothing could be more unethical than critical judgment in this field made by persons who have not studied the biology of the field or the patient."[2] At this same meeting, Albert Sabin (1906–1993), the developer of the polio vaccine—after listening to bioethicist Jay Katz (1922–2008) argue that the individual conscience of the investigator was not enough—sarcastically said, "While Dr. Katz was talking, I was looking around the audience to see how many of my colleagues whom I know to be engaged . . . in human medical research had horns sticking out of their foreheads."[3]

There are other objections to IRBs. Many experimenters complain about the extra burden and expense IRBs place on them. The IRB process can also be time-consuming for researchers, who say that the IRBs slow down the pace of medical discovery.

A new development is the commercialized IRB. In the 1990s, pharmaceutical companies began to conduct more drug trials outside of academic centers, so independent for-profit IRBs were established. Commercial IRBs are paid by the companies whose research protocols they are reviewing, so there is pressure on them to approve the proposals.

Since the formation of IRBs, the number of experiments in which subjects have been hurt has probably decreased. However, the death of Jesse Gelsinger (1981–1999) following a gene-therapy trial shocked the medical research community and raised questions about the nature of the research and the adequacy of his informed consent. Following his death, the DHHS mandated the NIH and FDA to improve education and training of IRB members and staff (as well as of clinical investigators). The NIH and FDA now expect research institutions and sponsors to audit records for evidence of compliance with the required guidelines for informed consent. NIH requires investigators conducting Phase 1 and Phase 2 trials to submit monitoring plans along with the grant applications and to share these with the IRBs. The FDA also established Data and Safety Monitoring Boards (DSMBs) to work with the IRBs.

IRBs themselves face a number of problems. They are asked to review many proposals, some of which they may have difficulty understanding. In addition, Katz pointed out that IRBs located in the institutions in which the research takes place may feel pressure to approve research proposals from their colleagues or those that fund their own institution. Katz noted that many IRBs fail to understand the importance of consent and suggested the need for a national board to oversee human experimentation. On the other hand, researchers complain that some IRBs can become overly zealous.

There is concern about regulation of the IRBs themselves and whether IRBs in different institutions operate in the same way. Multisite studies, which are increasingly common, raise problems. If every site where an experiment takes place has its own IRB approve the study, there is the risk of different sites having to answer different concerns raised by IRBs, as well as no one IRB taking responsibility for the entire study. Accreditation of IRBs has been suggested but is not mandatory. Some IRBs are accredited by the Association for the Accreditation of Human Research Protection Programs (AAHRPP), established in 2001.

Frances R. Frankenburg

References

1. Jonsen, *The Birth of Bioethics*, 93 and 143.
2. Ibid., 145.
3. Ibid., 145–146.

PROFESSIONAL GUINEA PIGS

Guinea pigs are a species of rodent native to the Andes in South America. Because of their use in some important medical experiments in the past, their name has been co-opted to describe human experimental subjects, some of whom now make a living from participating in studies.

Guinea pigs (*Cavia porcellus*) are often used in experiments because they are small, docile, and breed rapidly. French chemist Antoine Lavoisier (1743–1794) used them in experiments on respiration as early as 1780. They were particularly helpful in experiments on scurvy, a disease caused by a dietary deficiency of vitamin C. This disease does not occur in most animals because they can synthesize their own vitamin C. However, guinea pigs and humans (and a few other animals) are unable to synthesize the vitamin and so are susceptible to scurvy.

Robert Koch (1843–1910), the renowned German physician and microbiologist, used new staining techniques to identify tuberculosis bacilli. To prove that these bacilli caused the illness, he infected guinea pigs with material taken from apes, cattle, and humans ill with tuberculosis. The bacteria taken from the newly ill guinea pigs were identical to those taken from the other infected animals. His 1882 lecture describing these findings has been cited as one of the most important in medical history. He subsequently was awarded the Nobel Prize in Physiology or Medicine in 1905, in large part for this work.

John Cade (1912–1980), an Australian psychiatrist, injected uric acid and other possibly toxic components of urine into guinea pigs. In one experiment in the

1940s, he used lithium urate, and the guinea pigs became relaxed and placid. Cade guessed that lithium salts might therefore be beneficial in the treatment of mania in humans, a theory that proved to be correct.

Some experiments on human health and illness can be done in petri dishes or test tubes, but many need animals or humans as subjects. These people are sometimes called, colloquially, guinea pigs. Some people who have volunteered to be subjects have done so for altruistic reasons or to help out with a particular experiment or researcher. Another group of people, now known as professional guinea pigs, support themselves by becoming subjects in paid experiments or clinical trials.

The origin of the professional guinea pig lies in recent history, as the number of clinical trials has increased along with the need for large numbers of subjects. Until the early 1970s, much medical research was carried out in prisons. Growing concern about the exploitation of vulnerable people, including prisoners, led to the recommendations by the National Commission for the Protection of Human Subjects of Biomedical and Behavioral Research that highly regulated research on prisoners, greatly diminishing the numbers of prisoners involved in research. But the need for human subjects has continued to grow, and therefore professional guinea pigs are in demand to participate in clinical trials of various sorts, particularly Phase 1 trials.

Phase 1 trials, the first time that a new medication is used in more than a few humans, require the recruitment of healthy subjects. The trials sometimes involve following a careful diet and being subjected to repeated blood tests or other more invasive procedures. Those who volunteer to take part may not participate in other trials at the same time. (On a practical note, the professional guinea pig cannot have too many commitments or a full-time job because some trials, particularly those that pay generously, may involve staying in research housing for days or weeks at a time.) Because of the complexity of these trials, professional organizations, contract research organizations (CROs), often organize the study. Some CROs may maintain their own trial sites, housing and feeding the subjects during the trial.

There are two problems with the use of professional guinea pigs in clinical trials. One problem is that their commitment to the science may take second place to their interest in being paid. For example, some subjects, eager to participate in the study, may deceive study personnel about their qualifications for the research. They may claim to be healthier than they are or say that they have the condition of interest (if the trial involves people with a particular condition or illness). They may also be enrolled in another study at the same time. They may not adhere to the study diet or take the experimental drugs properly. These deceptions can harm both the subjects and the integrity of the research.

The other problem is that research subjects face risks when they participate in studies. For example, in 1996, the University of Rochester Medical Center conducted an experiment that involved bronchoscopy (the insertion of a tube through the subject's mouth into the lungs to collect cells). Hoiyan (Nicole) Wan, a young university student, agreed to participate in the study for a fee of $150. She died after the researchers used excessive lidocaine, a topical anesthetic agent.

To prove the safety of new drugs or procedures, some humans must be the first to try them. In the past, vulnerable people, such as prisoners, were the subjects. Because that practice has been made more difficult, an entirely different type of subject has emerged.

Frances R. Frankenburg

TROVAN IN NIGERIA

Pharmaceutical companies often carry out clinical trials in third-world countries. They have been accused of doing this to take advantage of easier access to patients and fewer regulations. In one case involving trials conducted in Nigeria in 1996, a court in the United States ruled that the principles of voluntary informed consent are international and that companies must follow them wherever they work.

In 1996, a meningitis epidemic broke out in northern Nigeria. Pfizer, a large international pharmaceutical company, sent physicians to the Kano Infectious Diseases Hospital in that county to compare the effectiveness of their new broad-spectrum antibiotic, trovafloxacin (brand name Trovan), to a low dose of ceftriaxone (brand name Rocephin). Rocephin was the standard treatment for meningitis, although usually given in higher doses than what was given in the Pfizer study. Trovan can be taken by mouth, but Rocephin has to be administered by an intramuscular injection. Five of the children who were treated with Trovan died, and six who were treated with the low doses of Rocephin died. A number of children were left with neurological damage, presumably due to the meningitis itself.

The families sued Pfizer in both Nigeria and in the United States, claiming that neither the children nor their guardians had been told about the study nor had given informed consent. They claimed that Médecins Sans Frontières (MSF), or Doctors Without Borders, an international nongovernmental organization, was treating children ill with meningitis with chloramphenicol (another antibiotic) without charge and more effectively.

Whether the children in Nigeria were put at risk or harmed by the study is difficult to determine. The low doses of Rocephin have been criticized as inadequate and designed to make Trovan look more effective than it actually was. In their defense, Pfizer noted that their study had been approved by all the relevant authorities. They claimed that they put no children at risk and had chosen low doses of Rocephin only to minimize pain to the children. They also argued that these low doses of Rocephin were more effective than the chloramphenicol given by MSF. (Later, Trovan was withdrawn from the market because of hepatotoxicity, but this was not an issue in the trials.)

The Nigerian minors and their guardians claimed that Pfizer's conduct of the study violated the Nuremberg Code, the Declaration of Helsinki, and the International Covenant on Civil and Political Rights. The legal issues became complicated because two countries were involved, and it was not clear whether the codes mentioned above could be used in a court case or in which country the suits should be filed. In one suit, the Nigerian government sued Pfizer in Nigeria. In another case, the Nigerian minors and their families sued Pfizer in the United States. This latter suit was at first dismissed, but in January 2009, the United States Court of Appeals for the Second Circuit (covering New York, Connecticut, and Vermont) ruled that this suit could proceed. The court ruled that the principles of voluntary informed consent are international and must be followed by pharmaceutical companies wherever they work. The codes and ethical guidelines cannot be ignored.

Whether Pfizer obtained informed consent from the children or their families will likely never be known. The final settlement was achieved out of court, so no information about the consent process was released. Pfizer resolved the case with a $75 million settlement. Case details of the involved children have disappeared.

Frances R. Frankenburg

DOCUMENTS

RADIATION EXPERIMENTATION VICTIMS ACT (1994)

In November 1986, Massachusetts congressman Ed Markey released a report titled American Nuclear Guinea Pigs: Three Decades of Radiation Experiments on U.S. Citizens *that describes 31 human radiation experiments involving nearly 700 people. This report received little coverage, and the Department of Energy (DOE) did not follow Markey's recommendations to locate the subjects to compensate them. Journalist Eileen Welsome was more successful in publicizing these and other experiments. Her 1993 work reached Energy Secretary Hazel O'Leary, who as a result, in December 1993, declassified over 30 million pages of documents, reversing a long-standing departmental policy of secrecy. It turned out that ionizing radiation experiments on humans were more widespread than previously acknowledged. In January 1994, President Bill Clinton created the Advisory Committee on Human Radiation Experiments (ACHRE) to further investigate. In this 1994 speech, Markey again asks that these subjects be compensated.*

HON. EDWARD J. MARKEY of Massachusetts, in the House of Representatives, Thursday, April 21, 1994

Mr. MARKEY. Mr. Speaker, I am today introducing the Radiation Experimentation Victims Act of 1994. The recent acknowledgement by Federal officials that the Government conducted radiation experiments with human guinea pigs grabbed the attention of all U.S. citizens, and the reason is that most people assumed that our country would not engage in this kind of activity. I think the fact that the Federal Government—our Government—funded or engaged in this kind of activity is the most disturbing aspect of this whole story. Most Americans thought that our country would not take that kind of action. To close the door on this regrettable legacy, we should focus on the proper remedies to respond to past wrongs, make certain these things can never happen again, and do the right thing today by compensating those who suffered injury. Accordingly, today I am introducing legislation to address past wrongs. My focus is on the Department of Energy, because that is the agency with which I have the most experience. My legislation has three goals. It is my hope that the administration will accomplish these goals before legislation is enacted, but I desire to have the force of legislation if the executive branch should falter in meeting these goals:

Require full disclosure from the Department of Energy, while protecting the privacy of subjects and their families, on experiments with ionizing radiation that provided little or no benefit to the subjects and were funded by the Department or its predecessor agencies;

Require the Department of Energy to formulate a plan to conduct proper medical follow-up of subjects where it seems feasible and indicated; and to provide free medical care for injuries related to experiments;

Require the Secretary of Energy, after consultation with other appropriate Federal officials, to recommend appropriate compensation for those subjects or their families who have suffered damages, and make any other recommendation for appropriate compensation for those who have been wronged.

The legislation I am introducing does not impose a particular compensation plan, but rather directs the Secretary of Energy to report to Congress in 6 months on what should be the appropriate scheme. I recognize that there is some debate on the effectiveness of existing legislation for exposed atomic veterans and for downwinders from atomic tests. In light of that debate, I think it is appropriate for the administration to review these and other compensation systems and then develop an appropriate system for the victims identified here today. The best system would merge science with compassion in determining standards for compassion. Provision should also be made for appropriate remedies other than monetary compensation to unwitting subjects who suffered dignity injury.

I would like to briefly describe my involvement with these issues. In October 1986, I released "American Nuclear Guinea Pigs: Three Decades of Radiation Experiments on U.S. Citizens," a staff reports of the House Subcommittee on Energy Conservation and Power. This report revealed the frequent and systematic use of human subjects as guinea pigs, describing 31 experiments in which nearly 700 persons were exposed to ionizing radiation that provided little or no medical benefit to the subjects.

The 1986 report also discussed some of the more repugnant or bizarre experiments. At the top of this list were the plutonium injection experiments, in which patients designated terminal within 10 years were given plutonium to determine how the body handled this radioactive material. This experiment provided no medical benefits to the subjects, and is marred by a lack of informed consent, since even the word plutonium was classified during the 1940's. Moreover, as my staff report documents, when the Atomic Energy Commission conducted a follow-up study in 1973 to determine the amounts of plutonium remaining in subjects' bodies, informed consent was not obtained from patients who were still alive, nor from families who were asked for permission to exhume the bodies of deceased subjects. Sadly, 30 years later, the word plutonium was still too explosive for the Federal Government to tell the victims.

The response of the Reagan administration to my 1986 staff report can be described as, "Thanks for the information, we're not going to do anything," and the report languished on a shelf at the Department of Energy until recently. Then in November 1993, a series of articles by Eileen Welsome, a reporter at the *Albuquerque Tribune*, identified some victims of the plutonium injection experiments and their families, and put a human face on the issue. Last week, Eileen Welsome was awarded the Pulitzer Prize for these articles. When Secretary of Energy Hazel O'Leary learned of these experiments and my 1986 staff report, she decided that the appropriate course of action was full disclosure of all information on experiments with human subjects. In January 1994, President Clinton formed the Human Radiation Interagency Working Group, and announced that he would establish an Advisory Committee for the Working Group. The Advisory Committee is meeting for the first time today. I commend the President for his leadership, and I commend Secretary O'Leary for her efforts to lift the shroud of secrecy on her Department, and bring the questionable past of the Department and its predecessor agencies into the sunshine of public scrutiny.

In another set of experiments which came to light in late 1993, at the Fernald School in Massachusetts during the 1940s and 1950s, schoolboys classified as mentally retarded were fed radioactive calcium and iron with their breakfast meals. Yet parents of these children were deceived about the nature of the experiments when they gave their consent. With at least one experiment, the letter from the school requesting consent never mentioned that radioactive material would be fed, noted that experimental subjects were selected from a "group of our brighter patients," and implied that the experiment might result in "gains in weight and other improvements."

These experiments were funded by the Atomic Energy Commission, the National Institutes of Health, and the Quaker Oats Company, and research was conducted by faculty at MIT and Harvard. These experiments clearly fit within the scope of the documents that I requested from the Department of Energy in the mid-1980s, yet they were not reported then. With the revelation of the Fernald School experiments, I began to question whether we know the full scope of human experimentation; whether the 1986 staff report provided a reasonably accurate picture or whether the extent of testing was larger.

This question has been reinforced by findings of the Massachusetts Department of Mental Retardation (DMR), which after the revelation of the Fernald School experiments launched its own investigation for full disclosure. With the assistance of Harvard University, the DMR identified additional experiments during the 1960s at the Wrentham School, where tiny children as young as two years old were administered radioactive iodine to test potential countermeasures to atomic fallout, in work funded by the U.S. Public Health Service, Division of Radiological Health.

One reason why I find these experiments so repugnant is because of the vulnerable nature of the subjects used. It was no accident that students at the Fernald and Wrentham Schools were fed radioactive material, and not university students. It is no accident that the terminally ill were experimental subjects, including some who were comatose. It is no accident that the elderly, soldiers, and prisoners were used for testing with radioactive material. Such members of society are not fully enfranchised and lack control over their lives. They deserve protection, not exploitation as human guinea pigs. Certainly, experimental drugs or treatments intended to make the patient better may be used. But that was not the case with these experiments. We must again look at our ethical guidelines to make certain they protect the vulnerable.

When I released my staff report in 1986, I had assumed that experiments of such nature were the product of the arrogance of the early atomic age, and the paranoia of the cold war. But as these experiments have gained new attention, I have been shocked and dismayed to find that individual scientists feel compelled even today to defend these experiments of years ago. Some have stepped forward to claim that such experiments should not be judged according to today's standards, and besides, the doses given were low. To these attitudes, I have two responses: First, contrary to such opinions, the 1940s and 1950s were not devoid of patient knowledge or ethical standards. Radiation and its health effects were widely discussed in the era of bomb shelters and air raid drills. Moreover, the Nuremberg Code was in effect, written by the United States and the Allies in the aftermath of World War II, and it established guidelines on obtaining informed consent for experiments. Clearly, the Fernald School experiments violate this basic human rights standard.

In this regard, I commend the recent statement of Charles Vest, president of MIT, who acknowledged that while doses at the Fernald School may have been relatively low, he was sorry for the experiments, because of the children selected and the lack of informed consent. MIT explained that President Vest issued his statement because "it seemed the decent thing to do," and I applaud his decency.

I wish to make clear that I consider such ethically questionable experiments to be aberrations, and I do not desire to cast doubt upon the overwhelming majority of biomedical research, representing laboratory experiments, legitimate nuclear medicine for treatment and diagnosis, and ethical clinical trials. I have long been a strong advocate of public funding for basic research, and I commend those investigators who work daily to understand, prevent, and treat disease.

Nor is it my desire to blame present leaders of organizations and institutions for past mistakes. My concern is that institutions work with Congress today to do the right thing to address past abuses. I therefore welcome the leadership by the Clinton administration, and I look forward to working with my colleagues in Congress, the administration and its Advisory Committee, and the scientific community in formulating proper responses today.

In March 1994, as part of the administration's commitment to full disclosure, Secretary of Energy O'Leary released two boxes of documents related to the plutonium injection experiments. I reiterate my commendation of Secretary O'Leary, and note that her efforts have already produced results not seen previously from the Department of Energy. Nonetheless, an analysis by my staff concludes that these plutonium papers raise some issues which have not yet been resolved. Matters identified, and their relevance to the ongoing work of the Interagency Working Group, or of the Advisory Committee, as it sees fit, are as follows:

The precise number of persons exposed to plutonium in experiments remains an open question. On this matter, the Working Group is already committed to full disclosure on all experiments.

The plutonium papers indicate, more clearly than material provided to my subcommittee in the 1980s, the coordinated nature of the plutonium injection experiments, and their connection to other experiments with human subjects, specifically injection of plutonium and uranium. It seems appropriate for the Working Group to determine to what extent experiments represent a coordinated Federal effort rather than a collection of isolated studies.

The plutonium papers suggest that for a brief period of time in the late 1940s, the Atomic Energy Commission required that experiments with ionizing radiation and human subjects should be conducted only if the subjects received medical benefits—a standard similar to those by which such experiments are being judged today. If this in fact was AEC policy, it must have been overturned or violated by many later experiments. It seems appropriate for the Working Group to determine what standards were in place in the late 1940s, and whether they deteriorated over time.

In February 1987, the Department of Energy notified me that they would not conduct further follow-up of experimental subjects. However, at the same time, the Department was desperately trying to conduct follow-up with the family of a deceased patient, an Australian national injected with plutonium before his fifth birthday. It seems appropriate for the Working Group to determine the full extent of any follow-up conducted in the 1980s, and evaluate whether the efforts then might facilitate follow-up of subjects now.

In addition, I want to emphasize the need to maintain the integrity of Government records during the search for documents on radiation experiments with human subjects. I have recommended that steps be taken to avoid review of files by individuals who may have direct conflicts of interest.

In summary, what has been revealed is no less than the frequent and systematic use of U.S. citizens as guinea pigs during experiments with ionizing radiation. These experiments shock the conscience and demand a response. I look forward to working with my colleagues and the administration to gain full disclosure of this shameful past, to provide the medical follow-up and treatment that experimental subjects deserve, and to take other measures as necessary for restitution to those citizens who have suffered injury.

Source: Congressional Record Volume 140, Number 45 (Thursday, April 21, 1994), page E.

PROBLEMS FACING INSTITUTIONAL REVIEW BOARDS (1998)

The purpose of the institutional review boards (IRBs) is to ensure the rights and welfare of research subjects. IRBs are regulated by the FDA and by the Office for Human Research Protections (OHRP), which is part of Human Health and Human Services (HHS). In 1998, the Office of the Inspector General investigated the effectiveness of IRBs. This passage is the summary of their findings. Following the release of this report, HHS responded by agreeing that the IRB system is stressed. HHS urged research institutions to strengthen their commitments to the protection of human research subjects as suggested by the Office of the Inspector General and to elevate the standing and resources of their IRBs. HHS noted that research institutions receive "overhead" payments and that the protection of human subjects is a high priority for the use of this money.

They Face Major Changes in the Research Environment. The current framework of IRB practices was shaped in the 1970s in an environment where research typically was carried out by a single investigator working under government funding with a small cohort of human subjects in a university teaching hospital. In recent years, that environment has been changing dramatically as a result of the expansion of managed care, the increased commercialization of research, the proliferation of multi-site trials, new types of research, the increased number of research proposals, and the rise of patient consumerism. Each of these developments has presented major disruptions and challenges for IRBs. "Never before," concluded one recent review, "has such a pressure-cooker atmosphere prevailed within the IRB system."

They Review Too Much, Too Quickly, with Too Little Expertise. This is especially apparent in many of the larger institutions. Expanded workloads, resource constraints, and extensive Federal mandates contribute to a rushed atmosphere where sufficient deliberation often is not possible. At the same time, the IRBs frequently are hard-pressed to gain access to the scientific expertise they need to reach informed judgments about the research taking place under their jurisdiction.

They Conduct Minimal Continuing Review of Approved Research. In the environment described above, continuing review often loses out. Even where there is the will, there often is not the time to go beyond the perfunctory obligations. A lack of feedback from other entities that oversee multi-site trials contributes to the problem. The result is that IRBs have all too little information about how the informed consent process really works and about how well the interests of subjects are being protected during the course of research.

They Face Conflicts That Threaten Their Independence. Clinical research provides revenue and prestige to the institutions to which many IRBs belong. The institutions expect IRBs to support these interests at the same time that they protect human subjects. The resulting tension can lessen the IRBs' focus on their basic mission. The minimal "outside" representation that typically exists on IRBs deprives them of an important counterbalance to the institutional interests. For independent IRBs, the dependence on revenue from industry sponsors exerts similar possibilities for conflict.

They Provide Little Training for Investigators and Board Members. The IRB system depends heavily on research investigators' commitment to uphold human-subject protections. But as that system now operates, it offers little educational outreach to investigators to help them become informed and sensitized about these protections. Similarly, it provides minimal orientation and continuing education for IRB members—a deficiency that is especially detrimental to nonscientific and noninstitutional members.

Neither IRBs nor HHS Devote Much Attention to Evaluating IRB Effectiveness. IRBs rarely conduct inquiries to determine how well they are accomplishing their mission; their judgments of effectiveness rely mainly on the number of protection lapses or complaints that are brought to their attention. The HHS agencies conducting oversight seldom go any further. The Office for Protection from Research Risks, in the National Institutes of Health, focuses almost entirely on up-front assurances. The Food and Drug Administration relies on compliance-focused inspections.

Recommendations

With the above findings, we do not claim that there are widespread abuses of human research subjects. The current system of protections is supported by many conscientious research investigators committed to protecting human subjects and by many dedicated IRB members and staff doing their best under trying circumstances. A reviewer of this system can not help but be impressed by the contributions of these individuals, and the important function that IRBs have fulfilled over the past quarter of a century.

But our findings present an important warning signal. The capacity of IRBs to accomplish all that is expected of them is strained. In the years ahead, this difficult situation could become even worse in view of Federal plans to increase significantly the numbers of subjects in clinical trials and various proposals to give IRBs added responsibility in the areas of genetics and confidentiality. It is time, we believe, for reform.

Our recommendations offer a framework for such a response. We direct them jointly to the two HHS agencies responsible for IRB oversight: the Office of Protection from Research Risks (OPRR), which is located within the National Institutes of Health (NIH), and the Food and Drug Administration (FDA). These agencies oversee IRBs with different jurisdictions and operational approaches. It is essential, therefore, for them to collaborate closely if HHS as a whole is to respond effectively to the serious concerns that emerge from our inquiry. Below we present our general recommendations for the two agencies. In the text, we offer more explicit elaborations directed, as appropriate, to the particular agencies.

Recast Federal IRB Requirements So That They Grant IRBs Greater Flexibility and Hold Them More Accountable for Results.

- Eliminate or lessen some of the procedural requirements directed to IRBs.
- Require that IRBs undergo regular performance-focused evaluations.

Strengthen Continuing Protections for Human Subjects Participating in Research.

- Require Data Safety Monitoring Boards for some multi-site trials.
- Provide IRBs with feedback on developments concerning multi-site trials.
- Routinely provide IRBs with feedback about FDA actions against investigators.
- Require sponsors and investigators to notify IRBs of prior reviews of research plans.
- Call for increased IRB awareness of on-site research practices.

Enact Federal Requirements That Help Ensure That Investigators and IRB Members Are Adequately Educated About and Sensitized to Human-Subject Protections.

- Require that research institutions have a program for educating its investigators on human-subject protections.
- Require that investigators provide a written attestation of their familiarity with and commitment to human-subject protections.
- Require that IRBs have an educational program for board members.

Help Insulate IRBs from Conflicts That Can Compromise Their Mission in Protecting Human Subjects.

- Require more representation on IRBs of nonscientific and noninstitutional members.
- Require more representation of IRBs of nonscientific and noninstitutional members.
- Reinforce to IRB institutions the importance of IRBs having sufficient independence.
- Prohibit IRB equity owners from participating in the IRB review process.

Recognize the Seriousness of the Workload Pressures That Many IRBs Face and Take Actions That Aim to Moderate Them.

- Require that IRBs have access to adequate resources.

Reengineer the Federal Oversight Process.

- Revamp the NIH/OPRR assurance process.
- Revamp the FDA on-site inspection process.
- Require the registration of IRBs.

Source: Office of Inspector General, *Institutional Review Boards: A Time for Reform.* OEI-01-97-00193. Department of Health and Human Services. June 1998.

Further Reading

Abadie, Roberto. 2010. *The Professional Guinea Pig: Big Pharma and the Risky World of Human Subjects.* Durham, NC: Duke University Press.

Angell, Marcia. 1997. "The Ethics of Clinical Research in the Third World." *New England Journal of Medicine* 337 (12): 847–849. doi:10.1056/NEJM199709183371209.

Annas, George J. 2009. "Globalized Clinical Trials and Informed Consent." *New England Journal of Medicine* 360 (20): 2,050–2,053. doi:10.1056/NEJMp0901474.

Annas, George J., and Michael A. Grodin.1992. *The Nazi Doctors and the Nuremberg Code: Human Rights in Human Experimentation.* New York: Oxford University Press.

Beecher, Henry K. 1955. "The Powerful Placebo." *Journal of the American Association* 159 (17): 1,602–1,606.

Cochrane, A. L. 1984. "Sickness in Salonica: My First, Worst, and Most Successful Clinical Trial." *British Medical Journal* 289 (6460) (December): 1,726–1,727. doi:10.1136/bmj.289.6460.1726.

Cochrane, A. L., and Max Blythe. 1989. *One Man's Medicine: An Autobiography of Professor Archie Cochrane.* London: British Medical Journal.

Eig, Jonathan. 2014. *The Birth of the Pill: How Four Crusaders Reinvented Sex and Launched a Revolution.* New York: W. W. Norton & Company.

Emanuel, Ezekiel J. 2011. *The Oxford Textbook of Clinical Research Ethics.* Oxford: Oxford University Press.

Frankenburg, Frances Rachel. 2009. *Vitamin Discoveries and Disasters: History, Science, and Controversies.* Santa Barbara, CA: Praeger/ABC-CLIO.

Glanz, James. 2001. "1978 Study Had Troubles Like a Fatal Hopkins Test." *New York Times,* July 26. http://www.nytimes.com/2001/07/26/us/1978-study-had-troubles-like-a-fatal-hopkins-test.html.

Harkness, Jon, Susan E. Lederer, and Daniel Wikler. 2001. "Laying Ethical Foundations for Clinical Research." *Bulletin of the World Health Organization* 79 (4): 365–372.

Helms, Robert. 2002. *Guinea Pig Zero: An Anthology of the Journal for Human Research Subjects.* New Orleans, LA: Garrett County Press.

Hill, A. B. 1952. "The Clinical Trial." *New England Journal of Medicine* 247 (4) (July): 113–119. doi:10.1056/nejm195207242470401.

Johns Hopkins University. 2001. "Report of Internal Investigation into the Death of a Volunteer Research Subject." (July). www.hopkinsmedicine.org/press/2001/JULY.

Jonsen, Albert R. 1998. *The Birth of Bioethics.* New York: Oxford University Press.

Jonsen, Albert R., Robert M. Veatch, and LeRoy Walters. 1998. *Source Book in Bioethics.* Washington, D.C.: Georgetown University Press.

Kelsey, Frances O. n.d. "Autobiographical Reflections." FDA History Office. http://www
.fda.gov/downloads/AboutFDA/WhatWeDo/History/OralHistories/SelectedOral
HistoryTranscripts/UCM406132.pdf.

Lederer, Susan E. 1995. *Subjected to Science: Human Experimentation in America before the
Second World War.* Baltimore: Johns Hopkins University Press.

Lurie, Peter, and Sidney M. Wolfe. 1997. "Unethical Trials of Interventions to Reduce
Perinatal Transmission of the Human Immunodeficiency Virus in Developing Countries." *New England Journal of Medicine* 337 (12): 853–856. doi:10.1056/NEJM1997
09183371212.

Meldrum, M. 1998. "'A Calculated Risk': The Salk Polio Vaccine Field Trials of 1954." *British
Medical Journal* 317 (7167) (October): 1,233–1,236. doi:10.1136/bmj.317.7167.1233.

Pappworth, M. H. 1967. *Human Guinea Pigs: Experimentation on Man.* London: Rutledge
and Kegan Paul.

Resnik, David B., and David J. McCann. 2015. "Deception by Research Participants." *New
England Journal of Medicine* 373 (13): 1,192–1,193. doi:10.1056/nejmp1506985.

Sackett, D. L., W. M. Rosenberg, J. A. Gray, R. B. Haynes, and W. S. Richardson. 1996.
"Evidence Based Medicine: What It Is and What It Isn't." *British Medical Journal* 312
(7023) (January): 71–72. doi:10.1136/bmj.312.7023.71.

Savulescu, J., and M. Spriggs. 2002. "The Hexamethonium Asthma Study and the Death of
a Normal Volunteer in Research." *Journal of Medical Ethics* 28: 3–4.

Steinbrook, Robert. 2002. "Improving Protection for Research Subjects." *New England
Journal of Medicine* 346 (18): 1,425–1,430. doi:10.1056/nejm200205023461828.

United States. 1996. *Final Report of the Advisory Committee on Human Radiation Experiments.*
New York: Oxford University Press.

Varmus, Harold, and David Satcher. 1997. "Ethical Complexities of Conducting Research
in Developing Countries." *New England Journal of Medicine* 337 (14) (October):
1,003–1,005.

Welsome, Eileen. 1999. *The Plutonium Files: America's Secret Medical Experiments in the Cold
War.* New York: Dial Press.

Wilson, James M. 2009. "Lessons Learned from the Gene Therapy Trial for Ornithine
Transcarbamylase Deficiency." *Molecular Genetics and Metabolism.* doi:10.1016/j.
ymgme.2008.12.016.

Conclusion

For most of human history, we have understood little about our bodies and the illnesses that affect them. It has largely been through experimentation that researchers have pushed back the borders of ignorance, revealing many of the human body's secrets and pioneering incredible advances in medicine, and yet, sometimes the subject of the experiment has suffered greatly as a result.

The researcher has on occasion experimented on the person who is more willing than the average person to suffer for the sake of science: himself. In most cases, however, the researcher needs subjects other than himself, and one area of research where that is particularly true is surgery, especially when it involves the transplantation of organs. The mid-1800s inventions of anesthesia and antisepsis allowed the pace of discovery of new surgical treatments to become rapid, and in the late 1900s, successful organ transplants became possible. The first transplants were therapeutic experiments, in the sense that they were designed to further expertise and knowledge in the field. For people with a poorly functioning kidney, liver, lung, or heart, an experimental transplant was often the last resort and eagerly welcomed, even though the outcome, in most of the early transplants, was likely to be poor.

Sometimes researchers have used different kinds of subjects to achieve their result. Anesthesiologists Peter Safar (1924–2003) and James Elam (1918–1995) organized experiments to work out the details of cardiopulmonary resuscitation using two sets of subjects. Untrained volunteers were the rescuers who used different resuscitation techniques. They were subjects in that their abilities, as well as the resuscitation techniques, were being tested. Medical personnel served as the other set of subjects; they were paralyzed and anesthetized so that they could mimic the state of the person needing to be revived. All subjects knew the details and the goals of the experiment. The rescuers did all of the work, but the medical personnel were taking serious risks in what they had agreed to undergo. Other subjects who have taken an active role in experiments were those with HIV-AIDS at the beginning of the HIV-AIDS epidemic, who, through the organization ACT-UP, volunteered to take unproven medications.

Despite advances due to the work of many researchers, the public has been suspicious about human experimentation, and often with good reason. When European physicians in the 1800s were interested in studying venereal diseases, they did so by transmitting contagious matter from people with venereal diseases to the blind and to prostitutes. Similarly, in the 1900s, when American physicians wanted to study syphilis, they did so by not treating it (or undertreating it) in poor black Americans, and even actually transmitted venereal diseases to uninformed subjects in Guatemala. Physicians Henry Beecher (1904–1976) and Maurice Pappworth (1910–1994) documented many such examples of how researchers can ignore the rights of their subjects in their zeal to make discoveries.

In some cases, the reputations of well-known and respected researchers of the past become tarnished when we look at their work through modern eyes. French biochemist Louis Pasteur (1822–1895) was celebrated throughout the world after successfully vaccinating a boy bitten by a rabid dog. But historian Gerald Geison (1943–2001) found inconsistencies between Pasteur's laboratory notes and his public announcements. The American Sexually Transmitted Diseases Association (ASTDA) named its lifetime achievement award after Thomas Parran (1892–1968), a distinguished physician who had contributed to the understanding and treatment of venereal diseases. After the historian Susan Reverby (b. 1946) discovered the details about the venereal disease experiments in Guatemala, in which Parran had played a part, the award's name was changed from the Thomas Parran Award to the "The ASTDA Distinguished Career Award." In a similar way, an award named after Cornelius "Dusty" Rhoads (1898–1959), a leading cancer researcher, was renamed after publicity about some of his insulting comments about his patients in Puerto Rico. (He said that the comments were meant as a parody.) Saul Krugman (1911–1995), who was awarded the Lasker Prize for his important discoveries about hepatitis, is now sometimes seen as a researcher who exploited children at the Willowbrook State School.

Many of the physician-researchers who have been criticized did not think that they were doing anything wrong and would have been astonished to be censured by today's standards, or even the standards of their own day. But others were more aware of how their work would look to others. For example, the American physicians who carried out the experiments in Guatemala joked to each other about being harshly judged if the public discovered the details of their experiments.

The publicity about the Tuskegee study, the regular use of prisoners and institutionalized children as subjects, and the Cold War–era experiments with radiation and plutonium have led to vastly increased regulation of research in the United States. Research projects have to be approved by institutional review boards (IRBs) in a time-consuming process. (This is not at all what Beecher would have wanted.) The requirement for researchers to have detailed protocols before beginning their work and then disclose all their data is burdensome but might have forestalled some of the disastrous experiments in the past, including Tuskegee and Guatemala. But regulation would probably not have stopped the experiments carried out by the Nazi physicians and Unit 731 in Japan. Indeed, Germany already had regulations in place, which were ignored.

Many scientists resent the paperwork burden and claim that the regulations are excessive and slow them down. Critics, notably physician and ethicist Jay Katz (1922–2008), claimed that the IRBs were insufficiently rigorous in protecting the subjects and ensuring that the subjects of experiments could give truly informed consent.

In a recollection of D. Ewen Cameron (1901–1967), a Central Intelligence Agency–funded psychiatrist who experimented with brainwashing, his successor writes about what happens when someone experiments by himself without collaboration or regulation: "[Cameron] was inclined to be stubborn, oppositional, and competitive with figures of authority, and was not given to emphasize collaboration. His intelligence, vigor, and drive to reach new horizons left him little time to dally with his peers. . . . His own personality became his own worst enemy as he could not tap the scientifically restraining milieu provided by a congenial group of colleagues in evaluating ideas and experiments."[1]

As the technology in experiments becomes more complicated, experiments become more difficult to understand. Some of the experimenters of the past were amateurs, in that they were not professionally trained, were not necessarily paid, and did what they did for the love of the work. Experimentation in the 21st century, on the other hand, is almost entirely the pursuit of those with doctoral degrees, often funded by laboriously obtained grants and beyond the comprehension of most. One of the consequences of this is that the gap in knowledge between subject and researcher widens. In the past, an intelligent member of the public without any particular medical training could be expected to understand much of medicine. This is becoming less true. This discrepancy should, in theory, be lessened by the presence of the informed consent, which was meant to educate the subject about the risks and benefits of the experiment. But informed consent is now used more to protect the researcher and his or her institution. The length and complexity of the forms often make them unintelligible to the layperson.

Another consequence of the complexity of studies today is that many people and committees become involved in the planning and execution of experiments. This provides extra safeguards, but it can also lead to a diffusion of responsibility or uncertainty about who is in charge. If mistakes are made, the blame is likely to be shared. For example, after the death of Ellen Roche, a young research assistant who volunteered to participate in an asthma study at Johns Hopkins, both the researcher and the IRB were accused of not sufficiently investigating the risks of inhaled hexamethonium.

Intelligence and imagination on the part of the researcher continue to be essential in making medical advances, but an ability to work as a member of a team and a willingness to cope with the burdens of regulations, grant writing, laboratory administration, and academic politics are also needed.

Research on human bodies has shed light on the personal qualities of the researchers. In some cases, as in Nazi Germany and Unit 731, it has revealed individuals at their worst, ready to exploit those with little power and cause much suffering. Yet, other researchers have shown talent, bravery, and altruism in abundance. The selflessness shown by the British father-and-son team John Scott Haldane (1860–1936) and John Burdon Sanderson Haldane (1892–1964)—who subjected themselves to extreme environmental conditions—and the perseverance of the vaccine developers, such as Edward Jenner (1749–1823), Louis Pasteur (1822–1895), Waldemar Haffkine (1860–1930), Albert Sabin (1906–1993), Jonas

Salk (1914–1995), and Hilary Koprowski (1916–2014), inspire others to continue to experiment to improve the lives of others. Perhaps some equally brilliant experimenters in the 21st century will be able to come up with discoveries that will lessen the misery caused by infectious illnesses, cancer, and the depredations of aging.

Note

1. Robert A. Cleghorn. 1990. "The McGill Experience of Robert A. Cleghorn, MD: Recollections of D. Ewen Cameron." *Canadian Bulletin of Medical History* 7: 73.

About the Editor and Contributors

EDITOR

Frances R. Frankenburg, MD, is a professor of psychiatry at the Boston University School of Medicine and chief of inpatient psychiatry at the Edith Nourse Rogers Memorial Veterans Hospital in Bedford, Massachusetts. Her published works include ABC-CLIO's *Vitamin Discoveries and Disasters: History, Science, and Controversies* and *Brain Robbers: How Alcohol, Cocaine, Nicotine, and Opiates Have Changed the World.* She received her medical education at the University of Toronto.

CONTRIBUTORS

Waitman W. Beorn, PhD, is an assistant professor of history as well as Louis and Frances Blumkin Professor of Holocaust and Genocide Studies at the University of Nebraska, Omaha. He has also taught as visiting assistant professor of history at Loyola University; adjunct professor of history at Campbell University, Fort Bragg; and an instructor of history at the University of North Carolina, Chapel Hill. Boern received his PhD in 2011 in history from the University of North Carolina, Chapel Hill.

Norbert C. Brockman, PhD, is Professor Emeritus of International Relations at St. Mary's University in San Antonio, Texas. He is the author of *Encyclopedia of Sacred Places,* second edition (2011), and *An African Biographical Dictionary* (1994).

Bernard A. Cook, PhD, is Provost Distinguished Professor of History at Loyola University New Orleans. There, he teaches courses on the Holocaust, Nazi Germany, historiography, and World War I. After studying at the Gregorian University in Rome and at the University of Marburg on a Fulbright Fellowship, he received his PhD in modern European history from Saint Louis University. He is the author of *Belgium: A History* (Peter Lang, 2002) and editor of *Europe since 1945: An Encyclopedia* (Garland, 2001).

Ken Kotani, PhD, has held positions as a visiting fellow at the Royal United Services Institute, a senior fellow at the Center for Military History, and a lecturer at the Japanese National Institute of Defense Studies. He received the 2007 Yamamota Shichihei Award for his book *Intelligence of the Imperial Japanese Army and Navy* (Koundansha, 2007). Kotani is also the author of *Japanese Intelligence in World War II* (Osprey Publishing, 2009) and the article "Could Japan Read Allied Signal

Traffic?" in *Intelligence and National Security*. He received his PhD in international history from Kyoto University in 2004.

Robert W. Malick, PhD, is adjunct professor of history at Harrisburg Area Community College. He earned his MA at Shippensburg University. He is the author of *Prussian Military and Civilian Educational Reforms, 1806–1815* (Shippensburg University of Pennsylvania, 2002).

Jack E. McCallum, PhD, MD, practiced adult and pediatric neurosurgery in Fort Worth, Texas, from 1977 to 2005. He earned a doctorate in history in 2001 and has taught American history, history of medicine, and the ethics of science at Texas Christian University since that time. His published works include a biography of Leonard Wood as well as *Military Medicine: From Ancient Times to the 21st Century* (ABC-CLIO, 2008).

Martin Moll, PhD, received his doctorate in 1987 from the University of Graz. He worked as a historian, becoming the Universität dozent for Modern and Contemporary History at his alma mater in 2003. Moll has contributed to a number of publications, including *World War I: A Student Encyclopedia* (ABC-CLIO, 2005) and *World War II at Sea: An Encyclopedia* (ABC-CLIO, 2011).

Jason Newman, PhD, is a professor of history and president of the Los Rios California Federation of Teachers at Consumnes River College. He attended UC Davis for his BA, MA, and PhD in Native American History. He contributed to *American Civil War: The Essential Reference Guide* (ABC-CLIO, 2011).

Paul G. Pierpaoli Jr., PhD, is a fellow in Military History at ABC-CLIO and the associate editor of ABC-CLIO's Military History series. A recipient of the Harry S. Truman Dissertation Fellowship, he received his MA and PhD degrees from the Ohio State University. He has also served on the faculties of numerous schools, including Hampden-Sydney College and the University of Arizona. Dr. Pierpaoli has been the assistant editor for *Diplomatic History* as well as the *Journal of Military History* and has been the associate editor of numerous ABC-CLIO projects, including *The Encyclopedia of the Korean War* (ABC-CLIO, 2010), *The Encyclopedia of the Cold War* (ABC-CLIO, 2007), and *The Encyclopedia of the Arab-Israeli Conflict* (ABC-CLIO, 2008).

Index